CORNELL UNIVERSITY
MEDICAL COLLEGE
LIBRARY

NEW YORK, NY

Clinical Handbook of

CHILD
PSYCHIATRY
and the LAW

Clinical Handbook of
CHILD
PSYCHIATRY
and the LAW

Edited by

Diane H. Schetky, M.D.
Private Practice
Rockport, Maine

Elissa P. Benedek, M.D.
Director, Department of Training and Research
Center for Forensic Psychiatry
Ann Arbor, Michigan

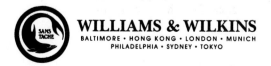
WILLIAMS & WILKINS
BALTIMORE · HONG KONG · LONDON · MUNICH
PHILADELPHIA · SYDNEY · TOKYO

Editor: Michael G. Fisher
Managing Editor: Carol Eckhart
Copy Editor: Mary Kidd
Designer: Norman W. Och
Illustration Planner: Ray Lowman
Production Coordinator: Barbara J. Felton
Cover Designer: Wilma E. Rosenberger

Copyright © 1992
Williams & Wilkins
428 East Preston Street
Baltimore, Maryland 21202, USA

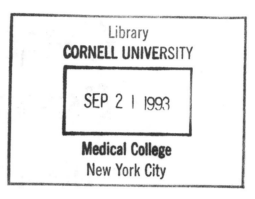

Printed in the United States of America

Library of Congress Cataloging-in-Publication Data

Clinical handbook of child psychiatry and the law / edited by Diane H. Schetky,
  Elissa P. Benedek.
     p.   cm.
  Includes bibliographical references and index.
  ISBN 0-683-07589-6
  1. Forensic psychiatry—Handbooks, manuals, etc.   2. Child psychiatry—Hand-
books, manuals, etc.   3. Juvenile justice. Administration of—Handbooks, manuals,
etc.   I. Schetky, Diane H., 1940–   . II. Benedek, Elissa P.
  [DNLM: 1. Child Psychiatry. 2. Forensic Psychiatry—in infancy & childhood.
  W 740 C641]
RA1151.C76   1992
614′.1–dc20
DNLM/DLC
for Library of Congress   91-30650
                                                                    CIP

                                         91 92 93 94 95
                         1   2   3   4   5   6   7   8   9   10

To our children:
David, Joel, Sarah, and Dina Benedek
James and Scott Browning

We first met while picking up our children at an APA daycare center in 1976. Our children have grown up with our books in progress and have survived our busy careers. We appreciate their ongoing support and encouragement, and it pleases us that they share our interests in writing, medicine, and law. Several of them are following in our footsteps, and they all share our concern for people who suffer.

Diane H. Schetky, M.D.
Elissa P. Benedek, M.D.

Foreword

The courtroom has rapidly emerged as the main stage upon which the serious strains on American family life are enacted. Disordered parental functioning, chronic relentless conflict, and the dissolution of families represent the largest identifiable pathogenic influence contributing to the various psychiatric disorders of childhood and adolescence. The coming together of these psychosocial stressors within the legal setting poses substantial tasks for the child mental health professional who must now utilize and master both clinical and forensic knowledge and skills to be competent in the field.

This book, edited by renowned forensic child and adolescent pychiatrists, stands out as the most comprehensive and up-to-date text available. The breadth and depth of its content are impressive but its style and format are "user-friendly." The *Clinical Handbook of Child Psychiatry and the Law* should become the basic textbook for training in child and adolescent psychiatry and related fields. Furthermore, this book provides an invaluable reference text for law students, practicing attorneys, and judges.

The standards of training in child forensic mental health are variable if not in many instances nonexistent, as in the evaluation of alleged sexual abuse. The number of "expert" service providers involved in such work continues to expand. Substandard work in this field is often damaging to both children and their families. Drs. Schetky and Benedek's book sets the "gold standard" for every area of child psychiatry and the law.

Kenneth S. Robson, M.D.
Professor and Director
Division of Child and Adolescent Psychiatry
Institute of Living/University of Connecticut
Hartford, Connecticut

Preface

Forensic child psychiatry is a subspecialty of child psychiatry that applies scientific and clinical experience to legal issues affecting children. Demands for service in this area have clearly outpaced training. Most child psychiatrists with expertise in this area are self-taught or have learned from mentors. As of this writing, there are no fellowships available in child forensic psychiatry. In contrast, there are 20 accredited fellowship training programs in forensic psychiatry in the United States and four in Canada. It is our position that the basics of child forensic psychiatry should be included in all child psychiatry training programs. For those desiring more in-depth experience, we would encourage the development of child forensic fellowships in selected locations.

Forensic child psychiatry utilizes all of the requisite skills of a child psychiatrist, including knowledge of child development, family and individual psychodynamics, child psychotherapy, psychopharmacology, consultation, teaching, and child advocacy. However, inasmuch as these skills are to be applied in an arena alien to most child psychiatrists, additional knowledge of the legal process and functions of expert witnesses are required. Given the frequency with which the law has an impact on the practice of child psychiatry, no clinician can afford to practice in ignorance of the law.

This book updates our earlier book, *Child Psychiatry and the Law*. Since the writing of that book, it has been gratifying to see the *Journal of the American Academy of Child and Adolescent Psychiatry* regularly publish articles related to forensic issues and the American Academy of Child and Adolescent Psychiatry sponsor numerous programs and institutes in this area. Interest in child forensic psychiatry continues to grow. Trainees express frustration regarding the lack of training materials and programs in the area. The field is becoming increasingly complex, and hardly a day goes by when child forensic issues are not major news stories.

This book is designed to consolidate the current state of knowledge in child forensic psychiatry, to provide principles to which we may turn as we tackle increasingly complex issues, and to foster interest in the area among trainees and clinicians. It is also intended to help those in law and child protection to better understand how the child psychiatrist approaches issues at the interface of child psychiatry and law. Hopefully, the book may promote better communication among the many disciplines involved in these difficult but fascinating cases. By taking the reader through the basic principles involved in child forensic psychiatry and by using didactic and clinical material, we will try to demystify the field.

Part I provides an overview of forensic child psychiatry and basic principles. Part II deals with clinical assessment in forensic settings. Part III deals with special issues, many of which have only come into focus within the past 10 years. This book is designed as a handbook, and the emphasis is practical, not scholarly.

Additional readings are provided, and suggested readings follow each chapter for those who wish to explore the issues in more depth.

We are indebted to Paul Appelbaum, M.D., Thomas Gutheil, M.D., and Michael Fisher of Williams & Wilkins, who suggested that we model this book after Appelbaum and Gutheil's highly successful *Clinical Handbook of Psychiatry and the Law*. Drs. Appelbaum and Gutheil have been leaders in the field of forensic psychiatry and have provided inspiration to many. In addition, we wish to thank attorneys Jean Anderson and Robert Walzer for their thoughtful comments on selected chapters.

Diane H. Schetky, M.D.
Elissa P. Benedek, M.D.

Contributors

Marcelino Amaya, M.D.
Director, Children's Psychiatric
  Institute
John Umstead Hospital
Butner, North Carolina
Assistant Professor of Psychiatry
Duke University Medical Center
Durham, North Carolina
Clinical Associate Professor of
  Psychiatry
University of North Carolina
Chapel Hill, North Carolina

Elissa P. Benedek, M.D.
Director of Research and Training
Center for Forensic Psychiatry
Clinical Professor of Psychiatry
University of Michigan Medical
  Center
Ann Arbor, Michigan

W. V. Burlingame, Ph.D.
Director, Adolescent Unit
John Umstead Hospital
Butner, North Carolina
Clinical Professor of Psychology
University of North Carolina
Chapel Hill, North Carolina

Beth K. Clark, Ph.D.
Private Practice
Ann Arbor, Michigan

Charles R. Clark, Ph.D.
Private Practice
Ann Arbor, Michigan

Catherine DeAngelis, M.D.
Professor of Pediatrics
Associate Dean for Academic Affairs
The Johns Hopkins University School
  of Medicine
Baltimore, Maryland

Lesley Devoe, M.S.W.
Private Practice
Rockland, Maine

James C. Harris, M.D.
Director, Developmental
  Neuropsychiatry
Associate Professor of Psychiatry,
  Mental Hygiene, and Pediatrics
The Johns Hopkins University
Baltimore, Maryland

Stephen P. Herman, M.D.
Associate Clinical Professor of
  Psychiatry
Yale Child Study Center
New Haven, Connecticut

Michael G. Kalogerakis, M.D.
Clinical Professor of Psychiatry
New York University School of
  Medicine
New York, New York

JoAnn E. Macbeth, J.D.
Crowell & Moring
Washington, DC

Eli H. Newberger, M.D.
Senior Associate in Medicine
Director, Family Development
   Program
The Children's Hospital
Boston, Massachusetts

Kathleen M. Quinn, M.D.
Associate Professor of Psychiatry
Case Western Reserve University
Cleveland, Ohio

Miriam B. Rosenthal, M.D.
Associate Professor of Psychiatry and
   Reproductive Biology
Case Western Reserve University
Division Chief of Behavioral
   Medicine
Department of Obstetrics and
   Gynecology
University MacDonald Womens
   Hospital
Cleveland, Ohio

Diane H. Schetky, M.D.
Private Practice
Rockport, Maine

Sue White, Ph.D.
Associate Professor of Psychology
Metro Health Center and Case
   Western Reserve University
Cleveland, Ohio

Contents

Section Three

SPECIAL ISSUES

SECTION ONE

OVERVIEW

1

History of Child Forensic Psychiatry

DIANE H. SCHETKY, M.D., AND ELISSA P. BENEDEK, M.D.

The roots of child forensic psychiatry go back to the early 20th century and the founding of the first juvenile court in Chicago. Before the creation of the juvenile court, children were considered property of their parents. They could be fully exploited in the labor market and, if charged with misconduct, were subject to the same criminal proceedings and sanctions as adults. The concept of childhood as a special period of life did not emerge until the 16th century, and only recently have children been recognized as having any special needs or rights.

Various forces converged in the early 20th century to impact on the way in which children were viewed. These included creation of the juvenile court, child labor laws, children's aid societies, The Children's Bureau, and interest in public education. In 1922, the court, in the case of *Finlay v. Finlay* (148 NE 624, NY, 1925), recognized that children were no longer mere property and might have interests separate from and beyond their parents, at least in matters of custody.

The first juvenile court was created in Chicago in 1899, and by the late 1920s all but two states had enacted laws founded on the Illinois model. The philosophy of the early juvenile court was one of benevolence. It sought to understand the total child and respond to him "as a wise, merciful father handles his own child whose errors are not discovered by the authorities" (Mack 1909). The juvenile court viewed its role as preventive, helping the child and protecting him from criminal proceedings. Julian Mack, an early juvenile court justice, pleaded that "there be attached to the court as there have been in a few cities, a child study department where every child, before hearing, shall be subjected to thorough psycho-physical examination. In hundreds of cases, the discovery and remedy of defective eyesight or hearing or some slight surgical operation will effectuate a complete change in the character of the lad" (Mack 1909, 120).

The mental health profession began to embrace the problem of juvenile delinquency. Clinics developed that approached delinquency through multidisciplinary evaluations. William Healy, a neurologist, stressed the need for obtaining an adequate medical history and physical exam on each child and understanding the child's total life situation. In 1924, the American Orthopsychiatric Association formed as an interdiscplinary forum for understanding the causes and treatment of delinquency. The publication of Aichhorn's *Wayward Youth* (1925) with its psychoanalytic interpretation of delinquent behavior had significant impact on the treatment of delinquents. Various researchers such as the Gluecks, Robins, and Lewis have since conducted epidemiological, genetic, and biological studies on delinquents. In spite of newer developments, we continue to go back to the wisdom of Healy who stressed getting a total picture of the child.

The early juvenile court did not live up to its promises. Dispositional and treatment components of clinics were severely lagging, and the benign atmosphere of the court failed to curb more hardened delinquents. Justice Fortas charged that "in most juvenile courts the child receives the worst of both worlds: that he gets neither the protection accorded to adults nor the solicitous care and regenerative treatment postulated for children" (*In re Gault*, 387, U.S. I). Years later, Stone lamented that "the court's only function in many cases is to funnel children from unsuitable homes to unsuitable placements" (1976, 156). In the 1960s President Johnson's Commission on Law Enforcement attempted to improve the juvenile justice system. The ensuing report by The Administration of Justice noted that juvenile courts were failing to meet the needs of delinquent youths and emphasized the need for prevention through community-based diversion programs aimed at predelinquents. These efforts failed and were felt to merely widen the net and be responsive to crises with little in the way of offering long-term help to hard core delinquents.

Two significant changes have affected the way in which the juvenile court functions. *In re Gault* (1967) afforded due process to juveniles in delinquency proceedings, thereby strengthening their rights. In the 1970s the use of waiver to the adult courts for seriously delinquent juveniles went into effect, subjecting these delinquents to harsher sanctions without the protections of the juvenile court.

The second interface of child psychiatry with the law occurred around custody issues. *Finlay v. Finlay* (1925) introduced the concept of making decisions in accord with "the child's best interests." Years later this concept was elaborated upon by Goldstein, Freud, and Solnit (1973) in *Beyond the Best Interests of the Child*, in which they applied psychoanalytic principles to the resolution of custody disputes. Mental health professionals continue to be involved in helping the court arrive at custody determinations. The issues have become far more complex as one is faced with a menu of parenting options as well as with high tech reproductive technologies that impinge on custody issues.

A third area of involvement has been with abused and neglected children. Sexual abuse of children has been documented since the 6th century BC, but only within the past two decades has society been willing to acknowledge the extent of the problem and develop treatment programs. It was not until 1974 that the U.S.A. enacted mandatory child abuse reporting laws. This, combined with increased media attention to the problems of child abuse, resulted in escalating reports of child abuse. In the 1980s reports of child sexual abuse began to eclipse reports of physical abuse and they continue to soar although many remain unsubstantiated. Currently we face the problem that there are simply not enough well-trained mental health professionals to evaluate the burgeoning number of allegations of sexual abuse. As less well-trained persons attempt to fill the void, we risk creating a whole new set of iatrogenic problems, i.e., failure to diagnose abuse or erroneous diagnoses of abuse made prematurely on inadequate data bases.

Foster care emerged in the early 20th century as an alternative to institutional care for children. Often these children were destitute, and in most cases they were white. Polier (1989) notes that racial discrimination in institutions and public agencies was rampant. When children were placed, little effort was made to find adoptive homes for them. In the last two decades, we have seen increased attention paid to all children in foster care. Whereas in the past it was not unusual for children to languish in foster care for 5 years or more, it is now recognized that multiple and extended placements have adverse consequences on children. In turn, there has been a new emphasis on permanency planning and periodic judicial review of all children in placement. Adoption agencies have become more aggressive in locating homes for hard to place children and are in turn relaxing their standards for adoptive parents. Child mental health clinicians are often called upon to determine a child's needs, including issues of termination of parental rights and adoption.

A relatively new area of involvement in forensic child psychiatry is civil litigation. This has paralleled emerging interest in post-traumatic stress disorder and the seminal work of Lenore Terr on psychic trauma in children. Currently there is much interest on research in the area of children's responses to trauma. The area of children as witnesses has stimulated research in the area of children's cognitive development, but research can scarcely keep pace with the court's demand for scientific data bases. More rigorous demands for evidence that is scientifically based has greatly altered how we may testify in courts on sexual abuse cases.

Heightened interest in ethics has emerged in the 90s and cuts across all areas of child psychiatry. There is no way the trainee of today can anticipate the ethical problems he will face in 10 years given the rapid evolution of technology and life styles. Surrogacy issues raised in the 1980s pale as we now worry about issues such as whether to press criminal charges against a pregnant woman whose substance abuse threatens her fetus; custody battles waged over frozen embryos; visitation disputes between a separating lesbian couple whose child was conceived by a sperm donation from a gay friend, who along with his lover wants equal time with the child; and the question of whether a teenager is competent to request the discontinuation of life supports. On a more mundane level we must daily confront the risks associated with boundary violations in our practices and increasingly practice defensive psychiatry to avoid the prospect of malpractice litigation. Therefore it behooves training programs to offer solid foundations in ethical and legal issues that will help future clinicians to keep their heads safely above water. Of most importance is the ability to recognize potential conflicts of interest and to have the tools for decision making that may be applied to the ever-changing array of clinical issues that will confront us down the road.

I. SUGGESTED READINGS

Aichorn, A. (1925), Wayward Youth. New York: Viking Press.

Aries, P. (1962), Centuries of Childhood: A Social History of Family Life. New York: Vintage Books.

Derdeyn, A. (1976), Child custody contests in historical perspective. Am J Psychiatry 133 (12) 1369–1376.

Glueck, S. and Glueck, E. (1930), Five Hundred Criminal Careers. New York: Knopf.

Goldstein, J., Freud, A., and Solnit, A. (1973), Beyond the Best Interests of the Child. New York: Free Press.

Healy, W. (1915), The Individual Delinquent. A Textbook of Diagnosis and Prognosis. Boston: Little Brown.

Lewis, D. and Ballas, D. (1976), Delinquency and Psychopathology. New York: Grune and Stratton.

Mack, J. (1909), The juvenile court. Harvard Law Rev 23:104–122.

Platt, A. M. (1969), The Child Savers: The Invention of Delinquency. Chicago: University of Chicago Press.

Polier, J. W. (1989), Juvenile Justice in Double Jeopardy. Hillsdale, N.Y.: Lawrence Erlbaum Association Publishers.

Postman, N. (1982), The Disappearance of Childhood. New York: Delacorte Press.

Robins, L. (1966), Deviant Children Grown Up. Baltimore: Williams & Wilkins.

Stone, A. (1976), Mental Health and the Law: A System in Transition. New York: Jason Aronson.

Terr, L. (1990), Too Scared to Cry: Psychic Trauma in Childhood. New York: Harper and Row.

2

The Child Forensic Evaluation

DIANE H. SCHETKY, M.D.

I. CASE EXAMPLES
II. LEGAL ISSUES
  A. Dealing with attorneys
    1. SOURCE OF REFERRAL
    2. DETERMINING PURPOSE OF EVALUATION
    3. CRITERIA FOR ACCEPTING CASE
      a. Merits of the case
      b. Your qualifications
      c. Time and distance limitations
      d. Avoiding conflicts of interest
      e. Is the attorney someone with whom you can work?
    4. STRUCTURING THE EVALUATION
      a. Access to parties and information
      b. Deadlines
      c. Fees
      d. Background material
      e. Determining the need for further consultations
  B. Obtaining consent
    1. CLARIFYING YOUR ROLE AND PURPOSE OF EVALUATION
    2. INFORMED CONSENT AND WAIVER
    3. ASSENT FROM A MINOR
  C. Liability of the expert witness
    1. PROTECTION
    2. NEW TRENDS IN SEXUAL ABUSE LITIGATION
III. THE CLINICAL EVALUATION
  A. Meeting with the parents
  B. Meeting with the child
  C. Observations of parent-child relationship
  D. Ancillary information
  E. The written evaluation
    1. FUNCTIONS OF WRITTEN REPORT
    2. LANGUAGE OF THE REPORT
    3. ORGANIZATION
      a. Circumstance of the evaluation
      b. Sources of information
      c. History
      d. Observations and foundations for opinions
      e. Impressions and recommendations
        i. *Reasonable*
        ii. *Feasible*
        iii. *Do data support conclusions?*

IV. PITFALLS
   A. Psychiatrist-related pitfalls
      1. Bias
      2. Double agentry
      3. Rigidity
      4. Inadequate data base
      5. Faulty methods
      6. Quoting the literature
      7. The hired gun
      8. Puffery
   B. Patient-related pitfalls
      1. The con man
      2. Nonpayment
      3. Harassment
      4. Litigious parents
   C Attorney-related pitfalls
      1. Flattery
      2. Coercive tactics
      3. Withholding of information
      4. Boundary violations
      5. Muddled thinking
      6. The unprepared
      7. Communication problems
V. CASE EXAMPLE EPILOGUES
VI. ACTION GUIDELINES
   A. Strive for honesty and objectivity.
   B. Maintain control of the evaluation.
   C. Be selective and take steps to protect self and family members.
   D. Hold the middle ground and learn to live with ambiguity.
   E. Learn to critique your report from the standpoint of the other side.
   F. Contrary quotients and validity percentages.
   G. Know your limitations.
   H. Seek consultation.
   I. Keep current and stay involved.
VII. SUGGESTED READINGS

I. CASE EXAMPLES

A. Case Example 1

An attorney requests that you see her client, a 17-year-old girl, who is suing her father for sexual abuse. She requests that you treat the girl, support her during the litigation process, and testify about damages. The client has limited funds and her attorney asks if you would defer payment for your services until after the settlement.

B. Case Example 2

An attorney refers his client to a child psychiatry clinic for a forensic evaluation of her parenting skills. The state has filed a petition to terminate her parental rights and he wants an independent evaluation. He insists his main concern is with the best interests of her children. The trainee who is assigned to the case spends hours reviewing records, meeting with the mother, and observing her with her young children. He produces a very comprehensive report in which he raises serious concerns about her ability to parent. He is irate because the attorney does not like his findings and has chosen not to use his evaluation. He wants to know if he can make his report available to the prosecution.

C. Case Example 3

An attorney requests an urgent evaluation of his client's three children. They are refusing to return to their mother after a two month summer visitation with their father. The children allege physical abuse by their mother and verbal abuse by their stepfather.

II. LEGAL ISSUES

A. Dealing with attorneys

1. SOURCE OF REFERRAL

In most forensic evaluations, the request for evaluation will come directly from an involved attorney or the guardian ad litem for the child. The expert may also be court appointed. The latter conveys more neutrality, but it is not always feasible and does not apply in cases of tort litigation. In the latter, requests for evaluation also may come from the insurance company that is defending the case.

If the request for evaluation comes directly from the patient, it is critical to clarify the legal issues with his or her attorney before proceeding. In contrast to most psychiatric evaluations, forensic evaluations are for the attorney or the court, not the patient. The forensic evaluation is directed toward answering a specific legal issue in question, not toward providing relief to the patient. Time spent initially with the referring attorney framing the evaluation will help to avoid problems down the road. This should include clarifying what you can and cannot do, and spelling out the terms of the evaluation.

2. DETERMINING PURPOSE OF THE EVALUATION

Attorneys may not be clear about what they want from you. Some will launch into a long description of the case before asking if you are available. It is helpful to try to get them to frame the legal question at the onset; then clarify what you might be able to offer. For instance, they may be wanting psychological testing and be unaware that psychiatrists do not perform psychometrics. If a case seems complex, a face-to-face meeting with the attorney may be helpful. Often after a cursory review of the case, the psychiatrist can point out the relevant psychological issues. This in turn helps the attorney develop his defense.

3. CRITERIA FOR ACCEPTING CASE

a. Merits of the case

Considering the time and energy that goes into a forensic evaluation, it is useful at the onset to ask whether the case merits such an investment on your part. Is this an issue you feel strongly about? Are there enough data available to enable you to reach a decision? If a party claims he is being falsely accused of sexual abuse is there sufficient doubt to warrant reexamining the parties?

b. Your qualifications

Credentials are carefully reviewed in court as part of qualifying an expert witness to testify. It is important to consider whether you have sufficient expertise in the area in question. The novice might wish to accrue forensic experience with custody and abuse cases before branching out into other civil cases and criminal litigation. Attorneys may be of great help in providing relevant literature and explaining the legal issues. For instance, you may have never testified in a toxic waste suit before, but if you understand the principles of civil litigation and are willing to do some reading you may soon be in command of the issues. Another example would be the child psychiatrist experienced in child sexual abuse who becomes involved with cases of patient-therapist sex as an expert witness for the plaintiff. The dynamic issues are similar, as are the damages, but one needs to become conversant with the burgeoning literature in the area and understand the relevant legal issues.

The neophyte should not be embarrassed by paucity of credentials. He can anticipate that the other side may try to use this to impeach him if they are not able to impeach his testimony. Sometimes inexperience in court can be an advantage in countering the image of being a hired gun.

c. Time and distance limitations

Some attorneys may frantically call an expert one week before trial date. This may occur when an expert he had lined up is unavailable or has withdrawn from the case or because the attorney is disorganized. A forensic evaluation done in haste is likely to be a sloppy one. The expert is advised not to jump in on such short notice as there is too much at stake. The expert should not agree to do a forensic evaluation unless he or she has sufficient time in which to do a thorough evaluation and report and can see the case through to the end. Civil litigation cases may linger for years and may require updating as the trial date approaches. Cases are likely to come to trial on short notice, and one needs to anticipate the disruptive effect this may have on one's practice.

Given the paucity of child forensic psychiatrists it is not unusual to be asked to consult on out-of-state cases, particularly if one has developed some area of expertise. One needs to weigh the effect of time lost in travel on one's practice and family as well. Travel time need not be lost time and can be put to good use in catching up on reading and writing. Geographical desirability also may be an issue, e.g., Florida in the winter holds more appeal than does Alaska. Given the likelihood of postponements, one could end up in Florida in the heat of the summer and wish it had been Alaska.

d. Avoiding conflicts of interest

Deal with conflicts of interest by recognizing their potential and avoiding them from the start. Conflicts of interest may arise when an attorney asks a psychiatrist to provide forensic testimony on a case she is treating. The therapist loses a certain degree of objectivity upon entering into a treatment relationship. This occurs because the patient's needs become foremost, and one is likely to be optimistic about the efficacy of therapy and one's skills as a therapist. In addition, there is no confidentiality in forensic evaluations, and this in itself undermines the therapeutic process. We therefore recommend a policy of separating the roles of therapist and forensic evaluator.

Similar conflicts may arise if one decides to treat a child after having done the custody evaluation. Some exceptions may exist, as when a custody evaluation is settled out of court and parents have maintained a good rapport with the child psychiatrist and would like him to treat their child. However, there is always the risk of relitigation and of having one's records subpoenaed.

The psychiatrist should avoid doing forensic evaluations on any parties with whom she has previous ties or is likely to deal with professionally or socially. For example, a child psychiatrist was reprimanded for doing a custody evaluation on a member of his clinical faculty with whom he had no previous relationship. Ties of that sort could be mistaken by some as grounds for bias. Sometimes these situations cannot be anticipated, and if one is living in a small community one might wish to think twice about evaluating someone who lives in close proximity.

Significant ties to the referring attorney, be they of friendship, legal, or even romantic nature, may affect the opinion rendered, and such potential conflicts should be carefully assessed.

e. Is the attorney someone with whom you can work?

Unfortunately, it is not always possible to answer this question until one has embarked upon the evaluation. It may be possible to inquire about the reputation of the attorney and his firm or to speak with others who have worked with him. Qualities to look out for include legal acumen, ethical conduct, treatment of the client, and willingness to communicate with you.

4. STRUCTURING THE EVALUATION

a. Access to parties and information

Having agreed to participate in the case, the psychiatrist should state which parties he wishes to see and approximately how much time will be involved. If you are entering a case at the request of one parent, it is critical to ensure that you have access to the other parent at the onset. A unilateral evaluation is of very limited value but there may be times when the other parent is truly not available. In such instances, one should state the limiting conditions of the evaluation and qualify any conclusions or recommendations. In evaluating children of divorced parents consent to evaluate the child must be obtained from the custodial parent. If custody is joint, usually permission from one parent suffices, though the intent of joint custody arrangements is to share decision making. If in doubt about a custody decree one may ask to see a copy of it.

Lawyers can be very helpful in amassing and indexing records related to a case. The psychiatrist needs to be certain that nothing is being withheld because it is unfavorable to the client. The psychiatrist will need to use discretion in determining what records to review and in how much depth to review them. In some cases of civil litigation it is not unusual for records to reach the height of 6 feet or more. The psychiatrist may wonder whether to charge for review time by the pound, inch, or hour.

b. Deadlines

One should clarify the time frame in which one is working, often working backward from the anticipated date of trial. Reports need to be submitted in time for them to be reviewed by both sides. In civil litigation one must meet a discovery date and allow time for depositions.

c. Fees

Fees need to be discussed at the onset. Rates vary regionally but customarily are higher than one's usual treatment fee. Most experts charge by the hour, as it is difficult to anticipate at the onset exactly how much time will be involved. In out-of-state cases one may choose to charge a *per diem* rate to cover travel, pretrial conferences, and testimony. The psychiatrist is advised to request a retainer fee at the onset. This should cover time to be spent interviewing, reviewing records, conferring with the attorney, and preparing a report. Attorneys operate with retainer fees and rarely object to this arrangement. If parents object to the cost of the evaluation, one may point out that good surgery is also expensive, and that it is better to do it right the first time. Further, the psychiatric evaluation is often pivotal to the outcome of the case, and one cannot afford to take shortcuts. Some psychiatrists may choose to request payment at the time of service, but this does not protect one from bounced checks or "I forgot my check book."

It is always unethical to take a case on a contingency fee. A contingency arrangement causes the expert to have too much invested in the outcome of the case and leads to a loss of objectivity.

d. Background material

One of the exciting aspects of forensic psychiatry is the opportunity to expand one's knowledge base. Attorneys and psychiatrists can share articles and knowledge related to the issues in the case and can learn from one another. For instance, discussing how a client has been affected by sexual abuse may enable her attorney to work more effectively with her and to better prepare her for trial.

e. Determining the need for further consultations

Early into the evaluation it is usually possible to determine what additional consultations will be needed. For instance, psychological testing often helps document damages and bolster the psychiatrist's opinions. The attorney and psychiatrist need to decide who is the best person to do the consult and schedule it well in advance of the court date.

B. Obtaining consent

At the onset the psychiatrist needs to clarify with the family who retained him and for what purpose. It is helpful to clarify that the evaluation, in contrast to therapy, is not confidential and that what they say and do will likely appear in your report. This becomes the basis for informed consent for the release of information. Waivers should be signed permitting release of the forensic report to the attorneys on each side before beginning the evaluation. Additional consent forms may be needed for request of information from other parties.

Sometimes there may be a question about a parent's capacity to give consent, for example, if one is psychotic or mentally retarded. In such instances one may need to refer to the court or to counsel for the parent and have a guardian ad litem appointed.

How much to tell a child about the evaluation is a function of the child's age. Although school-age children are not capable of giving informed consent, one may ask them for their assent.

C. Liability of the expert witness

Can the witness be sued for what he says in a report or on the witness stand? In most jurisdictions if the child psychiatrist is court appointed, he is considered to be acting in a quasi-judicial capacity and accordingly is entitled to the protection of absolute immunity (*Williams v. Rappeport*; DC Md, No. K–87–292, 6/9/88; *Lalonde v. Eissner*, Mass Sup Jud Ct, 405 Mass 207, 6/19/89). Courts have expanded the doctrine of absolute judicial immunity to include those persons involved in an integral part of the judicial process. This enables them to act freely without the threat of a lawsuit and encourages them to act with disinterested objectivity. In *Lalonde v. Eissner*, the expert was appointed not by the court but by the probation department pursuant to a court order and he was granted protection.

Less clear is the liability of the expert who is acting without court order. The author was sued in a custody case by angry grandparents who alleged, unsuccessfully, that, as a state employee, she must be in collusion with the state's adoption agency and that both had acted with malfeasance in depriving them of their right to adopt their grandchildren. Recently, several child psychologists and child psychiatrists have been sued for failure to diagnose child sexual abuse and one was sued by the alleged perpetrator for diagnosing sexual abuse. Even when these suits are dropped, as is often the case, they put the expert through unnecessary stress and harassment.

III. THE CLINICAL EVALUATION

A. Meeting with the parents

In doing an ordinary diagnostic evaluation one usually assumes that parents are being straightforward and acting out of concern for the child. In the forensic examination, how a parent presents may be colored by what the legal issue is. If custody is at stake, the parent is likely to put his or her best foot forward and be defensive. Parents in the throes of crisis or divorce may demonstrate regressive behavior that is not representative of usual levels of functioning. Where large sums of money are at stake, parents may consciously or unconsciously exaggerate their claims for secondary gain. Psychiatrists tend to be trusting, but in forensics it pays to be a bit of a skeptic. We often need to be more aggressive than in therapeutic settings, to look for contradictions and inconsistencies, and to probe for more detail.

Meeting with parents allows the examiner to gather history and to determine something about their functioning, parenting, and relationships with the child in question. How much one goes into these respective areas will depend on the purpose of the evaluation and will be explored in more depth in later chapters. If parents are not living together it may be necessary to obtain history from a child's parents separately. Contradictions may abound and can leave the evaluator feeling as if on a seesaw. It is critical to hear both sides in order to obtain a balanced picture of what is going on, particularly where parents are hurling accusations at one another. The psychiatrist needs to remember that the court, not he, is the ultimate finder of fact and that he is a clinician, not a detective.

B. Meeting with the child

The interview needs to be tailored to the legal question at hand. Interview tools such as the use of play, puppets, and drawings remain the same as in any diagnostic evaluation. However, it may also be necessary to take a more structured approach to answer specific questions relative to whether the child was abused and if so how it has affected her. Documentation becomes important and may take the form of written notes, audiotape, or videotape. If one chooses to record an interview it should only be done with the child's permission. One must consider how the process of recording affects the interviewer and child. The child's verbatim statements become very important, and it may be necessary to record them during an interview. It is also important to note how questions were put to the child. This will be discussed in more detail in Chapter 9.

Most forensic evaluations of children can be completed within two to four 1-hour visits with the child. The risk of going beyond this amount of time is that the child may perceive the interviews as interrogations and start to confabulate if repeatedly asked the same question. Another danger is that the evaluation may become treatment. With some very young or developmentally delayed children the evaluator may not be able to answer the ultimate questions. In such cases one must make do with presenting one's findings and recommending a course that will protect the child while trying to preserve the parent-child relationship if custody is at issue.

C. Observations of parent-child relationship

In custody and abuse cases it may be helpful to observe young children with their parents as long as this does not pose any risk to the child and the child does not object. The evaluator may choose to be in the room with them or watch from behind a one-way mirror. The evaluator should try to be unobtrusive and allow the parent and child to interact with one another as naturally as possible. This may be in a free play situation, or one may assign them a project to work on together. This type of evaluation is also useful for the unconscious material that emerges that a parent does not ordinarily volunteer, e.g., the parent is overcontrolling, intimidating, or rejecting; doesn't know how to play or parent; or has age-inappropriate expectations for the child. Observing parent and child together also sheds light on bonding.

D. Ancillary information

More effort needs to go into corroborating information in a forensic evaluation than in an ordinary diagnostic evaluation. If we err in the initial diagnosis of a patient we are treating, we have the opportunity to reassess and make adjustments in our treatment plan, and usually no serious harm ensues. In contrast, we do not have the luxury of time in forensic evaluations, and much more is at stake concerning the outcome of the legal proceedings. For instance, if a father is wrongfully acquitted of child sexual abuse, the victim and other potential victims remain at risk. On the other hand, if a father is erroneously convicted of sexual abuse, irreparable harm is done to his child's relationship with him, not to mention to his reputation and career.

Because credibility may be an issue in forensic evaluations, care needs to be taken, where possible, in cross-checking what the child has said to others. Police reports obtained immediately after disclosure are helpful. While children's descriptions of abuse may shift over time, the core features usually remain consistent, and their ability to give discrete detail enhances credibility. Results of physical examinations are helpful in determining whether injuries are consistent with allegations. However, one should heed the dictum that absence of physical findings does not mean absence of sexual abuse. The significance of physical findings will be discussed more in Chapter 8.

Other sources of valuable data include school reports, past psychological testing, and any previous psychiatric evaluations. These may be used to document prior levels of functioning relevant to a particular trauma or event.

Verbal reports from teachers, day care providers, and baby sitters also help complete the picture of how a child is functioning. For instance, the prosecution in an alleged sexual abuse case at a daycare center argued that a 5-year-old alleged victim was showing signs of post-traumatic stress disorder. This was based largely on a history obtained from the child's mother. Reports from the current daycare provider described a totally asymptomatic child. The defense successfully argued that had the child been traumatized during naptime at a daycare center she would likely show fears associated with going to her new daycare center and associated with taking naps there.

E. The written evaluation

1. FUNCTION OF THE WRITTEN REPORT

The well written report will often be a bargaining chip in reaching out-of-court settlement. Should the case go to court, the report becomes the basis for your testimony, and the opposing side will attempt to discredit it on cross-examination. The written report is also your work product and should not contain anything that might embarrass you in years to come.

The report should be directed toward the legal question at issue. How extensive the report is will depend on how complex the issues are. At a minimum the report must contain the building blocks that provide the foundation for one's opinion. It should also demonstrate that one has ruled out other possible causes for the patient's behaviors or symptoms. Psychodynamic formulations and speculations should be kept to a minimum as they are difficult to prove in court. A carefully documented history of child neglect and its impact on the child will go further in building a case for termination of parental rights than will psychoanalytic speculations about the mother's ambivalence toward her child.

2. LANGUAGE OF THE REPORT

The report is likely to be read by attorneys involved, their clients, the judge, and experts for the other side. The challenge in writing a good forensic report is to avoid psychiatric jargon and to render it fully intelligible to a lay person. The writer needs to strive for objectivity and avoid pejorative statements. For example, it is easy to substitute "he states" for "he claims" and "he seemed unduly suspicious" for "he showed paranoid traits." Avoiding the use of the first person also conveys more objectivity.

A tactfully worded report is less likely to inflame and put the subject of the report on the defensive. Direct quotes speak for themselves and supplant the need to make any value judgments, e.g., a father states he "never loses control" yet both children attest that he has tried to strangle them. Direct statements also serve to aid recall when months or years elapse between evaluation and testimony.

Vague or speculative statements should be avoided, also statements such as "clearly" or "obviously." Just because something is obvious to you does not mean it is to others.

Reports should be carefully proofread for content and typographical errors. The author once used a new typist who sent a report to "The Horrible Judge Gil." Fortunately, Judge Gil had a sense of humor.

3. ORGANIZATION

a. Circumstances of the evaluation

The report should reflect who retained your services and for what purposes.

b. Sources of information

Sources of information should include both firsthand and secondary information that was relied upon in reaching your recommendations. The report should state when, where, and for how long you saw the various parties. Information received by telephone, e.g., discussion with a therapist should also be noted. If records were requested but not received that should be so noted.

c. History

In relating the history it should be clear from whose perspective it is coming, e.g., "according to the mother," rather than stating something as factual. Often histories have to be presented from several perspectives. The psychiatrist may be selective in terms of what relevant history goes into the report. For example, toilet training has little bearing on the development of post-traumatic stress disorder in an adolescent who was in a building that caught on fire. In contrast, if the plaintiff is a 4-year-old who suddenly develops nightmares and enuresis after being bitten by a dog, it is more relevant.

d. Observations and foundations for opinions

Direct observations provide a strong bulwark for opinions and should be carefully described. It is helpful to note that the purpose of the evaluation was discussed with the patient. Some attorneys, desperate to suppress an unfavorable court ordered report, have tried to argue that the patient was being seen in therapy and that the communication was privileged.

The patient's manner should be described in terms of degree of cooperation, defensiveness, rapport, etc., which may have bearing on the material elicited. Which parent brought a child to an appointment may affect the child's behavior and comments that day and should therefore be noted. It may be necessary to interview very young children in the presence of a parent, and this should be noted in the event that it might influence the child's responses.

Children's productions and art work should be described and may be amended to the report. Copies should be made for your own files since the originals will be admitted as evidence.

e. Impressions and recommendations

Impressions and recommendations should be supported by data in the report. The court is likely to ask whether they are reasonable and feasible. A model the author learned to adopt in working with children in rural areas that have limited resources is to suggest 1) what is optimal, 2) what is feasible, and 3) having a backup plan when the feasible one falls through.

Whether one chooses to use DSM-III-R diagnoses will depend on the nature of the evaluation. Often they are not pertinent in custody matters, but they are quite relevant if one is claiming psychic harm in civil litigation. If diagnoses are used, one should be prepared to define and defend them.

IV. PITFALLS

A. Psychiatrist-related pitfalls

1. BIAS

Bias can occur in a variety of situations. Perhaps the worst sort of bias is the expert who is convinced that he is unbiased. As noted by Judge Bazelon, "Like any other man, a physician acquires an emotional identification with an opinion that comes down on one side of a conflict; he has an inescapable, prideful conviction in the accuracy of his own findings" (1974). Because of the nature of the adversary system, pressures inevitably arise to take sides and these may distort our views.

The evaluator needs to pay close attention to countertransference reactions that occur in forensic settings. For instance, we may favor adoption by a foster parent because her upper middle class status affords the child better educational opportunities than does return to a welfare mother who is a high school dropout. A psychiatrist with homophobic attitudes may balk at the request of a lesbian couple to adopt a disabled 5-year-old boy. Countertransference issues will be discussed further in Chapter 15.

2. DOUBLE AGENTRY

Double agentry occurs when one attempts to serve two masters or when conflicts of interest interfere with one's duty to act solely in the best interest of the person being evaluated. If one is consulting to a school and sees a student who discloses that he is dealing drugs in school, is one's duty to protect the patient or the school? Exploitation of a patient by writing a book about him is another example of double agentry. As noted by Simon (1987), it may result in the psychiatrist seeking out sensational material instead of acting in the patient's best interest.

3. RIGIDITY

Cognitive rigidity may occur when the psychiatrist is convinced of the accuracy of his own findings and is unwilling to consider other explanations for a patient's behavior or to alter his opinion in the face of new and contradictory information. Humility and admitting that one does not have all the answers is the preferred stance in court.

4. INADEQUATE DATA BASE

This pitfall may occur in experienced clinicians who owing to the pressures of a busy schedule or their cumulative experience try to take shortcuts. A child psychiatrist who boasted that she saw 100 cases per year of sexual abuse was convinced after spending only 30 minutes with a 2-year-old that the toddler had been sexually abused by his father. She apparently relied heavily on the mother's interpretations and erroneous report that sperm had been detected on the child's underpants. A corollary worth considering is that often the more we know/see the less we know. The inexperienced clinician needs to avoid premature conclusions and to consider other possible explanations for a child's behavior.

Another trap is failure to examine all the parties where custody is at issue and when sexual abuse allegations are alleged in this context.

Nonphysicians may misinterpret or fail to inquire about medical findings or confuse their significance. Urinary tract infections may become equated with vaginitis and diaper rash with sexual molestation. These problems will be discussed further in Chapter 8.

There may be times when all the data we would like to have are simply not available. In such instances, one may state the limiting factors of the evaluation and what attempts were made to obtain the information.

5. FAULTY METHODS

Evaluators may use idiosyncratic methods to determine a child's preference in custody cases or to diagnose sexual abuse. Increasingly, courts are demanding that in order for evidence to be accepted in court it must be based on scientific methods accepted within the community.

6. QUOTING THE LITERATURE

The novice in forensic psychiatry may be tempted to bolster her opinions by citing the literature. This is hazardous, as it invites the other side to come forth with literature countering your sources. Further, they manage to make the expert look foolish when she admits she's never heard of an arcane reference they dug up.

7. THE HIRED GUN

A few, but not many, child psychiatrists and psychologists have made bad names for themselves by traveling about the country and always appearing either on the side of the plaintiff or defendant. Not too surprisingly, this has led people to question whether these experts are being bought for their opinions regardless of the facts of the case.

8. PUFFERY

This occurs when the inexperienced or insecure expert attempts to inflate his credentials. He may infer that he is Board Certified when he is not, and bolster his credentials with inconsequential courses or seminars he has attended. Also, some may mislead the public in advertisements in terms of the services they offer and their qualifications.

B. Patient-related pitfalls

1. THE CON MAN

The con man is smooth, charming, and adept with words. He may try to convince you that his wife is hysterical, conniving, or man-hating. Rarely does he speak to his role in domestic difficulties, or if he does it may be with an air of contriteness. If sexual abuse is alleged he finds it "abhorrent" and thinks his wife has been watching too many TV shows on it. In an effort to come across as Mr. Nice Guy he may take in the psychiatrist. The psychiatrist needs to counter these tactics by reading between the lines, corroborating, and gently confronting.

2. NONPAYMENT

It is easy, but a mistake, to assume that because you render a favorable opinion that patients will gratefully pay you after the fact. Many other people may be trying to collect from them, and because you are so understanding they may decide to keep you waiting. Those who dislike your findings have even more reason not to pay. The best antidote is payment up front, which further enforces the message that your time, not your opinion, is being bought.

3. HARASSMENT

Harassment may occasionally occur in the form of threats to one's person, obscene phone calls, or calls in the middle of the night with no one on the other end. A more likely scenario is that of threats made in the form of groundless complaints by disgruntled patients to the licensing board, or to ethics committees of one's hospital, medical, or psychiatric society.

4. LITIGIOUS PARENTS

A history of repeated litigation and suits pending is often a tip-off that one is dealing with a litigious party. A psychologist evaluated a lady regarding her claim that her depression ensued from a motel fire in which she had been involved. When she told her patient that her depression seemed to precede the fire, the patient replied, "Well, I guess we'll have to go for the auto accident then." Her husband was simultaneously suing a physician for an allergic reaction to penicillin. They had also had their son evaluated in regard to symptoms of post-traumatic stress disorder related to an auto accident. While there was some reality base for their claims, their litigiousness would likely have undermined their credibility in the eyes of a jury.

Other clues to the litigious include vindictiveness, tendencies to externalize conflict, blame others for their mishaps, and not take responsibility for their own actions.

C. Attorney-related pitfalls

1. FLATTERY

"Doc, I'm told you are the best in the field," the attorney on the other end of the phone tells you. "We can't win our case without you," and so it goes. The assumption is that you are willing to rally to their defense regardless of what the issue is. Sometimes they may have a good case, but their come-on is an immediate turn-off.

2. COERCIVE TACTICS

This lawyer has trouble hearing "no" and aggressively pursues you. He may say, "money is no obstacle," insinuating that perhaps you can be had for a price.

3. WITHHOLDING OF INFORMATION

In an attempt to enlist your services, the attorney may withhold certain information such as his client's prior conviction for sexual abuse. If an attorney is behaving dishonestly or unethically this is grounds for withdrawing from the case.

4. BOUNDARY VIOLATIONS

An attorney, whom you've never met, calls you at home on a Saturday afternoon and addresses you by your first name. Such undue familiarity should raise concern as to other boundary violations and give pause for thought as to whether this attorney is one with whom you care to work.

5. MUDDLED THINKING

"Doc, I've got this client who drowned her kid in the river, and I don't know what the h—— is going on," says the inarticulate attorney on the other end of a long distance call. He is even more vague concerning the history and is befuddled as to what he wants from you. Unless you are eager for this type of case, this is one you might choose to avoid.

6. THE UNPREPARED

An attorney claimed that he couldn't work with his client, who was suing her physician for sexual abuse, because the client did not trust him. The psychiatrist repeatedly explained that mistrust was a common sequela of sexual abuse. She suggested that he do some basic reading in the area of patient-therapist sex and gave him references. One year into the case, the attorney knew no more about sexual abuse or mental illness even though he was claiming mental illness as grounds for tolling the statute of limitations. The client found that she could not work with this attorney, discharged him, and had to start anew. The experience left her feeling revictimized.

7. COMMUNICATION PROBLEMS

If an attorney is too busy to return phone calls one must wonder whether he has adequate time to devote to the case. Such lack of consideration does not promote a harmonious working relationship. The attorney who gives you 24 hours notice of a hearing, when he's known about it for a week, is also one you might not choose to work with in the future.

A related problem is the attorney who never bothers to give you a follow-up on the legal outcome of a case. Follow-up is a common courtesy and also is a chance for the expert to get constructive feedback on his testimony. It is also important to know whether or not the court agreed with your findings and recommendations.

V. CASE EXAMPLE EPILOGUES

A. Case Example 1

The psychiatrist explains to the attorney that she can either do a forensic evaluation or treatment, but not both. She remains firm about her policy of payment up front. The attorney agrees that her firm will pay for the forensic evaluation and that she will refer her client to a local mental health center for therapy.

B. Case Example 2

The trainee has become too invested in his evaluation. He has forgotten that he did the evaluation for the attorney, not the patient, and that it is protected as the attorney's work product. This case illustrates one of the risks of not being court-appointed.

C. Case Example 3

The psychiatrist first asks which parent has custody and learns that the mother, who lives out of state, does. The psychiatrist refuses to see the children without permission from the mother. The attorney does not see what the problem is and continues to press regarding the urgency of the situation. The psychiatrist recommends that he either 1) get the consent and cooperation of the mother, 2) contact protective services if he feels the children are truly at risk, or 3) petition the court for an order of change of custody. She does not hear from the attorney again.

VI. ACTION GUIDELINES

A. Strive for honesty and objectivity

Don't be afraid to admit that you don't know something. Take time to self-reflect and examine what you are basing your opinions upon.

B. Maintain control of the evaluation

Be firm in setting your terms and don't allow an attorney to push you into doing something that you feel is unethical or against the law.

C. Be selective and take steps to protect self and family members

If you are in solo practice or have a home office, it pays to think twice about evaluating potentially violent or vindictive patients. If you choose to see these patients, opt for a more protective setting and take steps to protect your privacy.

For instance, the author was referred an 8-year-old who had set several fires. His mother was notoriously litigious and was suing another doctor for injuries incurred when she fell down his office stairs. She agreed to see the child and his mother only if she could use the offices of Protective Services, where the case was active, rather than see him in her home office. She takes similar precautions in evaluating parents who may be headed for termination of parental rights.

D. Hold the middle ground and learn to live with ambiguity

Avoid premature closure and wait for the pieces of the puzzle to fall in place. Try to look at the issues from all sides, then steer a middle course based on what seems most reasonable. Reconcile yourself to not being able to resolve all contradictions.

E. Learn to critique your report from the standpoint of the other side

A helpful exercise is to go through your report from the vantage point of the opposing attorney and ask yourself, "How well will this statement hold up under cross-examination?" Try to anticipate where you are vulnerable and consider how you will deal with the weaknesses in the case.

F. Contrary quotients and validity percentages

Colbach (Schetky and Colbach, 1982) introduced these terms to help the clinician check his integrity. Although these concepts are designed for adult forensic psychiatry, they have some relevance to certain child forensic cases. The Contrary Quotient asks, "How often do I not give the side that hires me what they want?" The Validity Percentage asks, "How often does the judge or jury agree with me?" If one is consistently giving attorneys what they want, this should be cause for concern. If the courts repeatedly disagree with your stance, this should raise questions about the positions you are taking and/or your ability to communicate your findings.

G. Know your limitations

Do not overload yourself with too many forensic cases or too many cases of one kind. Pace yourself and your practice and take good care of yourself (see Chapter 15 on countertransference).

Avoid exceeding the limits of your data base when making conclusions and recommendations.

Don't be afraid to admit you don't know something.

Be cautious about making predictions and recognize that past behavior is usually the best predictor of future behavior.

H. Seek consultation

When in doubt turn to a more experienced colleague for consultation. Another useful avenue of consultation is the American Psychiatric Association Legal Consultation Plan which provides consultation with attorneys for issues related to practice. Hospital attorneys are also available to discuss issues related to patient management. Effective use of consultation on a case also provides some protection in the event that one is sued.

I. Keep current and stay involved

Don't allow fears of the legal system or malpractice litigation to keep you out of forensic child psychiatry. Keep informed, read, take courses, and stay involved. Each case is inevitably a learning experience.

VII. SUGGESTED READINGS

American Psychiatric Association (1988), Child Custody Consultation. A Report of the Task Force on Clinical Assessment in Child Custody. Washington, DC.: APA.

Bazelon, D. (1974), Psychiatrists and the Adversary Process. Scientific American 230 (6) 21.

Gutheil, T. G. and Appelbaum, P. S. (1991), 2nd ed. The Forensic Evaluation. In: Gutheil, T. G. and Appelbaum, P. S.: Clinical Handbook of Psychiatry and the Law. Baltimore: Williams & Wilkins.

Schetky, D. H. and Colbach, E. M. (1982), Countertransference on the witness stand: A flight from self? Bull Am Acad Psychiatry Law 10(2) 115–122.

Simon, R. I. (1987), The Psychiatrist as a Fiduciary: Avoiding the Role of the Double Agent. In: Simon, R. I.: Clinical Psychiatry and the Law. Washington, D.C.: APPI.

3

Testifying: The Expert Witness in Court

ELISSA P. BENEDEK, M.D.

The involvement of psychiatrists, psychologists, and other mental health clinicians in the legal arena continues to grow rapidly and remains highly controversial. Expert testimony of mental health professionals at depositions, administrative hearings, and trials alters many lives. It has been estimated that mental health clinicians participate in up to one million legal cases per year. The appropriate role of the mental health profession in the courtroom as an expert witness has been debated by numerous authors. While the debate rages, mental health professionals continue to participate as expert witnesses in administrative hearings and courts and as consultants. This chapter addresses the broad role of the expert witness from the psychiatrist's point of view.

I. CASE EXAMPLES

A. Case Example 1

An attorney requests that you review the documents of his client, a 16-year-old girl who has been severely burned after her flannel nightgown caught on fire. The attorney requests that you review the record (including mental health records) and render an opinion as to the extent of the psychiatric damages. The attorney claims that there is no need to see his client and indicates to you that the medical records will speak for themselves.

B. Case Example 2

An attorney requests your consultation with regard to the effect a below-the-knee amputation in a young schizophrenic boy has had on his psychosis and mental functioning. After reviewing the history and seeing the client/patient, there is no support for the theory that the amputation precipitated the patient's first psychotic episode. In fact, the episode occurred before the injury and amputation. In discussing the case with the attorney, she insists that "common sense" would make it clear that an amputation in a young boy would affect mental functioning and might precipitate another psychotic episode.

C. Case Example 3

A psychiatrist who has written extensively on child custody and divorce is testifying with regard to appropriate placement of two minor children. During the course of testimony, he is asked about a colleague's reputation, skill, and integrity by an attorney. He personally believes there were gross inadequacies in the conduct of the other expert's evaluation but declined to offer an opinion. He consults you as to whether he is "doing the right thing."

II. LEGAL ISSUES

A. The basis of expert testimony

Mental health professionals may be called to testify as fact witnesses or as expert witnesses. As fact witnesses, they are treated as other witnesses and may be asked to provide information from their practice (e.g., what is the diagnosis, what is the treatment, what is the prognosis, etc.). If a patient puts his mental health into the record as a possible cause of damage, the treating physician is at risk for being called as a fact witness. The physician may attempt to persuade an attorney from calling him by suggesting that treatment goals and objectives, response to treatment, and diagnosis may not be helpful to the patient/client. This tactic is ordinarily more persuasive than suggesting to an attorney that testifying in court will disrupt the doctor/patient relationship or may be harmful therapeutically to a patient. If an attorney insists on the treating physician's testimony, the physician might either call his or her own attorney and ask for advice or attempt to contact the judge personally.

An expert witness differs from a fact witness in that an expert witness may testify to matters of special learning or knowledge and opinion. A mental health clinician may be qualified as an expert on the basis of special training or education (a degree or seminar) or less commonly, special experience, skill, or information. The expert's testimony must be relevant to the matter in dispute, be reliable (have a significant scientific basis), and be based on some special expertise not otherwise available to a judge or jury. The testimony must be deemed to do more good than harm (probative value should be greater than its prejudicial value).

The expert may present an opinion or conclusion to the court. He or she may utilize facts gathered by others in forming the opinion. For example, the expert may review school records, past medical records, and past therapy records, or may speak with family members and with schoolteachers about the behavior of a patient and request that psychological testing be performed. Information gathered by others and communicated to the expert via medical records, interviews, psychological testing, and other laboratory testing may be used in formulating a final opinion. After reviewing and analyzing the findings of others, the expert may be allowed to formulate an opinion using "hearsay" material or material that has not been gleaned from a firsthand discussion with the patient.

The underlying theory of the American legal system and adversary system is that each side presents its best version of a case without perjury or manufactured evidence, subject to cross-examination and rebuttal. In many cases, expert testimony is helpful. In others, it is essential and required. Without expert testimony, a court will not entertain certain forms of litigation. For example, in Michigan, in medical malpractice cases, without an expert agreeing that there is ground for a suit (in a written opinion), court will not entertain a malpractice action. Additionally, the advent of advanced technology in the mental health field has resulted in increasingly complex litigation and has intensified the use of psychiatrists to explain to the court sophisticated tests and their meaning, e.g., CT scan, MRI. In criminal cases, failure to engage an expert may constitute ineffective assistance of counsel and may result in the reversal of a conviction. According to Slovenko, in *Ake v. Oklahoma*, a murder case where no psychiatrist was called to testify, the U.S. Supreme Court overturned a conviction on the grounds that the defendant, Ake, an indigent, should have had access to psychiatrist assistance in preparing an insanity defense. The court stated: "We hold that when a defendant has made a preliminary showing that his insanity at the time of the offense is likely to be a significant factor at trial, the Constitution requires that a state provide access to a psychiatrist's assistance on this issue if the defendant cannot otherwise afford one."

B. Tort reform

With recent tort reform, there has been an attempt made to control the use of professional experts or "hired guns." A Michigan Senate Bill, Number 24, would have required an expert to "devote not less than 75 percent of his professional time to the active clinical practice in the same specialty as the physician with the defendant in a medical malpractice action or to instruction of that specialty in the required medical school or to both clinical practice and instruction." Unfortunately, based on a consultant's recommendation, that Senate proposal did not pass. However, it appears as if 50% of a proposed expert's time must be devoted to teaching or clinical work for her to be qualified as an expert in Michigan courts (Personal Communication, Nels Carlson).

Most states require that experts state their opinions as being of "reasonable medical certainty," and others require only that testimony of an expert be something more than just speculation. A relaxation of the "reasonable certainty" standard suggests that judges and juries will be able to determine what probative weight should be given opinions and information once they are admitted into evidence.

C. Exceptions to expert testimony

The three most common exceptions to the broad admissibility of expert testimony are: (1) eyewitness reliability; (2) truthfulness of witness; and (3) syndrome of profiles. For the most part, psychologists have testified with regard to eyewitness reliability. This testimony generally focuses on psychological research with regard to the fallibility of eyewitness memory and the role of such factors as the effects of stress on witnesses, the problems associated with cross-racial identification, and the effects of post-event misinformation. The legal arguments that have been offered against expert testimony on eyewitness evidence include the following:

1. Mental health professionals do not have special expertise concerning eyewitness behavior.
2. The evaluation of the credibility of testimony by a witness is the province of the trier of fact and therefore not appropriate testimony from an expert.
3. A finding of eyewitness research has not "gained general acceptance in the particular field to which it belongs"—(the Frye Test, to be discussed later).
4. The findings of eyewitness researchers are common sense, and there is no need for an expert to inform the court of results.
5. An expert may have undue influence on a jury.

In eyewitness identification cases, it is generally the defense that wishes to use the expert. In the United States, the legal opinion is currently divided about the value of expert evidence on eyewitness testimony, but case law has been moving in the direction of admitting such evidence. In Canada, courts have been consistent in rejecting such testimony.

The second area where expert testimony is disputed is the area of truthfulness or credibility of other witnesses. Ordinarily, testimony regarding credibility of other witnesses is offered in child abuse, sexual abuse, malingering, or feigning. Traditional common law did not permit direct testimony on the truthfulness of another witness.

D. The Frye Test

The third area which is generally disputed is that area of syndromes or profiles. There is still considerable resistance in courts to accept syndromes not included in the *Diagnostic and Statistical Manual of Mental Disorders*, such as battered wife syndrome, rape trauma syndrome, battering parent profile, brainwashing, and sexually abused child. Here, again, courts have held that these profiles do not meet the Frye Test. This standard or test is derived from language in *Frye v. United States* and has been come to be known as the "general acceptance rule." It suggests that a test or syndrome must meet general acceptance in the scientific community at large. It is not enough that an expert is prepared to testify that a technique or procedure is valid or that the court believes that evidence is helpful or reliable.

The evidence must meet a standard of general scientific acceptance in the community.

The Frye Test has allowed radar evidence, public opinion surveys, breathalizers, psycholinguistics, trace metal detection, bite mark comparison, and blood splatter analysis into the courtroom but has denied on occasion polygraph test results, spectrographic voice identification, voice stress test, electrophoresis, microphobic analysis of hair, and the use of hypnosis as a means of refreshing a witnesses' memory. With regard to the *Frye* case, the Court of Appeals for the District of Columbia wrote: "Just when a scientific principle or discovery crosses the line between the experimental and demonstrable stages is difficult to define. Somewhere in this twilight zone, the evidential force of the principle must be recognized and while courts will go a long way in admitting expert testimony deduced from a well-recognized scientific principle or discovery, the thing from which the deduction is made must be sufficiently established to have gained general acceptance in the particular field in which it belongs."

The previous chapter mentioned the necessity for conducting a forensic clinical evaluation before agreeing to participate in a case as an expert witness. It is clear that the process of becoming an expert witness begins the moment one accepts a telephone call from an attorney or court and agrees to become involved in litigation. It continues through report writing and may culminate in testifying in court. However, in its broadest definition, then, being an expert witness involves evaluation, consultation, and testifying despite the fact that this chapter deals predominantly with testifying.

It must be emphasized that when a clinician agrees to participate with an attorney in a consultation, certain ground rules must be clearly articulated. Those ground rules can include the following.

1. The clinician will evaluate all materials in an objective manner. It is entirely possible that the opinion rendered by the clinician will not be favorable to the attorney's position. The clinician must make it clear from the onset that his or her objectivity and ethics will not be compromised.

2. The attorney must be willing to send all available documents to the clinician, allowing the clinician to judge which documents are or are not relevant to formulating an opinion in the case. Physicians are not the best judges of what material is relevant legally, and attorneys are not the best judges of what material is relevant clinically. In addition, there may be both a conscious act or unconscious temptation to select and review only materials that will portray the attorney-client's position and omit important data that might not be favorable.

3. The physician must articulate that it is impossible and unethical to articulate certain kinds of opinions without personal contact with clients. The clinician might agree to be an expert in a discrete clinical area (e.g., sexual abuse of children or post-traumatic stress), but it is impossible and unethical to articulate an opinion about a particular client/patient without seeing that client.

4. If questions posed by the attorney are outside the area of expertise of the clinician, it is incumbent upon the clinician to make that fact known.

5. The clinician should reach an agreement with the attorney about fees for evaluation, court report, deposition, and testimony. Such an agreement *cannot be based* on a contingent fee.

6. The clinician should discuss what follow-up may be necessary after the initial evaluation, e.g., consultation with an attorney about written report, deposition, testimony, etc.

III. CLINICAL ISSUES

A. Preparation

Subsequent to a clinical evaluation, discussion with an attorney, and completion of a written report (discussed in other chapters), if the clinician becomes aware that testimony at a deposition or in a trial will be necessary, it is sensible to contact the attorney for a pretrial conference to review the written report and conclusions with the attorney. This formal meeting allows the clinician an opportunity to educate an attorney about the clinical issues in the case as the clinician sees them. Such a meeting allows attorney and clinician to define medical terminology and legal standards. Such a meeting is also valuable for planning a strategy, anticipating questions at a deposition, and a possible sequence of direct examination and cross-examination. In addition, both clinician and attorney have an opportunity to meet one another and to become apprised of the strengths and weaknesses of each other and of the case. The clinician has an opportunity to evaluate the attorney and vice versa. It is helpful to know and understand all the actors in the courtroom drama before the drama begins.

B. Deposition

A deposition has been described as a dress rehearsal for a trial. No judge or jury are present; however, a bevy of attorneys and a court reporter may be present. Depositions are taken in order to preserve testimony, for discovery purposes, or to use for cross-examination at the time of a trial to impeach the credibility of a witness. Originally, depositions were done solely and only for the purpose of preserving testimony for trial. For example, a potential witness may be unavailable at the time of the trial because of conflicting obligations, illness, or death. Deposition of an expert witness may be used "because of unavailability." Expert witness depositions are often "de bene esse" depositions and may be taken by videotape. This strategy may backfire, as many witnesses present more favorably live than they do on videotape.

The second purpose of a deposition, to discover what the witness will say at trial and how the information will be presented, is more common. Here, the expert's opinions and the basis for such opinions are explored by opposing counsel. Opposing counsel also has an opportunity to observe firsthand how a proposed witness will hold up under the stressful circumstances of a trial and long periods of questioning. Infrequently, experts change their opinions during the course of questioning during a deposition. This is, of course, always helpful to opposing counsel. Even more infrequently, after the rigors of a deposition, an expert may decide not to testify if called at trial.

The third purpose of a deposition, to impeach the credibility of a witness, is a situation in which an attorney uses material obtained at a deposition during trial. Here, the attorney will quote the expert's answer in a deposition back to the expert to suggest that the expert has changed his opinion between the time of deposition and trial. Statements from the deposition may be quoted out of context in order to support or bolster one side of the case. Clinicians should be aware that attorneys share old depositions and trial transcripts and it is not unusual to have one's opinion from an old deposition or trial used to impeach a new opinion in a similar but distinct case.

The site for a deposition is up to the expert, and it can be held in the clinician's office, an attorney's office, or at a court reporter's. The defendant/patient has the right to be present during deposition. The proceedings in a deposition are recorded by a court reporter or stenographer.

In preparing for a deposition, the expert should review all the materials that have been furnished previously and be familiar with them. They should all be brought to the deposition. These materials (minus any attorney work product such as letters) are open to opposing counsel and may be inspected by him and attached to the record of the deposition. This includes clinical notes and notes that the expert has taken on other medical records and depositions. An expert may be called upon to explain why he or she underlined material in a deposition, made a marginal comment, or changed the size of paper used in recording material and notes.

Because a judge is not present to rule on objections, attorneys do exercise more latitude in their range of questions. An attorney may offer an objection to a question, but such objections are infrequent. If the behavior of one attorney is too objectionable to another, too hostile, too demeaning, or ranges too far and wide, the opposing counsel may terminate the deposition and ask for a ruling by the judge with regard to whether to continue. Termination of a deposition is rare.

The expert may receive a copy of a deposition to be proofread for typographical errors and errors of content. This copy should be read carefully and corrected. It is always advisable to insist on a copy of the deposition for record so that one can review it prior to trial.

It is wise to clarify payment for a deposition prior to the taking of the deposition. On occasion, it is even wise to ask for a fee to be paid in advance if there is reason to believe opposing counsel will not be responsible for payment. The firm that deposes the expert usually pays for time at the deposition, although it is wise to clarify in advance who was responsible for payment.

C. The courtroom

If a clinician has never visited a courtroom before, either as an expert or a defendant, it is helpful to do so prior to testifying. A courtroom is a strange, bewildering, foreboding place to the uninitiated. The role and function of courtroom personnel are unclear, and the mere atmosphere is hostile to the novice. It is always helpful to ask a forensically sophisticated colleague to observe his/her testimony prior to an actual testifying experience or to view a videotape of testimony. It is also sensible to ask that colleague to identify various players in the courtroom—bailiff, court reporter, stenographer, defense attorney, prosecutor—and to define their functions and roles.

Dress and demeanor are important in testifying. It is grossly inappropriate to testify in blue jeans and a turtleneck shirt or to not remove overcoat and scarf and boots before testifying. It is important to dress in a neat and conservative, nonflamboyant fashion. Occasionally, attorneys are flamboyant (wearing cowboy hats and boots, for example) but they are allowed more latitude than expert witnesses, and drama and flamboyance may enhance rather than detract from their performance. Dress is a clear way of showing respect for one's self and for the legal process.

D. Qualification of experts

When one is called as an expert witness, the first step in the testimonial process is the voir dire. Here, the attorney leads the witness through a standard set of questions designed to provide the foundations for the expert's credentials. These questions include relevant aspects of education and training such as medical school, residency, and fellowships. They also cover any special qualifications, including membership and offices in local and national organizations, publications, presentations, and special consultations. Following the recital of credentials, the opposing counsel has an opportunity to voir dire further. Opposing counsel's emphasis will be on the weakest areas in the witness' experience and training such as his limited contact with a particular population or particular evaluation (child custody evaluation, evaluation or personal experience with a particular form of medication). Voir dire generally is not particularly difficult, traumatic, or challenging. Although it may feel similar to a personal attack, and in fact may be designed to embarrass or discomfort the expert, the best witness is calm and dispassionate and recognizes that an attempt to discredit is simply a tactic used by opposing counsel.

E. Direct examination

The next step following qualification is a direct examination of the witness. During this portion of the testimony, the witness will be asked first to identify the patient/defendant/plaintiff and to explain the facts and conclusions on which an opinion is based. It is important that the expert present all relevant data in an articulate, clear, logical, and coherent fashion. It is equally important that the expert avoid using technical jargon here. Terms such as illusions, delusions, hallucination, affect, loosening of associations, must be avoided, and nontechnical terms used. In addition, any lab tests or psychological tests and their significance must be explained. The judge or jury has no innate understanding of psychological tests, which test data might be elicited from each test, and which test might be relevant, valid, or reliable. Judges and juries tend to think of psychological tests as objective and clinical evaluations as subjective. On occasion, it is important to articulate that the interpretation of a psychological test is as subjective as the interpretation of a clinical evaluation.

As mentioned earlier, attorneys may attempt to use clinicians to establish the credibility of a child client. Most courts today do not allow testimony in regard to client credibility from experts, believing that this invades the province of a judge or jury. Questions about credibility generally raise valid legal objection. As with all objections, the clinician should allow counsel to argue the merits of an objection and the court to rule upon it. The clinician has no expertise in regard to the validity of a legal objection, and although it is tempting to engage in the legal debate, it is unadvisable.

Testimony is resumed when a judge rules upon an objection. Here too the novice finds it difficult to remember that the objection is not personal, is not an objection to the clinician or testimony. It is an objection based on legal precedent or grounds. If the objection is overruled, and thereafter witnesses do not attend to prior limits on testimony and objections they may be chastised from the bench. Needless to say, being chastised by a judge in open court does not make a favorable impression on a juror.

The attorney and clinician decide prior to the onset of trial whether to use a direct examination to elucidate material that is unfavorable to the client/patient and that may be inconsistent with the expert's findings. If such material does not come out on direct examination, it most likely will come out on cross-examination. The ultimate decision in regard to trial strategy is, of course, an attorney's. Despite the fact that an expert may feel that he is more experienced than a particular attorney in an area (and he may be) and an attorney's decisions will lead to disaster for a patient/client, the conduct of the case is ultimately the attorney's responsibility. Second guessing an attorney is poor clinical judgment.

F. Cross-examination

The behavior of attorneys that arouses the greatest anger and ire among mental health professionals is that exhibited during cross-examination. The stated purpose of cross-examination is laudable, that is, to contribute to the purpose of seeking truth. However, in practice, cross-examination may seem to the witness to be less concerned with elucidation than with obfuscation. The opposing attorney's primary objective in cross-examination ordinarily is to negate the impact of the testimony given by a witness on direct examination. Some attorneys go to great lengths to suggest bias or expose uncertainty in a witness' testimony. Other attorneys make deliberate attempts to malign or distort a witness' testimony so as to make it misunderstood by a judge or jury.

The primary goals for an expert on cross-examination seem simple but may be difficult to observe. The first rule is to always be honest. Remember that not only do we have an ethical responsibility to be honest, we are also under oath. The second rule is to admit weakness or to admit that you do not know information if you do not know information. That may include specific information about a patient or literature cited by an attorney. The third rule is to take time to think. Occasionally, attorneys during cross-examination tend to lead witnesses in a very hostile fashion, asking questions in a staccato, machine gun pace. The witness always has time to think and can request time from the court if being pushed to give an answer. Fourth, do not speak for other experts. An expert can only speak for himself and cannot elucidate what other experts might say. Fifth, do not be critical of other experts. Such criticism is not valid. It is impossible to know all the material, data, skills, and experience that the other expert took into consideration when formulating an opinion. Criticizing another expert is looked upon favorably by neither bench nor jury. Sixth, do not talk too much. On occasion it is tempting to elaborate or, rather, filibuster with the rationalization that one is educating the jury. Juries and judges can be bored easily by lengthy, ponderous explanations.

G. Redirect and recross-examination

At this stage of the trial, the expert's attorney and opposing counsel have a final opportunity to elaborate and challenge points that may have emerged during direct and cross. Only material that has emerged on direct and cross may be referred to during redirect and recross. Opposing counsel will object if new material is introduced during this stage of the proceeding.

Attorneys and psychiatrists are divided with regard to whether clinicians should answer the "so-called ultimate issue" in a case. This would mean directly addressing the depositive legal issue. For example, whether a person is or is not incompetent, insane, or committable, whether a child has been sexually abused, or whether parental rights should be terminated, or which parent serves the best interest of a child. Some commentators would suggest that mental health experts should only testify with regard to the relationship of the diagnosis to the legally relevant behavior, and still others would allow testimony with regard to the ultimate issue with the caveat that such testimony should be subject to cross-examination and the adversarial process. To date, no one has suggested that responding to a request for testimony on the ultimate issue is unethical.

When testimony is completed, the witness may be excused by a judge. The witness then must decide if he or she wishes to remain in the courtroom to listen to other expert testimony or leave. On occasion, the witness may be sequestered prior to testimony and asked to leave after testimony. Leaving does make a witness seem less involved, impartial, and less interested in the outcome of a case. On occasion, an attorney may request that the expert sit at the counsel's table and act as a personal coach to that attorney while other witnesses are questioned. Although on rare occasions this may be acceptable, it is better to prepare the attorney for cross-examination of other witnesses ahead of time and during pretrial conferences. Sitting at the counsel's table may make the expert witness appear too involved in the outcome of a case.

IV. ACTION GUIDE

If one contemplates testifying in court, preparation, as mentioned earlier, is to go to court with a skilled expert and to observe experts during testimony. Another useful training technique is to participate in a mock trial at a training institution or a law school. If a novice can survive the challenge of a mock trial in a collegial atmosphere, a real trial may seem tame in contrast. Videotapes of mock trials are useful for ongoing critique and training. Participants are often surprised at the performances during a mock trial and learn a great deal from them.

V. PITFALLS

A. Psychiatrist-related pitfalls

1. Bias and overinvolvement. The psychiatrist must attempt to be objective when evaluating forensic cases. Such objectivity needs to be carried over into the courtroom. The psychiatrist is not the advocate for the patient/client. He or she merely presents data and conclusions based on those data.
2. Inadequate data base. It is important to have access to and review all available data.
3. Literature. Relevant clinical literature must be reviewed before testimony. Although one cannot hope to review all literature in a given area, it is

prudent to review recent scientific material and any material that the expert may have written in the area.

4. Hired gun. A psychiatrist who always testifies for prosecution or defense, plaintiff or defendant, will become quickly known as nonobjective and a "hired gun." In addition, one who testifies regularly outside an area of expertise may also be tagged as a hired gun.

5. Testifying outside of one's area of expertise. It is seductive to be called an expert and easy to be trapped by that appellation into testifying outside of one's area of expertise.

B. Patient-related pitfalls

1. Dual agent. The clinician should decide which role he or she may accept with regard to patients. One cannot assume the role of a forensic expert and that of a treating clinician without falling into the trap of dual agency. It is difficult, if not impossible, to retain objectivity when treating a patient.

C. Attorney-related pitfalls

1. Coercion. Attorneys are experts at persuasion, and they may attempt to overtly or covertly coerce a clinician into changing an opinion. Remember that attorneys are prepared to evaluate and destroy the other side of a case.

2. Lack of preparation. Attorneys may come to court without adequate preparation. This is disconcerting for the expert. Pre-trial conferences with attorneys help the expert to determine the degree of the attorney's preparedness and to make suggestions regarding mental health areas that attorneys should know.

3. Communication. Attorneys may not be skilled in communicating legal standards in a nontechnical way. It is important to continue to ask for clarification.

VI. CASE EXAMPLE EPILOGUES

A. Case Example 1

It is difficult, if not impossible, to assess the clinician status of any patient with regard to psychiatric illness without actually seeing that patient. It is impossible to offer an opinion about mental health status without seeing the patient. The clinician in this case advised the attorney that it would be impossible to offer an opinion without seeing the patient. Arrangements were made to transport the patient to the clinician's office where an adequate evaluation could be conducted.

B. Case Example 2

The attorney in this case is attempting to coerce the potential expert to change an opinion. It is clear that the psychotic episode occurred before the injury and amputation, and the records seem to indicate that the young schizophrenic boy is not acutely psychotic now. The clinician offers to reevaluate the youngster but suggests that such a reevaluation would in all probability not be helpful to the attorney's case.

C. Case Example 3

Despite the fact that a psychiatrist may believe that there are gross inadequacies in another's evaluation, you advise the attorney that it might be helpful to testify with regard to how a particular evaluation should be conducted, allowing the judge or jury to make a determination about how another expert's evaluation was conducted. Here, you suggest to the consultee/psychiatrist that imputing a colleague's reputation, skill, and integrity in a courtroom may be inappropriate.

VII. SUGGESTED READING

Criminal Justice Standards. Approved by American Psychiatric Association House of Delegates, August 1984.

Bank, S. C. and Poythress, N. G (1982), The elements of persuasion in expert testimony. Psychiatry Law (Summer), 173–204.

Benedek, E. P. (1991), Testifying in court. In: M. Lewis (ed.): Child and Adolescent Psychiatry: A Comprehensive Textbook. Baltimore: Williams & Wilkins.

Benedek, R. S. and Benedek, E. P. (1980), The expert witness in child custody cases. In: Schetky, D. H. and Benedek, E. P. (eds.): Child Psychiatry and the Law. New York: Brunner/Mazel.

Brodsky, S. L. The mental health professional on the witness stand: A survival game.

Melton, G. B., Petrica, J., Poythress, N. G., and Slobodkin (1987), Consultation, report writing and expert testimony. In: Psychological Evaluations for the Court. New York: Guilford Press.

Poythress, N. G. (1980), Coping on the witness stand: learned responses to learned treatise. Prof Psychol.

Poythress, N. G. and Petrella, R. (1983), The quality of forensic evaluations: an interdisciplinary study. Consult Clin Psychol 31:76.

Resnick, P. J. (1986), Perceptions of psychiatric testimony: an historical perspective on an hysterical invective. Bull Am Acad Psychiatry Law 14(3) 203–219.

Simon, R. I. (1987), Clinical Psychiatry and the Law. Washington, D.C.: American Psychiatric Press, Inc.

Slobogin, C. (1989), The ultimate issue. Behav Sci Law 7(2) 259–266.

Smith, S. R. (1989), Mental health expert witnesses of science and crystal balls. Behav Sci Law 7(2) 144–180.

Stone, A. (1984), The ethical boundaries of forensic psychiatry: a view from the ivory tower. Bull Am Acad Psychiatry Law 12:209–219.

Watson, A. S. (1978), On the preparation and use of psychiatric expert testimony: some suggestions in an ongoing controversy. Bull Am Acad Psychiatry Law 6:226–246.

Weitzel, W. D. (1977), Public skepticism: forensic psychiatry's albatross. Bull Am Acad Psychiatry Law 5:456–463.

Ziskin, J. (1981), Coping with Psychiatric and Psychological Testimony. Venus, California: Law and Psychology Press.

Ziskin, J. and Faust, D. (1988), Coping with Psychiatric and Psychological Testimony. Venus, California: Law and Psychology Press.

Ziskin, J. and Faust, D. (1988), The expert witness in psychology and psychiatry. Science 241 (July) 31–35.

CASE CITATION:

Frye v. U.S. 293 F. 1013–1014 (D.C. Cir. 1923).

4

Psychological Testing in Child Forensic Evaluations

BETH K. CLARK, PH.D., AND CHARLES R. CLARK, PH.D.

I. CASE EXAMPLES

A. Case Example 1

The local department of social services contacts a psychologist requesting an evaluation of a single-parent family to determine whether to terminate parental rights. The children, a four-year-old boy and an eight-year-old girl, have been placed in foster care for about a year because of neglect. During this time they have had sporadic supervised visits with the mother. The children were described by their foster parents as "hyperactive" and undersocialized when they first came into their home. Though they have settled down, the foster parents are concerned that they revert back to their old behavior after each visit with the mother. The mother is described by the social services worker as seeming "spaced out," and the worker wonders whether she might be "a little crazy." However, she also describes her as attached to her children and wanting them back.

The psychologist conducts extensive interviews with the mother and the children, and they are observed interacting. The mother is given a battery of psychological tests, which includes an intelligence test, projective techniques, and standardized psychological inventories. She is also given a series of behavior rating scales in order to assess her perception of the adaptation and behavior of her children. The foster parents are interviewed and also given the same rating scales. Both children are given intelligence tests appropriate to their ages. The younger child is engaged in a structured play technique, and the older child is given age-appropriate projective tests and an instrument which measures academic functioning. Test data are integrated into interview data and history.

The data indicate that the mother may be impulsive and unable to tolerate stress, and they raise some question about her potential for alcohol or drug abuse. There are suggestions of antisocial attitudes and very poor interpersonal skills, accompanied by strong narcissistic needs; these appear to be long-standing, chronic problems. The mother gives an extremely different account of the children's behavior on the rating scales from that given by the foster parents. Test data on the children suggest significant intellectual deficits. The older child appears to be well behind her peers in academic skills. There are some alarming indications of cognitive disorganization and distortion of interpersonal relationships. The younger child appears withdrawn from adult figures and experiences them as unable to help him. The psychologist compares this test data with information received from her interviews, observations, and from external sources. Interview data confirm that the mother has a drug problem. The psychologist prepares to write her report.

B. Case Example 2

A bitter custody dispute is referred by the court for evaluation. Three children, ages two-and-a-half, five, and seven are involved. The psychologist has each child draw pictures of his or her family and gives the two older children a Wechsler IQ test. The mother and father are given the Rorschach. In light of complaints by the mother which raise questions of psychopathology or personality disorder in the father, the father is given the MMPI-2 (revised Minnesota Multiphasic Personality Inventory). In the report, the psychologist includes the computer printout from his scoring of the MMPI-2. He notes that the mother is the more nurturing parent, because she reported more people-oriented percepts on the Rorschach. He also notes that this test shows that she has healthily resolved her Oedipal conflict. The father, he notes, is not to be trusted and may be a sociopath because the MMPI-2 Scale 4 (Psychopathic Deviate) is elevated; he does not indicate the extent of the elevation. He also expresses concern that the father has seen human figures on Card III of the Rorschach as having both breasts and penises; he offers that this response is indicative of confusion in sexual identity and strongly suggests a propensity for sexual abuse when seen in an adult male. He also notes that one of the children has drawn a figure without hands, which he maintains indicates possible conflict over aggression or sexuality, which in turn suggests that this child has been a victim of sexual abuse. The examiner recommends that sole custody be awarded to the mother and recommends that visitation with the father be suspended until he has entered psychotherapy because of his clear potential for sexual abuse.

C. Case Example 3

An eleven-year-old boy and his nine-year-old sister are present when the boy's clothing is ignited by contact with an electric heater; the boy is severely burned on his face and hands. The parents sue the maker of the heater and the store that sold it. One of the claims of damages is the psychological trauma to the boy as a result of the burns and to his sister from witnessing the event. A psychiatrist/ psychologist team is asked to evaluate the children. Interviews are conducted with the children and their parents. The boy will say little about the injury and seems withdrawn; the parents are concerned about the withdrawal but say he was always a child who did not talk about his problems; he had been tested in school prior to the injury because of these concerns. The daughter freely discussed the experience without much difficulty and says that she feels sorry for her brother, but is not too worried about it. The parents indicated they have been able to talk at length with the daughter about the situation.

A battery of tests is given to each child. The daughter responds within normal limits on all of the tests. She shows healthy problem-solving abilities and good overall adjustment. The son's test results, on the other hand, show pervasive concerns about body integrity. Images of fire are everywhere and projective stories primarily consist of children being injured or in grave danger. There are test indications of marked social withdrawal and anxiety.

II. LEGAL ISSUES

Psychologists in the United States have testified on a variety of legal issues since the 1920s, either on the basis of research findings or on the results of psychological testing. Controversies concerning the admissibility of clinical psychological testimony based on testing have in almost all jurisdictions been resolved in favor of broad latitude to psychological expert testimony.

The chief issue before the courts in years past was whether medical training or methodology was necessary for expert testimony regarding mental and emotional conditions; the general response has been that it is not. Where psychologist qualifications have been mentioned in appellate decisions discussing the admissibility of testimony based on testing, they have included factors such as the possession of a doctorate, licensing, teaching experience, publication in professional journals, membership in the American Psychological Association, and certification by the American Board of Professional Psychology. Medical credentials as such have not been specified as necessary, nor has medical supervision of psychological work.

A secondary controversy regarding the admissibility of testimony based on psychological testing pertains to the scientific acceptability of test findings in general and of particular test instruments. As indicated below, all tests are not created equal in regard to reliability and validity, and some tests are more applicable to legal issues than are others. On this question, courts have generally upheld the admissibility of psychological testing, leaving open the question of the weight which might be accorded to it. Testing in general, and certain instruments in particular—those deficient in psychometric foundation—remain subject to challenge in court, in the voir dire of the proposed psychological witness, or in cross-examination. This is no different, however, from the legal challenges any mental health testimony is liable to face.

A related issue, and one which also concerns all expert testimony, is the extent to which psychological testimony should embrace opinions on the so-called ultimate issue—the factual and legal question on which the trier of fact must rule such as the best interests of the child or the presence of negligence and damages. Rules of evidence adopted by the federal and state courts differ in regard to the limits placed on the scope of expert opinion testimony. Where opinions on ultimate issues are permitted, the adequacy of claimed bases for those opinions, whether psychological test data or other evaluative information, are subject to legal challenge.

III. CLINICAL ISSUES

A. Indications for psychological testing

1. CONTRIBUTION TO THE OVERALL EVALUATION

Forensic questions about children can place clinicians in a position of tremendous responsibility. The difficulty and importance of helping the court to decide such things as how a child's life will be structured, whether to permanently terminate a parental relationship, or how damaged he or she might be from abuse require extensive and thorough evaluation. While psychological testing should never be used alone in making recommendations, it is often useful in evaluations.

Psychological testing permits observation of each subject under controlled conditions. Ideally, tests are given to each subject in a uniform fashion; the same questions are asked; and each subject is under the same expectations to respond. A relatively objective view of the subject is possible, in that the tests are constructed so as to minimize any influence or bias the examiner might bring to the evaluation.

Second, testing adds normative information to the picture. Psychological tests compare the performance of an individual to the performance of the general population or to a more specific population, such as psychiatric patients. Although clinicians are sometimes frustrated that tests cannot speak specifically enough to the issues that must be dealt with in child forensic work to dictate definitive answers to legal questions, testing can provide information that augments that gathered from other assessment methods.

Finally, the use of psychological tests permits the examiner to measure and evaluate the subject's approach to the assessment itself. Understanding an individual's set or general approach toward the evaluation—candor and insight, guardedness and deception, repression and denial—can be essential to accurately evaluating the assessment data as a whole. Some tests, such as the MMPI-2, used with adults and adolescents, have built-in measures that provide significant information about whether a subject may be trying to gloss over difficulties or may be trying to present himself or herself in a biased way. Close attention to a child's approach to testing can provide data regarding whether a child may have been coached or influenced by a parent. For example, in a custody dispute, if a child were to give rote answers to every card on the Rorschach, and these answers all had the theme of a bad man, one might wonder whether the child had been told to make sure that he or she conveyed that thought, especially if this was continued in a similar way throughout the interview, interaction, or observation portions of the evaluation.

2. Choice of tester

The administration and interpretation of psychological tests require specific training, not only in personality theory, psychological development, and psychopathology, but also in test construction and quantitative research methodology. While some tests can be administered by a technician, the interpretation should not be done by anyone other than a psychologist fully trained and experienced in all of the instruments given. As will be further explained below, responsibility for the interpretation of testing should also not be left with a computer program.

3. When to use testing

Many child evaluations can benefit from psychological testing. Its research base and standardized administration make it particularly useful in forensic settings where clinicians are called upon to carefully ground and explicate their findings. The only testing that is contraindicated is testing which, due to the instruments used or the manner in which they are administered or interpreted, serve to compound rather than resolve the clinical difficulties in the assessment of these most difficult questions. Properly employed tests can be a useful adjunct to the evaluation, providing information that converges with other sources of information, or which raises by itself useful hypotheses to be explored. Below is a list of particular forensic areas, with recommendations of whom to test and what type of questions testing may be of use in answering. More specific information about each type of test is in a subsequent section.

a. Abuse and neglect

There are three general issues in abuse where testing can be of particular help. First, especially in sexual abuse, there are often questions of the reliability of the child's report. Second are questions of the effects of the abuse and neglect on the child. Third, there may be questions pertaining to an adult involved, either as an alleged perpetrator of abuse or in terms of parenting ability in the case of neglect. It is important to note here that while testing should be used with caution in any forensic setting, it along with other assessment techniques should be used extremely carefully in the area of sexual abuse. Clinical Example 2 shows a situation where the misuse of testing created serious effects in a custody dispute. This point is further elucidated later in the chapter.

Testing can contribute to judgments of a child's reliability. Intelligence tests can provide information on whether the child is intellectually capable of being able to remember details and coherently tell about an incident. In addition, knowledge of the child's intellectual functioning, developmental level, and view of his or her world can provide a context for the clinician to evaluate the child's report. Specific references to abuse are not commonly encountered in the testing situation. However, comparison of less direct themes in the child's productions with interview data can help in assessing reliability.

Testing may also provide data on the effects of abuse and neglect. Physical abuse or neglect can in itself cause decrements in intellectual functioning or learning disabilities which testing can elucidate, for example, trauma- or anxiety-induced problems in attention and concentration. Thematic content of some tests can provide data on effects of abuse. A sexually abused child who tells many stories only about being physically damaged or terrorized by adults on the Roberts Apperception Test may require the evaluator to more strongly consider serious damage. Similarly, bland and affectless test responding from a child who suffered abuse may signal maladaptive emotional blunting and withdrawal. Information on the coping styles and interpersonal skills of the child can lend important information to the consideration of placement, when that is necessary.

With respect to cases in which the adult disputes an allegation of abuse or neglect, testing of the adult may have value in contributing to a clearer total picture of the individual, which may be helpful to the trier of fact. It is important to acknowledge, however, that psychological testing is not capable of identifying the guilty or the innocent, nor of establishing the credibility or truthfulness of a person. Any conclusion based on test data that an accused individual is or is not a sexual abuser, for instance, is a conclusion that goes beyond the data. As is true of other assessment strategies as well, there is no reliable test-based profile of offenders, nor any pattern of test results which would indicate truthfulness. Test indications of intentional distortion of the person's presentation—denial, exaggeration, guardedness, or malingering—may shed light on the individual, but cannot be brought to bear directly on a question of guilt or innocence.

b. Termination of parental rights

Evaluation of the adults involved in the question of parental rights termination is obviously as important as that of the children themselves. While there is often a long paper trail as well as data in social service records on both parents and children, frequently in cases of abuse or neglect the psychological evaluation is not considered until very late in the termination process. Often data of a mental health nature are from therapists who are in the difficult position of both treating the child or parent and providing evaluative information for the court or social services. An evaluation that includes concrete information from testing of the level of character problems or frank psychopathology of the parents, their intelligence and cognitive integrity, their social skills and personality can be of great use to the court. It can help to generate hypotheses about how insightful parents are and how able parents are to use psychotherapeutic or educational and social intervention. Treatment issues, goals, and impediments may be identified, increasing the likelihood of success when a strategy of intervention is attempted.

In addition, testing the children in cases in which termination of parental rights is at issue can provide information on their level of functioning and attachment to the parent, which can be woven together with interview, observation, and history to determine whether further contact with the parent would be beneficial or detrimental. The complex question of how the parent and child's temperaments, strengths, and weaknesses interact with each other can be addressed by considering test results. Clinical Example 1 describes a case in which relatively vague speculations by foster parents and social services workers were initially the only data regarding the psychological functioning of the children and mother in this case. The testing that accompanied the evaluation provided information on the chronicity of the mother's problems and her intellectual limitations, as well as finding a complexity in the problems of the children that might tax even the most able parent. This led to the synthesis and recommendation reported in the epilogue.

c. Delinquency and criminal proceedings

Testing is frequently used in cases of juvenile delinquency commitments to identify personality variables, treatment focuses, and academic and social skill levels. Increasingly assessments are being ordered by courts to determine whether adolescents charged with serious felonies, particularly murder and rape, ought to be tried, not as juveniles, but as adults, subject to the full range of adult sentencing provisions. Provisions for the waiver of juvenile court jurisdiction to adult courts differ across jurisdictions, and many considerations taken into account by the courts, such as the seriousness of the offense, the juvenile's criminal record, or the welfare of the community, are not assessment questions open to psychological or psychiatric assessment. Though in practice frequently outweighed by those considerations, juvenile waiver provisions commonly involve an assessment of the juvenile's amenability to treatment or rehabilitation in a juvenile facility and the juvenile's character. On those issues, psychological testing can serve as another source of information about personality functioning, insight, and treatment motivation.

At times in particular jurisdictions, questions of competency to stand trial and criminal responsibility or insanity are raised in respect to juveniles. A full discussion of the role of testing in regard to what are essentially adult issues goes beyond the scope of this chapter; juveniles are generally not accorded adult competency status in any event, and there is debate as to the pertinence of adult insanity provisions to juvenile offenders.

d. Child custody

As with termination of rights, child custody questions require thorough evaluation of both adults and children, including interview, observation of parent-child interaction, and consideration of testing. When a dispute has reached the level that a custody evaluation is required, parental animosity may be expected to be high, together with concern by the parents that their points of view be fully heard. Testing can contribute to the thoroughness of the evaluation as well as add an objective comparative standard to the process. They enhance the clinician's ability to compare and contrast parental strengths and weaknesses in relation to those of their children. Parent rating scales can be compared with interview data as a measure of how accurately a parent understands the children. Testing of the children can lend important information about how the child views adult figures, how they perceive the family, and whether and how the divorce process has affected them.

e. Civil damages

Civil suits brought because of injury to a child have more and more often required the evaluative services of a forensically trained clinician. These can include claims of psychological effects of a physical injury, emotional stress because of disasters, and psychological trauma resulting from sexual abuse. At times, parents are also named as plaintiffs in these suits. For example, in the case of preschool sexual abuse, a parent may enter the suit because of claims of psychological stress caused by having to deal with the trauma experienced by his or her child.

In assessing psychological damages to plaintiffs, testing may help identify or rule out preexisting conditions which may have continued unchanged or been exacerbated by the events in question. Testing can help answer questions of malingering or unreliability which unfortunately need to be considered in situations where large amounts of money are at stake. Comparisons of current and past testing, when that has been done, can point to changes in psychological functioning.

The intrusion of the traumatic event into test data, as mentioned above, may help to determine how pervasive the response to the injury is. For example, a sexually abused boy saw the word "sex" on the WISC-R on the part that notes identifying data. He became extremely anxious and asked "what is that there for, it's yucky!" A general picture of personality functioning and coping skills will aid in the difficult task of attempting to predict future effects of the trauma. It is worth considering testing parents of children involved in civil litigation even if the parents are not named plaintiffs. Emerging research is showing the importance of addressing the aftermath of trauma by adults and institutions. Information on parental functioning as well as that of the children provides a systemic picture of the experience by the family unit.

B. Selection of tests and their relative utility

Most often a battery of tests, rather than a single instrument, is administered. Individual tests should be selected for inclusion in an assessment strategy to provide information about specific problems at issue in the case. The most commonly used tests and their relative utility in child forensic work are listed below. Included are test instruments used with adults, who will be the focus of assessment in many cases involving children, particularly child custody questions.

1. ADULTS

a. Intelligence tests

The most common adult intelligence test in use today is the Wechsler Adult Intelligence Scale—Revised (WAIS-R), though the Stanford-Binet, which has a lower "floor" or more sensitive measurement of impaired intellectual functioning, is especially useful with the developmentally disabled. The WAIS-R, like its child counterparts, provides measures of a variety of abilities taken to be associated with what is commonly referred to as intelligence; it loads heavily for abilities important to academic and occupational achievement, rather than for social skills and creativity, and a variety of specific intellectual capabilities. Cognitive impairment of various types can be identified in WAIS-R performance, as can areas of strength and comparative skill. Many psychologists "mine" the WAIS-R for useful information regarding personality factors, similar to the information obtained from projective testing. While the Wechsler can be helpful in this way, tests of intelligence would usually not be administered unless there was some concern about the adult having an intellectual deficit.

b. Personality inventories

Well-researched personality inventories are very commonly given; they have considerable reliability and provide quantified results that may be readily interpreted in light of published norms. Such tests are "paper-and-pencil" instruments which require endorsement by the subject as true or false a variety of statements pertaining to beliefs, emotions, and behavior. Among the instruments developed for use with non-clinical or "normal" populations are the California Personality Inventory (CPI) and the Sixteen Personality Factors Questionnaire (16 PF). The recently revised Minnesota Multiphasic Personality Inventory (MMPI-2), for some years the most commonly administered psychological test, is designed to assess significant functional disorders in the neurotic, characterological, and psychotic spectra but is also sensitive to subclinical personality factors or traits. Although the MMPI was created for use with individuals 16 years old or older, interpretive strategies and normative data have been developed for younger adolescents.

The Millon Clinical Multiaxial Inventory (MCMI-II) was specifically designed to assess DSM-III-R personality disorders, though it is normed on individuals who are in the early stages of treatment, and may provide an overestimate of problems in other populations. Tests such as the MMPI-2 and the MCMI-II have the advantage in forensic settings of providing indications of test-taking attitude and test validity.

Although they are often called "objective" tests, the personality inventories, no less than other tests, require clinical skill and subjectivity for interpretation. Undue reliance on the score profile from such instruments in reaching diagnostic conclusions, let alone recommendations on matters such as custody or sexual abuse, without considering the psychometric properties of the instruments together with a variety of data obtained elsewhere, invites error. The instruments are "objective" in the relative sense that they sharply reduce subjective factors, particularly those produced in the interaction between examiner and subject, that are present in other assessment methods. While somewhat time-consuming for subjects to complete, they allow for efficient and inexpensive use of examiner time.

c. Projective tests

Projective tests require responses by the subject to ambiguous stimuli. A very wide variety of such instruments have been developed in past years, though relatively few are in common use. The Rorschach inkblot technique is perhaps the best known and most widely used of these instruments; ten cards are presented in sequence to the subject, who is asked to indicate what the inkblots on the cards might be; inquiry follows as to where on the card the percept was seen, and what made it appear to the subject in the way that it had. It can provide information on psychopathology or its absence. It is also used to examine the subject's usual response or coping style, how he or she approaches ambiguous situations, and how emotions are handled. Comparison of the Rorschach summaries of various members of families can help generate hypotheses about how the styles of various members might interact with those of others in the family.

A frequently used projective test with adults is the Thematic Apperception Test (TAT). The subject is presented with a number of ambiguous pictures, and is asked to relate a story about the picture—what is happening and what happened before, how the individuals in the pictures are thinking and feeling, and what the outcome will be.

Drawing tasks of different types are frequently used as projective techniques. The House-Tree-Person and Draw A Person techniques are the two such techniques most likely to be encountered. The Bender-Gestalt, developed for detection of organic impairment but abandoned for that purpose in standard neuropsychological assessment, is often interpreted projectively.

Projective tests vary in the extent to which they have been subjected to the empirical study of their psychometric properties. Generally when examined such instruments appear to have, relative to the "objective" personality measures of tests of ability and aptitude, poor reliability and uncertain validity. These problems are compounded by the frequent lack of standardization in administration, scoring, and interpretation; for example, there are five major systems for using the Rorschach, but some clinicians do not even formally score the protocol.

As test instruments, projective techniques are more vulnerable than other types of testing to examiner error and bias, since they typically require a great deal of subjectivity in interpretation if not in scoring and administration. Used carelessly, they may be more projective tests of the examiner than of the subject. In the case of the Rorschach at least, considerable work has been done by Exner and his associates on improving standardization and reliability, quantifying scoring, and identifying from empirical research personality and behavioral correlates of test data; as a result, Exner's Rorschach shares more in common with objective personality instruments than do other projectives.

Most clinical psychologists view projectives as adding information to the examination not otherwise available. Unlike the self-report inventories, the manifest content of projectives gives little clue as to what a "good" or desirable response might be; this aspect of these techniques is particularly valuable in forensic settings where subjects are not disinterested in the outcome and recommendations and in which they may feel strong needs to present themselves in particular ways. Projectives also permit an observation of a subject's response to an ambiguous and unfamiliar task. Weighing against the value of projectives in forensic settings is their vulnerability to cross-examination. This vulnerability increases with the extent to which diagnostic opinions or recommendations rest on the results of projective tests. The vulnerability is also greater with respect to particular instruments; drawing techniques are perhaps the most assailable.

2. CHILDREN

a. Intelligence

Intelligence testing for children can be helpful even if there is no question of serious intellectual difficulties. This testing can give significant information about the child's cognitive abilities, especially his or her ability to understand the current legal or familial situation, to report events accurately, or to interpret events. The revised Wechsler Intelligence Scale for Children (WISC-R), the revised Wechsler Preschool and Primary Scales of Intelligence (WPPSI-R), and the Kaufmann batteries are most commonly used.

In some evaluations, particularly those in the civil damages area, there may be concerns about attention deficit disorder or learning disabilities. Simple intelligence tests have little to say alone about these issues and should be combined with more specialized testing to help specifically elucidate these areas.

b. Projective testing

Discovering how children, especially young children, feel and think about events in their lives is not an easy task. In forensic evaluations the issue is particularly sensitive. Many would agree that it is not appropriate to directly ask young children about their preference for one parent or the other in a custody evaluation or to ask leading questions in an evaluation of sexual abuse. Most children, no matter what age, are exquisitely aware of why they are being evaluated and may feel anxious about what they say to an evaluator and how it may affect their parents or the decision of the court. Projective testing provides a forum a step removed from direct discourse and can skirt a child's conscious intentions and permit reasonable inferences about the child's needs and fears. Case Example 3 shows how a testing can reveal serious difficulties in a child who is uncomfortable in an interview situation.

An Exner Rorschach will give information about a child similar to that previously mentioned in regard to adults.

Also of utility are apperception tests for children, of which there are several in common use. As with the TAT, the child is asked to tell a story about a number of ambiguous pictures. The Children's Apperception Test (CAT) and the Make a Picture Story (MAPS) are frequently used examples of this type of test. The Roberts Apperception Test for Children (RATC) is particularly useful in forensic cases; its pictures pull for stories about family events and it has separate cards for boys, girls, and minority groups. In addition, the RATC can be quantitatively scored and compared to a general population of children.

c. Structured play and drawing techniques

While not psychological tests as such, structured play and drawing techniques can be used as additional sources of information about how the child perceives his or her family. They have the same advantages as the projective techniques listed above. They are particularly useful with very young children who are not able to easily tell stories or answer questions.

There are a number of structured play techniques in the literature (e.g., Gardner, 1976). One of the more helpful ones was developed by Lynn (1959, as found in Palmer, 1983) and was designed for children between the ages of two and six. It consists of a series of vignettes that the child plays out with props and dolls given him or her by the evaluator. The dolls chosen can be adapted to the particular situation of the child. The evaluator reads a scenario and the child plays it out and answers specific questions about it. For example, one scenario reads, "The dolly gets a bad ouch! Who is coming to care for him?" The child's answers, both verbally and through play, to this type of vignette often convey helpful information about family situations and impose little stress on the child.

Projective drawings may be used with children of any age. However, care should be taken in the selection and especially the interpretation of drawings. As is the case with adults as well, it has been charged that tests such as the House-Tree-Person and the Draw A Person are too far removed from the referral question and too indefensible in court to be of much utility. However, the Kinetic Family Drawing (KFD), which asks the child to draw a picture of his or her family doing something, appears to be quite directly related to the issues involved in much child forensic work. How the child describes the picture and answers questions about it provide provocative clinical information. Who is and is not included in the picture, the activity depicted, and the interaction among family members may help generate hypotheses about the child's view of the family.

Again, it is important to note that these techniques are not psychological tests in the way the WISC-R or MMPI-2 are. They may indeed be more properly considered as clinical observation tools. Inferences made from a child's performance on these tasks must be very cautiously made and be integrated with interview and other observational data. It would be inappropriate to base important conclusions or recommendations solely or largely on such inferences.

d. Tests of academic functioning

It is often helpful to determine whether and how a child's school performance has been affected by events at issue, such as sexual abuse or a custody or visitation dispute. The Wide Range Achievement Test-Revised (WRAT-R) is a quick test of word reading, spelling, and mathematics skills. For a broader picture of a child's academic abilities, the Woodcock-Johnson Psychoeducational Battery-Revised provides data on a number of skills in relation to the child's age and grade level. With these tests the evaluator can determine a child's academic rank relative to peers and can use this information in conjunction with the intelligence scales and teacher and parent reports to look at overall adaptation in this important area of functioning.

3. BEHAVIOR RATING SCALES AND PERSONALITY INVENTORIES

Unfortunately, there are no personality instruments for children with the strong research of adult tests; as noted above, the MMPI-2 may be used with younger adolescents. It is promising to note that research on MMPI-2 norms for adolescents is almost completed, and the test will be available for adolescents in the near future. However, there are a few scales and inventories that might be included in a child forensic evaluation. These instruments are completed by parents and thus must be used carefully, since in a forensic case a parent might be motivated to respond in a biased fashion about the child in hopes of minimizing or over-emphasizing pathology. The Child Behavior Checklist, the Connors Symptom Checklist, and the Personality Inventory for Children all provide profiles of how the parents' description of the child's behavior compares to normed populations of children.

While they have some utility in identifying the strengths and weaknesses of the child, scales may be more helpful in another way. Having each parent, for example, in a custody dispute independently fill out a scale permits a comparison of the way in which each parent sees the child and the extent to which this may or may not coincide with the evaluator's hypotheses about the child. Parents in custody disputes may be quite discrepant in their views of the child, and both may underestimate the effect of the dispute on their children. In other situations, such as termination of rights, the scales can be compared to those filled out by teachers or other significant adults such as foster parents. In cases of civil damage, comparisons of ratings by parents or others may indicate the reliability with which certain features of behavior appear. This type of concrete information about the parents' own assessment of their children and how it relates to those of others can be an asset in making recommendations.

4. INSTRUMENTS SPECIFICALLY DESIGNED FOR USE IN FORENSIC EVALUATIONS

There have been efforts on the part of some clinicians to develop tests that are designed specifically for use in child forensic evaluations. One such instrument is the Bricklin Perceptual Scales, which involves the child in responding nonverbally to questions "designed to assess a particular child's ability to profit from the particular parenting style of a given parent." Another, the Custody Quotient (Gordon and McPeek, 1987) is a structured interview that yields a score which is designed to reflect parental competency. Gardner has published a scale which he indicates helps to determine the validity of a child's accusation of sexual abuse. While such scales invite strong and even exclusive reliance by examiners on their results, empirical research to date does not justify such reliance. Some of the scales now available to the clinical community are more properly viewed as research instruments still undergoing development; none can be recommended as substitutes for full consideration of the wide variety of data obtained in standard evaluations.

C. Interpretation of test data

The results of psychological tests do not stand alone, but must be carefully interpreted in light of the information obtained in the rest of the evaluation. Test interpretation is inherently inferential, and care should be taken to stay as close to the actual data as possible. Although it may be interesting to make wide-ranging dynamically oriented hypotheses about test responses when evaluating a person for treatment planning, it is inappropriate to do so in the forensic arena where the evaluator must be able to clearly account for the basis on which conclusions and recommendations are made. Speculations about repressed Oedipal content as seen on the Rorschach are much less helpful to the court than clear statements about how such a conflict may be expressed in personality style, behavior, and parenting abilities. Misidentifying remote and speculative inferences from testing as "findings" and "indications" may be seen as a misuse of testing and a disservice to the individuals affected. The examiner bears grave responsibility for affecting the lives of others, and must strive to ground recommendations in actual data rather than in speculation.

1. INTEGRATION WITH OTHER EVALUATION DATA

In Case Example 2, the psychologist has made an important error in interpretation. He has taken several isolated responses from the test data and has extrapolated from them an accusation of sexual abuse. There are no single responses on any test instrument that warrant such an accusation; test data need to be considered as a whole, and individual responses have little significance by themselves.

Interpretations of test responses should not go beyond what the tests themselves can measure. In a thorough evaluation, each test should be carefully scored and interpreted. The information gained from the tests should be integrated into hypotheses about persons and how they interact with one another, if that is relevant to the legal question. These hypotheses can then be considered in light of the other data from the evaluation. Interpretive hypotheses from testing can help objectively confirm what the clinician has found and enrich an understanding of otherwise unexplained facts. They serve also to point up discrepancies or other avenues to pursue. As can be seen in Case Example 1, the MMPI-2 indicated that there could be substance abuse problems in the mother. This led the psychologist to interview her in depth about drug abuse, which she then admitted to. Rather than simply reporting an inference from test data, i.e., a scale score on the MMPI, the psychologist now had clear, direct evidence which could be used in her report.

2. USE OF COMPUTER-SCORED INTERPRETATIONS

Many of the personality inventories have computer programs available which not only score the tests, but also provide clinical interpretations based on the test data. It may be tempting for the clinician to consider these printouts as a finished interpretation and include them verbatim in reports. As most manuals for these tests point out, this is not the intended use for the automated interpretation. Computerized interpretation may help the clinician, especially one inexpert in testing, to generate hypotheses which again must be carefully integrated with other data. It is debatable whether these interpretations should be used at all in forensic work. Many of the statements generated by computer programs may not be accurate descriptions of the person being evaluated, since the programs fail to take into account the richness of the full evaluation and instead generate hypotheses on the basis of actuarial data. The resulting interpretive statements are derived from aggregate data; within normative groups, each individual's behavior, characteristics, or score occupies a place around a group average or other measure of group tendency. To conclude from an individual's score on an instrument that he or she is typical of the normative group neglects the fact of variance. Without referring to other data, the extent to which the person fits the picture of the group to which he or she is assigned by virtue of a score cannot be known. Computerized interpretations are in actuality more or less accurate for particular individuals, depending on a variety of factors. It is necessary that these factors be identified and considered by the examining clinician. The introduction into court proceedings of uninterpreted computerized interpretations may lend testing a false importance that leads to more attention by the court to the testing than the rest of the data because of a mistaken view that computerized assessments are somehow more objective.

D. Reporting of test data

One assumption that should always be made in reporting results in forensic work is that no matter how attorneys are cautioned that disclosure of the contents of a report may be harmful to their clients, the clients will have access to the report and read it. While this assumption should in no way alter or distort the actual findings or recommendations included in a report, it is tactful to employ some sensitivity in how findings are reported. In forensic work, there needs to be attention to accountability; nothing should be reported as opinion in reports or in testimony that cannot be supported by data and reasoned inference. It should be clear from the written report what the data were that were considered and the way in which conclusions were reached. Unlike consultation reports read by colleagues in the mental health field, results and opinions should be presented in clear language rather than in jargon. A treatment of testing results that is overly technical mystifies rather than elucidates the basis for recommendations and may mask an absence of any adequate basis for a recommendation. Excessive detailing of raw test data may indicate lack of expertise, as it is no substitute for clear and accurate summarization of the results of testing.

1. BALANCED REPORTING

Something at times forgotten by clinicians both in using psychological tests and in doing forensic evaluations is that attention needs to be paid to the relative strengths of each person being evaluated. Custody disputes in particular should not ordinarily be battles of pathology, with attempts to demonstrate which of the parties is the more disturbed. The court needs to know what they do well; it also needs to know not only how a child has been and might be affected but also the positive aspects of how he or she is coping with a stressful situation. Test findings need to be reported in a balanced manner, preferably with statements about strengths made first. For instance, in an evaluation for placement of a juvenile offender, the evaluator should be careful not to simply list negative test findings when there may be clear examples of intellectual strengths or ability to relate interpersonally. When reporting on deficit, psychopathology found, or personality problems, attention should be paid to the comparative extent of these problems, especially since children involved in forensic cases are often not from traditional clinical populations.

2. NONSELECTIVE REPORTING

It may be tempting for the clinician, who has already formed some hypotheses about a subject from interview, to report test findings that support these hypotheses only. In Case Example 2, the psychologist neglected to report his observations of the father and children, which had indicated a warm and loving relationship; also, he neglected to mention that he had never interviewed the children about possible abuse. Instead he had selectively used some test responses to confirm his hypothesis of sexual abuse.

Test data that are discrepant with the clinician's overall hypotheses should be reported and explained candidly. In the long run it will be left to the trier of fact and not the clinician to determine which of the data are most compelling.

IV. PITFALLS

A. Failure to test all parties

In Case Example 2, the MMPI-2 was administered to the father but not to the mother, supposedly because of concerns (raised by the mother's own report) about character disorder or other pathology in the father. The differential testing of the father permitted what would inevitably be viewed by him as invidious comparisons with the mother, who was not given the MMPI-2. When either negative characterizations which may damage an individual's custody claim, or positive characterizations which may enhance the claim, are made on the basis of test results, the same test had better be given to the competing party.

All parties need to be treated fairly but also need to feel they have been treated fairly. The probability of an indefinite contesting of custody or visitation after the initial adjudication is only increased by the perception of the "losing" side that they were subjected to procedural unfairness. If one party is to be tested, then all parties should be tested; the same tests should be given to each parent. Children should receive similar batteries, with modifications only to account for age differences. Failure to do so may, and frequently does, result in accusations of bias.

B. Failure to administer tests in a uniform fashion

Psychological tests should be administered in the standardized way they are intended to be given, as provided by the test manuals. Administering a few subscales of the WISC-R or a couple of Rorschach cards is poor practice in general, but never more so than in forensic settings. Such administrations outside testing protocols result in nonvalid findings that have no clear and interpretable relationship to group norms.

Anything that might allow the test taking to appear or be influenced by outside sources should not be permitted. Thus, tests should not be sent home with subjects for completion, nor should interested parties be present when tests are given. In some settings, attorneys or parents may want to monitor or observe the evaluation. This may be done through video- or audiotaping or through one-way mirrors. These methods reduce the chances of outside influence. Careless test administration leaves the clinician open to questions of the accuracy of conclusions and the quality of recommendations. Similarly, lack of control over choice of tester when testing is delegated, or over the way in which testing is conducted, damages the actual and perceived reliability of reported test findings.

C. Misuse of testing by attorneys or the court

Lay people may attempt to misuse or misinterpret psychological testing in court in several ways. First, testing can present an aura of complete objectivity and can be seen by the court as the most important piece of data, rather than an integrated part of a whole evaluation. Second, as mentioned above, computerized reports also give a false sense of scientific certainty which may be unduly impressive to a nonclinician. Third, attorneys often try to use individual responses or tests selectively. For example, a frequent line of questioning in testimony about the MMPI centers around taking each individual scale and asking what the elevation means or asking how a client responded to particular items. Clinicians who fail to correct this approach support a mistaken view that a single scale or score, taken out of context, can be considered meaningful. It is the clinician's responsibility to do his or her best to see that those involved understand the proper use of testing.

V. ACTION GUIDE

A. Know the law.

B. Use a qualified evaluator.

C. Select and administer appropriate tests.

1. Give a battery of tests.
2. Use tests appropriate to ages of children and to issues involved in the evaluation.
3. Administer tests uniformly to all parties.
4. Administer tests in a standardized fashion within protocols provided by manuals.
5. Use tests that are well-researched and documented.

D. Interpret cautiously.

1. Integrate data with other clinical findings.
2. Do not rely solely on computerized interpretations.
3. Avoid over-interpretation of single scores or responses.
4. Keep interpretations close to the data, avoiding remote inferences.

E. Report responsibly.

1. Provide a balanced view of each party.
2. Include all relevant data, even data which do not support conclusions and recommendations.
3. Assume subjects will have access to the report.

VI. CASE EXAMPLE EPILOGUES

A. Case Example 1

The psychologist prepares an extensive report which includes a separate section on test results and integrates the results with the rest of the information gathered. On the basis of her familiarity with the laws of her state regarding termination of parental rights, she concludes that the children have extensive, serious, and complicated problems which will require intensive attention and monitoring by a parent, as well as long-term treatment. She concludes that the mother's concern about her children seems only to reflect her own needs. Her drug problem and long-standing interpersonal difficulties do not allow her to be able to provide the level of care required by her children, and the psychologist recommends termination of parental rights.

B. Case Example 2

The psychologist in this case has gone far beyond the test data by making speculative statements which have little grounding in objective data. His use of interpretations of the projective tests and drawings as clear-cut signs of an actual event is inappropriate. On the basis of these insufficient and faulty data, the court moves to cut off the father's access to his children. The children are extremely upset at this and begin to show behavioral problems and school difficulties. The father's attorney calls in a new evaluator, who does extensive interviewing and testing of the father, but who is denied access to the mother or the children now in her custody. She concludes that there is an insufficient basis to arrive at a finding of sexual abuse in this case. The judge, having ruled, is not swayed; citing the earlier court-ordered evaluation of all parties, visitation with the father is not reinstated. The father files a malpractice suit and an ethics complaint against the first psychologist.

C. Case Example 3

The psychologist carefully reviews the previous test battery given to the son. She notes that there was some concern about the boy's social skills and that his level of anxiety appears to have increased. The concerns about body integrity and danger so prominent in the current assessment were not apparent in the earlier testing. Academic functioning has shown marked impairment; as tests show, he has fallen behind his classmates in most areas. She and the psychiatrist can determine no other life events that may have contributed to this change and conclude that what the child is experiencing is most likely due to the trauma caused by the burns. Neither interview nor test data support a claim of damage to the daughter, who appears to be dealing successfully with the accident and is functioning normally.

VII. SUGGESTED READINGS

Anastasi, A. (1988), Psychological Testing. 6th ed. New York: Macmillan.

Dahlstrom, W. G., Welsh, G. S., and Dahlstrom, L. E. (1972), An MMPI Handbook: Vol. I. Clinical Interpretation. Minneapolis: University of Minnesota Press.

Exner, J. E. (1986), The Rorschach: A Comprehensive System: Vol I. Basic Foundations. 2nd ed. New York: Wiley.

Exner, J. E. (1987), The Rorschach: A Comprehensive System: Vol. II. Current Research and Advanced Interpretations. New York: Wiley.

Exner, J. E. (1982), The Rorschach: A Comprehensive System: Vol. III. Assessment of Children and Adolescents. New York: Wiley.

Gardner, R. A. (1982), Family Evaluation in Child Custody Litigation. Caskill, N.J.: Creative Therapeutics.

Gass, R. (1979), The psychologist as expert witness: science in the courtroom? Comment. Maryland Law Review 38:539–621.

Goldman, J., L'Engle Stein, C., and Guerry, S. (1983), Psychological Methods of Child Assessment. New York: Brunner-Mazel.

Graham, J. R. (1990), MMPI-2: Assessing Personality and Psychopathology. New York: Oxford University Press.

Melton, G. B., Petrila, J., Poythress, N. G., and Slobogin, C. (1987), Psychological Evaluations for the Courts. New York: Guilford.

Palmer, J. O. (1983), The Psychological Assessment of Children. 2nd ed. New York: Wiley.

Weaver, S. J. (1984), Testing Children. Kansas City: Test Corporation of America.

Weiner, I. B. and Hess, A. K. (1987), Handbook of Forensic Psychology. New York: Wiley.

Weithorn, L. A. (ed.) (1987), Psychology and Child Custody Determinations. Lincoln: University of Nebraska Press.

Ziskin, J. and Faust, D. (1988), Coping with Psychiatric and Psychological Testimony. 4th ed., 3 vols. Marina del Rey: Law and Psychology Press.

5

Legal Issues in the Psychiatric Treatment of Minors

JOANN E. MACBETH, J.D.

Although many legal issues confronted by psychiatrists who treat children or adolescents are similar to those faced by other psychiatrists, certain problems—which derive from the patients' status as minors—are unique to this practice. This chapter focuses on these legal issues and problems and offers a framework for their resolution.

I. CASE EXAMPLES

A. Case Example 1

A woman calls a psychiatrist to make an appointment to discuss her 11-year-old son, Richard. When the psychiatrist meets with her, the mother explains that she is concerned about Richard because over the past several months he has begun to have terrible nightmares and on many days has adamantly refused to go to school. Upon questioning, the psychiatrist learns that he is also fighting more with his younger sister.

Richard's mother is not able to offer any explanation for this behavior. The psychiatrist agrees to see Richard for assessment and potential treatment. In his second session with Richard, it becomes clear that Richard's mother and father are not living together.

B. Case Example 2

A psychiatrist has been treating a 6-year-old girl, Rachel, for 9 months. The psychiatrist sees Rachel twice weekly and meets with her parents once every 2 weeks to discuss her treatment. The sessions with the parents frequently focus on their different parenting styles. This is particularly apparent in the area of discipline. Rachel's father is demanding; he believes that at 6 years old Rachel should obey her parents without question and should be punished when she does not. The punishment has become increasingly severe; her father often hits Rachel and restricts her to her room for extended periods. Rachel's mother believes that Rachel is still too young to be expected to behave and to consistently control her conduct. She is very reluctant to disagree with Rachel in any way. She is willing to use "time outs," but often retreats and does not impose them because of Rachel's promises and entreaties.

Rachel's mother expresses increasing concern about her husband's temper and his treatment of Rachel. Finally, near the end of a session, Rachel's mother tells the psychiatrist that she and Rachel's father are separated and that she wants the psychiatrist to testify in support of her attempt to obtain sole custody of Rachel.

Shortly thereafter, the mother's attorney calls the psychiatrist, asking for copies of Rachel's records and to schedule a time to talk with the psychiatrist about the case. This is followed by a subpoena sent by the father's attorney for records and a deposition.

C. Case Example 3

A psychiatrist is treating Linda, a 16-year-old who has a stormy relationship with her mother. It has been extremely difficult for the psychiatrist to establish a relationship with Linda, who is suspicious of him, partly because her mother arranged treatment. Linda repeatedly accuses the psychiatrist of "selling" information about her to her mother, who is paying for treatment. The psychiatrist repeatedly assures her that the relationship is a confidential one and that the information she gives the psychiatrist will not be shared with her mother. After a number of months and some testing around this issue, Linda appears to begin to trust the psychiatrist and starts to work in therapy, making significant progress. She then tells the psychiatrist about her plans to run away and marry her boyfriend. The boyfriend has been one of the main points of contention with her mother. He dropped out of school a year earlier, and Linda's mother strongly suspects that he supports himself by selling drugs. More than once, Linda has told the psychiatrist that her boyfriend has left town for a few days because people are "after him." He has bought a gun to protect himself.

II. LEGAL AND CLINICAL ISSUES[a]

A. Minority, custody, guardianship, and divorce

The law of minority, custody, and divorce is central to many of the legal issues facing child and adolescent psychiatrists. In most states, the age of majority is 16 or 18; in a few it is 21. Persons under the age of majority are minors and are considered by law to be incapable either of making important decisions affecting their welfare or, more generally, of managing their affairs in their own best interests[b]. In the traditional two-parent family, both parents are the child's natural guardians and, as such, have control over the child's property and person, just as they have a duty to provide for the child's basic needs.

---

[a] The focus of this chapter is the legal issues facing psychiatrists who treat children and adolescents. While clinical issues are not addressed separately, the discussion of legal issues focuses on the impact their resolution may have on the patient's treatment and clinical status.

[b] Minors may be "emancipated" from the control of their parents with their parents' consent. An emancipated minor is released from the legal restraints of minority and attains the rights (and responsibilities) he would otherwise not receive until the age of majority. Parental consent may be expressed or implied from the conduct of parent and child. Marriage or military enlistment will establish emancipation; a minor's self-support will be evidence thereof.

When a child's parents were divorced, only one parent traditionally was granted legal custody of the child, typically through the mechanism of a court decree. However, joint custody is increasingly more common. Generally speaking, the parent or parents who have legal custody of the child are empowered to make all decisions for the child. A parent without legal custody, in contrast, has no legally enforceable right to participate in these decisions, although he or she may have other rights, such as the right to visit the child at certain times. Indeed, he or she may have actual (i.e., physical) custody of the child. It is important to distinguish between these types of custody and to remember that only the parent or parents with legal custody may exercise the minor's legal rights. In certain legal proceedings, a special guardian—or guardian *ad litem*—may be appointed to represent the child even where one or both parents have legal custody.

Child psychiatrists frequently treat children whose parents are divorced or are in the process of separating or divorcing. This complicates matters significantly, not only because it may be unclear which parent has custody and thus the right to exercise many of the child's rights, but also because the psychiatrist may be drawn into an acrimonious custody dispute where his or her treatment role will be compromised.

B. Consent to treatment

Parents have significant power over decisions involving the medical treatment of their minor children. The parent or parents with legal custody are usually empowered to decide if a minor child will receive medical treatment, including psychiatric services. As a general rule a psychiatrist should not treat a minor patient without the consent of the custodial parent. To do so, in most jurisdictions, would create significant legal exposure. However, this general rule is subject to the following exceptions[c].

1. TREATMENT WITHOUT PARENTAL CONSENT

a. Emergencies

In most jurisdictions an exception is recognized for emergency situations. The rationale behind this exception is obvious: it is reasonable to assume that if there were sufficient time to consult a parent, the parent would consent to the provision of a child's emergency medical needs. Courts are especially willing to invoke this exception where obtaining or attempting to obtain consent will delay treatment and the delay will significantly increase the risk to the patient's life[d]. In some jurisdictions, the exception is broader, permitting treatment without parental consent when delay would endanger the health of the minor[e].

b. Emancipated minors

Parental consent is generally not needed for the treatment of an emancipated minor. The minor's status may be established in litigation contesting the physician's treatment. For example, in *Smith v. Selby*[f], the court held that an 18-year-old was

---

[c] *See generally* Annotation, *Medical Practitioner's Liability for Treatment Given Child Without Parent's Consent*, 67 A.L.R.4th 511 (1989 & Supp. 1990).

[d] *See, e.g., Luka v. Lowrie*, 171 Mich. 122, 136 N.W. 1106 (1912).

[e] *See, e.g., Sullivan v. Montgomery*, 279 N.Y.S. 575 (1935); *see generally*, Annotation, *supra* at 525–526.

[f] 431 P.2d 719 (Wash. 1967).

an emancipated minor capable of consenting to a vasectomy. The court focused on the minor's conduct, noting that he had completed high school, was "the head of his own family," and supported himself. It held that the jury could decide whether the minor was emancipated based on factors such as his "economic independence or lack thereof, general conduct as an adult and freedom from the control of parents"[g].

c. Mature minors

In a smaller number of states, a "mature minor" rule allows minors who demonstrate a certain level of comprehension and maturity to make medical decisions without parental consent. For example, in *Cardwell v. Bechtol*[h], the Supreme Court of Tennessee held that a 17½-year-old high school senior who was intelligent and had demonstrated significant maturity could give effective consent to osteopathic treatment. The *Cardwell* court explained that whether a minor is sufficiently mature, "depends upon the age, ability, experience, education, training, and degree of maturity or judgment obtained by the minor, as well as upon the conduct and demeanor of the minor at the time of the incident involved"[i].

This exception is not recognized in many states and varies considerably among those states that do recognize it. In some states, courts have been willing to apply the exception only when simple procedures were involved; in others, the courts have confined the exception to situations in which a parent has not been available. However, statutes that have codified the mature minor rule generally have not limited the rule in such ways. Even where the rule is available, it can be difficult to apply. The rule's subjective nature requires the psychiatrist to make judgments about the individual minor's capacity to comprehend the nature and purpose of the treatment in question. Psychiatrists who choose to rely on this exception must make sure of the contours of the rule in their state and should fully document the basis for their conclusions that the minor patient in question satisfies its requirements.

d. Specific consent statutes

Some states have granted minors the right to participate in, or make, certain kinds of treatment decisions. For example, some states allow minors to consent to treatment for chemical dependency and alcoholism, and to psychiatric counseling or treatment for mental illness. In many states minors may receive birth control counseling without parental consent. These statutes vary in terms of the critical age and should be consulted by psychiatrists who may plan to rely on them.

2. CONSENT IN CONTEXT OF SEPARATION

When a minor's parents are embroiled in a contentious divorce or custody proceeding, psychiatrists should be especially vigilant in obtaining effective consent to treat the child. The case of *Dymek v. Nyquist*[j] illustrates some potential risks of

---

[g] *Id.* at 723. *See also Carter v. Cangello*, 105 Cal. App.3d 348, 349–50, 164 Cal. Rptr. 361, 362 (Cal. Ct. App. 1980) (applying California statute authorizing minors 15 years or older who live apart from parents or grandparents and who manage their own financial affairs "regardless of the source of [their] income" to consent to medical treatment.)

[h] 724 S.W.2d 739 (Tenn. 1987).

[i] *Id.* at 748. *See also Younts v. St. Francis Hospital and School of Nursing, Inc.*, 469 P.2d 330 (Kan. 1970).

[j] 469 N.E.2d 659 (Ill. App. Ct., 1st Div. 1984).

not doing so. In that case, the noncustodial parent—the mother—took her 9-year-old son to see a psychiatrist twice a week for a year without the knowledge of the father, who had legal custody of the child. The mother later called the psychiatrist to testify in custody proceedings against the father. The father sued the mother and the psychiatrist on a variety of grounds, including the psychiatrist's failure to obtain the consent of the child's guardian prior to providing treatment. The court found this a legitimate basis for legal relief where there was no emergency situation necessitating immediate treatment.

When asked to treat a child whose parents are divorced, a psychiatrist will be maximally protected if he asks the parent requesting treatment for proof that he/she has *legal* custody of the child. When a patient's parents have both been involved in the minor's treatment but separate during the course of treatment, it is probably safe for a psychiatrist to continue treatment unless he is told by one of the parents that he is to stop treatment. If this occurs, the psychiatrist should consult the parent continuing to request treatment and ask for some confirmation of authority to consent to treatment.

3. INFORMED CONSENT

Consent to treatment—whether by the custodial parent or the child—is legally meaningless unless it is "informed." Consent is informed if it is based on adequate knowledge of the risks and benefits of the proposed treatment. One court has explained that the sufficiency of the information given to the patient will depend on "the nature of the treatment, the extent or the risks involved, and the standard of care of the treating physician," *Cardwell v. Bechtol*[k]. Generally speaking, there are at least three different approaches used to judge whether consent is informed: (1) the reasonable physician or national standard, (2) the community or local practice standard, and (3) the patient need standard[l]. Psychiatrists should familiarize themselves with the approach taken by courts in their state and its implications for effective consent.

C. Confidentiality and privilege

In addition to a psychiatrist's ethical duty not to disclose information learned from a patient[m], a psychiatrist has an independent *legal* duty to maintain a patient's confidences. That duty is reflected in two overlapping but distinct areas of law that are frequently confused: privilege and confidentiality. Privilege rules are rules of evidence; they govern disclosure of information learned through treatment in judicial, quasi-judicial, or administrative proceedings. Information disclosed to a psychiatrist during treatment is privileged, i.e., the patient may prevent the psychiatrist from disclosing it in such a proceeding. Confidentiality rules, by contrast, are much broader, barring disclosure of any information learned from the patient to any person not directly involved in the current patient's care. Privilege and confidentiality rules both apply not only to the oral disclosure of information

---

[k] 724 S.W. 2d at 749.

[l] *See Cross v. Trapp*, 294 S.E.2d 446, 450–55 (W. Va. 1982) (discussing various standards).

[m] *See e.g.*, American Psychiatric Association's *Principles of Medical Ethics with Annotations Especially Applicable to Psychiatry*, Section 4, Annotation 1, American Medical Association's *Principles of Medical Ethics*, Section 2.

learned from patients but also to the release of written notes, records, or other documents relating to the treatment of the patient.

1. CONFIDENTIALITY

Confidentiality is central to the therapeutic relationship; its importance is reflected in the double duty—ethical and legal—to maintain patient confidences. Unfortunately, the legal status of minors complicates the rather clear-cut rules that apply in the treatment of adults. When minors are involved, there are frequently countervailing duties running to different interested parties[n]. On one hand, it is clear both that a minor's parents generally are entitled to more information about the patient than family members of an adult patient would be and that they may make certain decisions about the release of information about the minor that would ordinarily only be made by the patient himself. On the other hand, it is also clear that minors possess an independent right of confidentiality, which must be considered and which will outweigh other rights in a variety of situations. Thus, psychiatrists are placed in a difficult situation when parents seek information and minor patients resist disclosure.

a. Risks of confidentiality breach

In most jurisdictions, what was solely an ethical obligation to keep patient information confidential is now a legal duty as well. Suits for breach of confidentiality have been brought under various theories[o]. In some cases, patients have sued for invasion of privacy, tortious breach of a duty of confidentiality, or breach of an implied contract to maintain confidentiality. In states where disclosure of patient information is barred by licensing statutes or rules of privilege, patients have sought, with mixed success, to bring a civil suit under these provisions. The trend is clearly in the direction of recognizing a legal duty and concomitant right of recovery, regardless of the legal theory on which this duty is based.

In addition to potential civil liability, a breach of confidentiality may form the basis of a complaint to a psychiatrist's professional organization. The resulting investigation is likely to be time-consuming, expensive, and anxiety-provoking; negative findings may have to be reported to the National Practitioner Data Bank, licensing boards, insurance carriers, etc. Similarly, in states where breach of confidentiality is included within the definition of unprofessional conduct by the licensing authority, the psychiatrist is potentially subject to a licensure action.

b. Release of information to parents

Generally. The rules regarding authority to consent to treatment of a minor are discussed above. Speaking generally, unless there is a statute to the contrary, it is fair to assume that if a parent is legally entitled to authorize treatment for a minor child, that parent has a legal right to full information about the treatment, including any confidential information disclosed by the minor.

This legal rule poses obvious clinical problems. Even when patients are young, many psychiatrists would feel uncomfortable if parents actually sought to exercise

---

[n] *See, e.g.*, American Psychiatric Association's *Principles of Medical Ethics with Annotations Especially Applicable to Psychiatry*, Section 4, Annotation 7.

[o] *See*, Annotation, *Physicians' Tort Liability for Unauthorized Disclosure of Confidential Information About Patient*, 48 A.L.R.4th 668 (1986 and 1990 Supp.)

their right of full access to information about the treatment. The potential damage to the therapeutic relationship with the minor is the most obvious risk. In addition, disclosures—particularly about one parent to the other—may well exacerbate family problems. To avoid such risks, it is advisable to lay out ground rules regarding confidentiality and disclosure at the outset of treatment. The psychiatrist should explain what he will tell the parents, what he will withhold, and his reasoning. Most parents will understand. In any event, if they elect to go forward with treatment, you may assume that they have agreed to those terms[p].

The problem of disclosure to parents assumes even greater importance with adolescent patients. Parents of adolescent children may well not be entitled to the same amount of information as are parents of very young minors. To begin with, as discussed above, it is likely that minors who are legally able to give effective consent to treatment will also be entitled to control the release of information about that treatment. The statutes of some states specifically link consent to treatment and disclosure authority. Even without such a statute, there is little risk in relying on an adolescent's consent to release confidential information when that adolescent was legally entitled to consent to the treatment in question.

When it is not clear that the adolescent controls consent to treatment, it is essential that the psychiatrist make disclosure rules clear to both minor and parents. The risks of not doing so are significant. If the matter is not discussed, the adolescent and parent each may well assume that he controls confidentiality. If, at some point during treatment, it becomes clear to one party or the other that he is mistaken, the therapeutic relationship may well be seriously damaged.

While an angry parent may refuse to continue to pay for treatment, from a clinical perspective, the adolescent's expectations are clearly more significant. For many adolescents, not only is confidentiality an absolute prerequisite to treatment, but the confidentiality that concerns them most is in relations to their parents. Learning that information they believed to be confidential has been shared with their parents could seriously impair their treatment.

Both adolescent and parent should be informed at the outset of treatment to what extent the adolescent will control the disclosure of information—including disclosure to the parents—and to what extent or in what situations information will be shared with the parents regardless of the adolescent's wishes.

The decision of where this line will be drawn should be informed by both ethical and legal considerations. The APA's *Principles of Medical Ethics with Annotations Especially Applicable to Psychiatry*, Section 4, Annotation 7, addresses the countervailing ethical interests as follows:

> Careful judgment must be exercised by the psychiatrist in order to include, when appropriate, the parents or guardian in the treatment of a minor. At the same time the psychiatrist must assure the minor proper confidentiality.

Legally, a psychiatrist will be at risk if he withholds information that could enable parents to protect their adolescents from serious harm. When the interests involved

---

[p] While obtaining written agreement to such conditions offers the greatest degree of protection, many psychiatrists are unwilling to go beyond an oral explanation to their patients' parents. An intermediate approach would be to develop a standard statement regarding confidentiality to go over with and provide to the parents.

are less vital, but the psychiatrist feels that certain information would benefit the family, he should attempt to arrange this disclosure without breaching confidentiality and, thus, endangering his relationship with the adolescent. First, the psychiatrist may be able to work with the adolescent, encouraging him to disclose the information to his parents himself. If the adolescent is unwilling to do this, he may be willing to permit the psychiatrist to do so. If the adolescent resists both options, the psychiatrist may be able to accomplish his purpose by discussing a general problem without disclosing anything the minor may have said about himself or any other specific information about the minor.

Parental separation or divorce. The divorce or separation of the parents of an adolescent patient further complicates the situation. Generally speaking, the principles discussed above apply; the parent(s) with legal custody enjoy whatever legal rights exist to obtain information about the minor's treatment, including information disclosed by the minor in the course of therapy. The law does not protect the interest of a noncustodial parent in such information.

Unfortunately, this relatively simple rule frequently breaks down in practice. This occurs because the parent who does not have legal custody often has actual custody of the child for certain periods[q]. In many cases, this may be addressed in the divorce decree, e.g., the decree may provide that the parent without legal custody is entitled to actual custody for 1 month each summer. In others, the arrangement develops informally or evolves over time as the child grows and/or the relative circumstances of his parents change.

However it occurs, a psychiatrist would be ill-advised to treat the parent with actual, but no legal, custody as an ordinary third party. Arrangements should be made to provide the noncustodial parent with any information the psychiatrist believes essential, e.g., information about medications, behavior that has signaled trouble in the past, concerns about the minor's safety, etc. If possible, consent should be obtained from the parent with legal custody. If the custodial parent is unwilling, the parent with the child can seek assistance from the court or guardian *ad litem*.

c. Release of information to third parties

The rules that govern the release of information about minors to unrelated third parties—schools, researchers, insurers, etc.—are somewhat less clear. The principles discussed above would clearly suggest that custodial parents may consent to such releases unless the minor controls the right to consent to the underlying treatment. However, both ethical and legal concerns suggest that this general rule needs to be tempered somewhat when the information is to be released to someone other than the minor's parents.

Regardless of the breadth of the authorization, a psychiatrist has an ethical obligation to limit disclosures to those necessary in the particular situation[r]. Psy-

---

[q] E.g., in *Dymek v. Nyquist, supra*, it was the mother, who did not have legal custody, who brought the patient for treatment twice every week for a year.

[r] The APA's *Principles of Medical Ethics with Annotations Especially Applicable to Psychiatry*, Section 4, Annotation 5 provides:

Ethically the psychiatrist may disclose only that information which is relevant to a given situation. He/she should avoid offering speculation as fact. Sensitive information such as an individual's sexual orientation or fantasy material is usually unnecessary.

chiatrists should be particularly sensitive to this obligation when the person authorizing the disclosure (the parent) is someone other than the person who may be harmed by the disclosures (the minor). Moreover, as indicated earlier, minors appear to possess some independent right of confidentiality. Although its contours are far from clear, courts may be less reluctant to protect this right when information is being withheld from third parties, rather than from the minor's parents.

Particular caution should be exercised when the disclosures are clearly to benefit someone other than the child. The psychiatrist who wants to write about the minor or use information about the patient in some other kind of research would be well-advised to obtain the consent both of the parents and of the minor himself.

Exceptions to consent requirement.   There are several important exceptions to the requirement that confidential information be disclosed to third parties only with consent. First, in virtually every state there is a statute *requiring* the psychiatrist to report child abuse[5]. Frequently, these statutes carry criminal penalties. Civil liability is less clear. At least one court has rejected an attempt to bring a civil action under such a penal statute. In *Fischer v. Metcalf*[6], the court dismissed a suit brought on behalf of two children against the psychiatrist who had treated their father but had failed to report their abuse by the father to the state department of rehabilitation services. Nonetheless, psychiatrists should expect that failure to report child abuse may subject them to civil liability in other jurisdictions.

Second, state confidentiality statutes sometimes authorize psychiatrists to breach confidentiality in order to warn of a danger posed by a patient. These statutes obviously apply to minors as well as to adults; although permissive in nature, they should be regarded as imposing a duty to warn.

Third, even in the absence of such statutes, in most jurisdictions a psychiatrist will be at risk if he does not appropriately disclose information that suggests that another person is endangered by his patient. Similarly, as with adult patients, where a psychiatrist possesses information about a minor's suicidal intent, it must be disclosed as necessary and appropriate to prevent suicide.

Fourth, some state statutes require the psychiatrist to report infectious diseases and a variety of other conditions that may affect children. The requirements vary significantly from state to state; psychiatrists should familiarize themselves with the law of the jurisdictions in which they practice.

d. Custody disputes

The sections above address how to proceed when a minor's custody has already been settled through a separation agreement or divorce decree. When parents decide to separate during the course of a minor's treatment, different problems may arise. It is not uncommon in such a situation for one or even both parents to seek the psychiatrist's assistance in the custody contest.

As is discussed in the next section, the physician-patient privilege may prevent this testimony. However, even if it does not and even if the psychiatrist has very clear opinions as to where the patient's custody interests lie, he should resist efforts to draw him into the case. The risks are many. If the minor is aware of his ap-

---

[5] *See generally*, Annotation, *Validity Construction and Application of State Statute Requiring Doctor or Other Person to Report Child Abuse*, 73 A.L.R.4th 782 (1989 and 1990 Supp.)

[6] 543 So.2d 785 (Fla. 3d Dist. Ct. App. 1989) (en banc).

pearances in court, particularly if it is "in support of" one parent and "against" the other, it may seriously undermine the treatment relationship. Nor are the risks confined to the child's reactions. One or both parents may resent the psychiatrist's expressed views and may refuse to continue to work with the psychiatrist or to pay for treatment. The psychiatrist should explain to the parent(s) seeking his help that the child is best served by the therapist remaining solely in a therapeutic role and that they can obtain an independent evaluation for purposes of the litigation. The following section on privilege will discuss how to proceed if the parent or his counsel persists and seeks to compel the psychiatrist's involvement.

e. Authorization to release information

In order to protect a psychiatrist who has disclosed confidential information, authorization to make the disclosure must be legally valid. A psychiatrist should make certain that the authorization actually extends to the information in question and that it satisfies state confidentiality law requirements. A number of states have enacted mental health confidentiality statutes that specify the form for a valid authorization[u].

These statutes generally require that authorization be written. Even when there is no such statutory requirement, it is advisable to use a consent form. The use of a form both encourages a patient to focus on the process and the rights being waived and serves as later documentation of consent. This is particularly useful when children and adolescents are involved and consent may become a contentious issue between parents and children.

Before releasing the information in question, a psychiatrist should satisfy himself that the patient's or parents' consent is informed[v]. Those authorizing the disclosure should be aware of the nature of the information sought as well as what will be included in the information released. If release of the patient's medical record is at issue, the patient should be informed of the types and sources of information in that record. This is particularly important when the consent of a minor is involved, as the record is likely to include significant information from parents and other sources of which the patient is unaware.

Authorization for the release of information frequently comes indirectly from third parties—such as insurance carriers or schools—who have obtained it from the patient or parent. If the psychiatrist believes that the patient or parent would not have consented if fully aware of the nature of the information involved or was not aware that the authorization would be used to obtain mental health information, the psychiatrist should contact the patient to discuss authorization and disclosure.

The most effective consent is that made with knowledge of exactly what the psychiatrist will be disclosing. This would require the psychiatrist to make all disclosures in writing and to provide the patient a copy to review and approve prior

---

[u] *See, e.g.,* Ill. Stat. Ann. Ch. 91 1/2 §805. These statutes should be consulted prior to the release of any patient information; they may preclude the release of certain information despite patient (or parent) consent.

[v] This is advisable for ethical as well as for legal reasons. Section 4, Annotation 2 of the APA's *Principles of Medical Ethics with Annotations Especially Applicable to Psychiatry* provides in part:

"The continuing duty of the psychiatrist to protect the patient includes fully apprising him/her of the annotations of 'waiving the privilege of privacy'."

to release. For both legal and clinical reasons, the psychiatrist should consider this approach if it would not compromise treatment.

2. Privilege

Privilege rules govern the disclosure of confidential information in judicial, quasi-judicial, or administrative proceedings. At common law, evidentiary privileges did not exist; the prevailing view was that courts were entitled to everyone's testimony. The later statutory creation of privileges reflected a recognition that certain societal values—namely, the protection of certain kinds of relationships—were more important than the need for full disclosure. Privileges were created in order to encourage full and frank communication in certain relationships, such as attorney-client and physician-patient. The rationale for the physician-patient privilege is that without full communication between doctors and patients, effective treatment cannot take place.

a. Scope of the privilege

Whether or not particular information from or about the patient will be found privileged—and therefore, subject to exclusion by the patient (or the person legally authorized to exercise the privilege on the patient's behalf)—depends on a variety of factors that vary considerably from jurisdiction to jurisdiction. The law of virtually every state includes a psychotherapist-patient or physician-patient privilege that applies to communications between psychiatrists and their patients, including minor patients. These state-law rules will apply in proceedings in state courts or state administrative bodies. Federal courts, however, apply both state and federal law, depending upon the nature of the claim at issue. When entertaining a federal claim, federal courts will apply the federal privilege rule. Unfortunately, federal courts in different parts of the country have developed different rules regarding the psychiatrist-patient privilege[w]. While federal courts in Michigan, Ohio, Kentucky, and Tennessee recognize a federal psychotherapist-patient privilege, those in Florida, Georgia, Alabama, Texas, Mississippi, and Louisiana do not[x]. In federal courts sitting in other states, the law is unclear.

Matters protected by privilege. In most jurisdictions, the privilege protects not only appropriate communications from the patient to the psychiatrist, but also any information learned in the course of examination and the psychiatrist's diagnosis and other conclusions about the patient and diagnosis. The privilege is usually held to apply only to communications between the psychiatrist and patient which relate to the patient's treatment. However, in psychiatry this should cover virtually all information learned from the patient[y].

---

[w] *See Dickson v. City of Lawton, Oklahoma*, 898 F.2d 1443, 1450 (10th Cir. 1990).

[x] *Compare In re Zuniga*, 714 F.2d 632, 639 (6th Cir.), *cert. denied*, 464 U.S. 983 (1983) (recognizing privilege) *with United States v. Corona*, 849 F.2d 562, 567 (11th Cir. 1988), *cert. denied*, 109 S.Ct. 1542 (1989) (declining to recognize privilege); *United States v. Meagher*, 531 F.2d 752, 753 (5th Cir.), *cert. denied*, 429 U.S. 853 (1976) (same). *See generally* annotation, *Psychotherapist-Patient Privilege Under Federal Common Law*, 72 A.L.R. Fed. 395 (1985 and 1990 Supp.).

[y] Communications made during the course of examinations undertaken for purposes other than treatment usually will not be protected. This exception would likely include examinations conducted pursuant to court order and evaluations requested by a school.

An important issue in the treatment of children and adolescents is whether information disclosed in the presence of another person is privileged. The traditional rule was that such communications were not privileged—that there could be no expectation of privacy when a third person, including a parent, was present. However, this rule is under modification as courts examine and acknowledge the reality of child and adolescent therapy and other family treatment situations.

Another issue of obvious importance in the treatment of children and adolescents is whether information received from a minor patient's parents, other family members, and third parties is protected by the privilege. Important interests are served by including this information within the privilege. Particularly in the treatment of young children, some of the most sensitive information about both the patient and the family may come from parents. This information may be critical to the successful treatment of the minor; if confidentiality is not assured, family members may not be willing to provide this information to the psychiatrist. To date, although some courts have understood the importance of extending the privilege to such third-party communications, there is no uniformity on this point[z].

b. Exceptions to the privilege

The privilege statutes of virtually every state contain significant exceptions. Commitment proceedings, will contests, and criminal matters are frequently excepted from the privilege. Particularly important to the psychiatrist who treats minors is the common abrogation of the privilege in proceedings relating to child abuse or neglect[aa]. The scope of this exception varies from state to state, depending on the language of the state's statute and subsequent judicial interpretations. In some states, such as Alaska, the privilege is abrogated only in proceedings brought under the state's child abuse acts[bb]. In other states, the exception has been drafted more broadly and courts have held that the privilege does not apply in civil proceedings unrelated to the state's child abuse act.

In *State ex rel D.U. v. Hoester*[cc] the court considered an exception to the privilege that applied in "*any* judicial proceeding relating to child abuse or neglect"[dd]. It held that the privilege had been abrogated in a damages action for intentional tort brought by a daughter against her adoptive father. The daughter alleged that she had been sexually molested and assaulted by the adoptive father. The father argued that the privilege should apply, i.e., that the exception was only relevant in proceedings under Missouri's child abuse statute. The court rejected this argument on the basis of the plain language of the statute[ee].

---

[z] *See Grosslight v. Superior Court*, 72 Cal. App. 3d 502, 140 Cal. Rptr. 278 (1977).

[aa] *See generally*, Annotation, *Validity, Construction, and Application of Statute Limiting Physician-Patient Privilege to Judicial Proceedings Relating to Child Abuse or Neglect*, 44 A.L.R.4th 649 (1986 and Supp. 1990).

[bb] *See State ex rel. D.M. v. Hoester*, 681 S.W.2d 449, 452 n.5 (Mo. 1984) (en banc); Alaska Statutes § 47.17.060 (1990).

[cc] 681 S.W.2d 449, 452 n.5 (Mo. 1984) (en banc).

[dd] Mo. Statutes § 210.140.

[ee] 681 S.W. 2d at 452. *See also Carson v. Jackson*, 466 So.2nd 1188 (Fla. 4th Dist. Ct. App. 1985) (in which a Florida court construed a Florida statute as abrogating the privilege in a civil suit brought by parents against a babysitter based on suspected abuse of the parent's child).

A number of courts have held similarly that the psychiatrist/patient privilege does not apply in criminal proceedings involving child abuse[ff].

Some states have created a specific exception for child custody cases. In these jurisdictions, a minor's treating psychiatrist can be compelled to provide testimony and disclose confidential information learned through treatment even over the objection of the minor patient and the minor's parents. However, some courts have recognized that there are countervailing interests involved and that the evidence can be obtained in other ways. These courts have upheld the privilege, requiring an independent psychiatrist examination instead. In Massachusetts the testimony will be permitted only if the judge determines after a hearing not only that the psychiatrist has significant evidence regarding the parent's ability to provide custody, but also that the disclosure of the evidence is more important to the child's welfare than is the protection of the therapeutic relationship[gg].

c. Waiver

Explicit waiver.   The privilege belongs to the patient. If the patient or the person authorized to act on his behalf waives the privilege (does not choose to exercise it), the confidential information may be introduced into the proceeding.

Psychiatrists who treat children and adolescents face the uncertainty of whether the patient is competent to exercise (and therefore to waive) the privilege. Although this depends on state statutes and case law, which differ from state to state, if the patient is a minor, the parent or legal guardian will ordinarily have the power to waive the privilege on behalf of the child[hh]. If the parents are divorced or separated, the parent with legal custody has traditionally controlled the exercise of the privilege.

The most difficult questions arise in the context of custody disputes, where the psychiatrist's testimony is likely to be central to the dispute, and the parents frequently disagree about whether the privilege should be exercised or waived. The law in this area varies dramatically from state to state. In *Nagle v. Hooks*[ii], Maryland's highest court held that when the child was too young to make decisions about the privilege himself the decision in a custody dispute could not be made by either parent or even by both together. The court explained that a custodial parent has an inherent conflict of interest in acting on the child's behalf in asserting or waiving the privilege in the context of a continuing custody contest. The court required that a neutral party be appointed to serve as guardian for the limited purpose of deciding whether or not to assert the privilege; the guardian was to be guided by what was in the child's best interest.

The lesson to be drawn from *Nagle* and similar cases is that care should be taken to determine who is entitled to exercise (and waive) the privilege for the

----

[ff] *See e.g. State v. Brydon*, 626 S.W. 2d 443 (Mo. App. 1981); *People v. Battaglia*, 156 Cal. App. 3d 1058, 203 Cal. Rptr. 370 (2d Dist. 1984); *State v. Fagalde*, 85 Wash. 2d. 730, 539 P.2d 86 (1975) (en banc) (doctor/patient privilege did not apply to communications between a patient and various clinic personnel concerning the patient's hostility toward a child who was later found to have been abused physically). But *see State v. R.H.*, 683 P.2d 269 (Alaska Ct. of App. 1984) (court declined to consider the privilege abrogated in grand jury proceedings, reasoning that such a construction might run afoul of the Alaska constitution's privilege against self-incrimination). *See generally* annotation 44 A.L.R. 4th at 658–63 (summarizing cases).

[gg] Mass. Gen. Laws. Ann. Ch. 233 § 20B(e).

[hh] *See Yancy v. Erman*, 99 N.E.2d 524, 532 (Ct. Common Pleas, Cuyahoga Cty. 1951).

[ii] 295 Md. 123, 460 A.2d 49 (Md. 1983).

minor patient. This will turn not only on state law rules of competency and minority, but also on who has legal custody of the child and on state statutory and decisional law. A psychiatrist should consult counsel before testifying or releasing medical records in a judicial proceeding.

Implied waiver.   Courts have also recognized implied waivers of the privilege in a variety of circumstances. These include cases in which the patient has testified about his treatment[jj], where the patient has testified about his condition at the time of the communications in question or has called another physician to testify about his condition at that time, and where there has been a waiver in another case or disclosure of the confidential information outside the courtroom.

The extent to which the privilege is held to be waived in these or other circumstances varies significantly from one jurisdiction to another. Because the applicability of the privilege is often unclear, a psychiatrist should never disclose information in reliance on a litigant's or lawyer's representation that the patient has waived the privilege or waived confidentiality. Unless the psychiatrist is provided with a signed release from the patient (or person authorized to act on his behalf), the psychiatrist should explain that he will not turn over any information without a subpoena and should follow the procedure outlined below for responding to a subpoena.

D. Responding to subpoena

1. NATURE OF SUBPOENA

A subpoena is a document issued by a court at the request of an attorney, which commands the recipient to appear at a particular proceeding and/or to produce particular documents. It is usually routinely issued by the clerk of the court without knowledge of the litigation in question or the role or potential evidence of the person to whom it will be issued. It does not reflect a judicial determination that the physician-patient privilege does not apply.

2. RESPONDING TO A SUBPOENA

a. General

In general, information sought by a subpoena can be provided if the patient consents to its release (i.e., waives the privilege) or if there has been a judicial determination that the privilege does not apply. Upon receiving a subpoena, a psychiatrist should determine whether either has occurred and, if not, should take appropriate steps to protect the privileged nature of the information within the context of responding to the subpoena. These steps will depend to a certain extent on whether the subpoena is for trial or for deposition and document production.

Deposition and/or document subpoena.   A subpoena for a deposition should first be reviewed to determine if authorization from the patient is included. This is not unusual; if it is clear that the patient must waive his privilege in order to pursue the litigation, opposing counsel will frequently request a release for this purpose. If an authorization is not included, a call or brief letter to the issuing attorney may result in one. If not, the psychiatrist can contact the patient's attorney to determine if the patient consents to the deposition and/or document prod-

---

[jj] *See e.g.,* *Giamanco v. Giamanco,* 57 A.D. 2d 564, 393 N.Y.S. 2d 453 (1977).

uction[kk]. Alternatively, the psychiatrist can contact the attorney who issued the subpoena to inform him that he will not be able to provide any substantive information in response to the subpoena without authorization from the patient or a court order. The attorney can then take steps to secure one or the other.

If patient consent is not forthcoming, the psychiatrist should make clear to the issuing attorney that without a court order he will be able to provide information about himself and his practice, but no information about any patient, including information as to whether a particular person is or has been his patient. Attorneys so notified are likely to take steps to secure consent or a court order before the deposition or to cancel the deposition. If an attorney insists on going forward with the deposition, the psychiatrist is obligated to appear unless he is taking steps to quash the subpoena himself[ll]. At such a deposition, the psychiatrist should remember that he should not provide any information about patients. If asked questions that seek such information, he should respond that the information sought is confidential and privileged. It is possible that another deposition will be held after the issuing attorney has obtained a court order or consent.

b. Trial subpoena

As with a subpoena for a deposition, when a psychiatrist receives a trial subpoena, he should attempt to determine whether the patient has authorized his testimony. (When the patient is an adult and the subpoena is from the patient's attorney, the psychiatrist can assume that the patient has consented[mm]. When the patient is a minor the situation may be somewhat more complicated; this situation is discussed below.)

If the situation has not been resolved before the date on which the psychiatrist has been ordered to appear for trial, he should appear as directed. As at deposition, he can testify about general matters (name, profession, etc.). When asked the first substantive question, there may be an objection on the grounds of physician-patient privilege. If this occurs, the psychiatrist may follow the judge's subsequent decision and direction. If there is no objection, but the psychiatrist does not feel that there has been adequate consent, he may raise this issue with the judge himself, simply stating his concern (that the material is confidential and privileged) and asking if he should testify.

c. Minor patient

The foregoing discussion has focused on issues all psychiatrists face when they receive a subpoena. As in other contexts, a minor patient presents a special challenge. An important issue is who may authorize trial and deposition testimony. The rules reviewed above control. Again, the greatest uncertainty will be in the

---

[kk] Although oral consent is sufficient, many psychiatrists feel more comfortable with written authorization, especially if they have never dealt with the attorney in question or they are no longer treating the patient. Oral consent should be documented in the psychiatrists' records.

[ll] Deposition scheduling is usually flexible. Although the subpoena may name a particular date and time, it is almost always possible to negotiate a more convenient time. The patient's attorney may be helpful in this process.

[mm] Trial counsel will frequently issue subpoenas even for supporting witnesses; such subpoenas permit the rescheduling of the testimony in question if for some reason the witness subpoenaed does not appear.

custody area. To begin with, it is very common in a custody case for one parent to "consent" to disclosure and for the other parent to adamantly oppose it. While a psychiatrist may usually rely on the consent of one parent, it clearly would be risky to do so in the custody context, unless the consenting parent already has sole legal custody. In any other case, consent of both parents or a court order is necessary. As the *Nagle* case demonstrates, even the former may not be sufficient.

For clinical reasons, even when there appears to be effective consent or waiver, the treating psychiatrist should attempt to limit his role to treatment. The psychiatrist may be able to convince the parents of the importance of protecting his treatment relationship with their child. Offering the parents assistance in locating another psychiatrist to evaluate the child may encourage them in this regard. It may also help to discuss these matters with the parents' attorneys, who are likely to prefer using experts who are not reluctant to testify. If parents and attorneys cannot be convinced, the psychiatrist may want to consider contacting the judge to urge the appointment of an independent psychiatrist to conduct an evaluation and to testify in the custody proceeding.

III. PITFALLS

A. Inappropriate guarantee of confidentiality

Adolescent patients may be particularly concerned about confidentiality and suspicious about their parents' participation and role in the treatment process. This attitude may prevent the formation of a therapeutic relationship and the beginning of effective treatment. The frustration inherent in attempting to help an adolescent under these circumstances may incline a psychiatrist to assure the adolescent that regardless of what the adolescent tells him, he will not share that information with the patient's parents.

This temptation should be resisted. It entails significant legal and treatment risks. As with an adult patient, there will be situations in which the psychiatrist will have to disclose information told to him in confidence in order to protect the patient or third parties. The psychiatrist cannot observe the promises made to the patient without unacceptably high legal risk, and breaching confidentiality after a specific promise to observe it will be particularly damaging to the treatment relationship.

B. Inappropriate maintenance of confidentiality

Even when an adolescent's parents have been told at the outset of treatment of the extent to which the adolescent will be accorded confidentiality (and information withheld), when the adolescent continues to express concerns about confidentiality and the parents' continuing request for information becomes a source of contention in dealing with them, the psychiatrist may begin to side with the adolescent in this contest to the extent that he refuses to provide any information to the parents. The risks in this are clear; information that may be necessary to protect the adolescent, his family members, or others from harm may be withheld inappropriately from the parents.

IV. CASE EXAMPLE EPILOGUES

A. Case Example 1

When a child lives with both natural parents, it is generally safe for a psychiatrist to rely on the consent of either one for treatment. Once the psychiatrist learns that the parents of a minor patient may be separated or divorced, however, the psychiatrist is on notice that one parent may not have any legal authority to consent to treatment and he should take steps to investigate who has legal custody.

In this case, after the second session, the psychiatrist called Richard's mother to inquire about the separation and legal custody. She told the psychiatrist that Richard's father had moved out several months earlier but that he remained in touch with both her and the children and that she hoped that he would return. Neither had taken any steps to obtain a legal separation or begin divorce proceedings.

The psychiatrist inquired whether Richard's father knew that Richard was in treatment. The mother hesitated, then admitted that she had not told him but that she was certain that he would not object. The psychiatrist explained that under the circumstances he would feel more comfortable if the boy's father also consented to treatment. He also told her that he felt that children obtained maximum benefit from treatment when both parents participated. Richard's mother reluctantly gave the psychiatrist the father's telephone number and address. When contacted by the psychiatrist, the father angrily said that he did not care whether Richard was in treatment or not, but that he was not going to pay for therapy, which he considered another of his wife's wasteful expenditures. The psychiatrist wrote the father a letter confirming his consent to the treatment in question.

B. Case Example 2

When Rachel's mother asked the psychiatrist to testify in support of her in the pending custody suit, the psychiatrist told the mother that his most important role in the trying months ahead was as therapist to Rachel and explained how his testifying in support of either parent could undermine Rachel's therapy and progress. Rachel's mother reacted angrily, reminding the psychiatrist that she paid for the treatment and that she felt that she should be able to have him testify if she wanted. She told the psychiatrist that he had a duty to protect Rachel from her father's increasingly harsh punishment by helping her obtain custody. The psychiatrist reiterated his earlier statements about the importance of protecting his treatment relationship with Rachel and asked her mother to think about this and to discuss the matter with him at their next appointment.

After she left, the psychiatrist reviewed the child abuse reporting statute in his state. He made a preliminary determination that none of the punishment he had heard about would qualify as "abuse" under the statute and, using no names, confirmed this interpretation with the state office that enforced the law.

The call from the mother's attorney arrived before the psychiatrist's next scheduled appointment with the mother. The psychiatrist told the attorney that he did not believe that it was in Rachel's best interests to have him appear as an expert in the custody case and offered to suggest the names of other psychiatrists who could serve solely as evaluators of Rachel. The attorney told the psychiatrist that he was willing to recommend this approach to Rachel's mother because he could tell that the psychiatrist was going to be uncooperative and therefore could hurt his case. However, he reiterated his request for copies of Rachel's records, expressing curiosity as to what was in them, in case they were released during the proceeding. The psychiatrist told the attorney that given the custody dispute, he did not feel comfortable disclosing any information—including what is in the records—without the consent of both parents. The attorney muttered something about a court order and hung up.

When the psychiatrist received the subpoena from the father's attorney, he called the attorney who issued it and indicated that he would need consent or waiver from both parents before he could provide any information without a court order. He also explained to the psychiatrist why he believed Rachel's interests would best be served by having psychiatric testimony provided by another psychiatrist who was not involved in Rachel's care. The attorney persisted, indicating he would get consent from Rachel's mother and that the psychiatrist should arrange to be at the deposition as scheduled.

When the psychiatrist had heard nothing further by the day before the deposition, he called the father's attorney again, asking whether he had obtained the mother's consent. The attorney responded angrily, telling the psychiatrist that the mother's consent was not needed, because the father had legal custody and he was waiving the privilege. The psychiatrist warned the attorney that if there was no consent before the deposition, he would not be able to answer any questions about Rachel or her treatment.

The psychiatrist then called the mother's attorney to ask if he were willing to take any steps to prevent the deposition. Her attorney asked that the psychiatrist refuse to provide the confidential information at the deposition and said that he would move to quash thereafter. The psychiatrist called the father's attorney again to make clear that he would be providing no substantive information. The attorney finally canceled the deposition. Three days later the psychiatrist received a copy of a motion to quash the subpoena. He heard nothing further until a session several weeks later with Rachel's mother when she told the psychiatrist that she and her husband had agreed on an independent psychiatrist to evaluate Rachel.

C. Case Example 3

The psychiatrist in this example gave Linda a flat promise that any information she gave him would not be shared with her mother, who had sole legal custody of Linda. Although the psychiatrist had not shared confidential information with the mother in the past, he had failed to explain to her that he was unwilling to provide full information about Linda. When Linda told him about her plans to run away, he was concerned about Linda's safety and future and wanted to alert the mother about this possibility and to discuss ways of defusing the tension between Linda and her mother about the boyfriend.

Assuming that the mother was legally entitled to this information, the psychiatrist discussed his possible disclosure with Linda at her next session. She was sufficiently agitated that he agreed to postpone any decision in this regard. After this session, he called his attorney who told him that there was a state statute authorizing consent to mental health treatment when the patient was 16 years old. The psychiatrist then considered whether informing the mother of Linda's plans was necessary because of the potential risk to Linda's safety. He decided that there was not a sufficient risk of serious injury to justify this disclosure.

In his next session with Linda, he discussed his decision, but informed her of the limits to confidentiality that would apply in the future. Linda discussed her feelings about the situation and after a number of sessions agreed that the psychiatrist could talk generally with her mother about the conflict regarding her boyfriend, but that he could not tell her mother of her plan to run away with him, as she had decided not to do so for the moment.

V. ACTION GUIDE

A. Checklist for providing nonemergency treatment requested by child/adolescent:

1. Determine if child/adolescent is authorized to consent by statute.
   a. Determine if prospective patient has reached age of majority.
   b. For patient who has not achieved majority, determine if any specialized consent statute applies to treatment in question.
2. If no statutory authority, explore possibility of parental/guardian consent with patient.
3. If parental consent cannot be obtained, determine if exception applies.
   a. Determine if child meets emancipation criteria.
   b. Determine if minor is "mature."
   c. If child urgently needs treatment, determine whether failure to consent may constitute abuse or neglect that should be reported to social welfare agency.

B. Checklist for providing emergency treatment to minors:

1. Determine severity of emergency, i.e., would delay in treatment significantly increase risk to patient's life? Would it endanger health of minor?
2. Determine if risks of delay meet requirements of applicable emergency exception.

C. Checklist for establishing confidentiality ground rules:

1. Determine what information should be disclosed to parents, based upon child's age, reasons for treatment, legal requirements.
2. Explain to parents necessity of confidentiality in treatment and what information will be shared, what information will be kept confidential (including information where minor controls consent to treatment).
3. Explain confidentiality ground rules to minor, making clear what will be shared with parents and the reasons for such potential disclosures.

D. Checklist for disclosing confidential information to minor's parents or parents with legal custody:

1. Responding to emergency situation:
   a. Document emergency, i.e., concerns about suicide, serious injury to patient or others.

    b. Discussion with minor patient:
       1) Attempt to obtain minor's consent.
       2) Explain need to report.
       3) Explore patient's reactions.
    c. Reveal minimum information to serve purposes of disclosure.
  2. Disclosures that serve other interests:
    a. Determine if minor controls consent to treatment.
    b. Determine if disclosures would be consistent with ground rules explained to minor at outset of treatment.
    c. If disclosure would be consistent with ground rules or no ground rules have been set:
       1) Discuss matter with minor patient;
         a) Encourage minor to make disclosure to parents.
         b) Request consent to make disclosure.
         c) If minor refuses (a) and (b), explain need for disclosure, remind patient of ground rules (or of fact that parents have legal right to information), and explore minor's feelings.
       2) Document discussions with minor.
       3) Disclose minimum information necessary to serve purposes of disclosure.
    d. If disclosure would not be consistent with ground rules:
       1) Discuss matter with minor patient:
         a) Encourage minor to make disclosure to parents.
         b) Request consent to make disclosure.
       2) If minor refuses 1) (a) and (b), limit information to general discussion or advice without disclosing anything specific about minor in question.
  3. Responding to specific requests for information from minor's parents:
    a. If disclosures would serve other important interests, respond as in D 2.
    b. For other disclosures, if disclosures would be consistent with ground rules or no ground rules have been set, respond as in D 2 b.
    c. For other disclosures, if disclosures would not be consistent with ground rules:
       1) Discuss parental request with minor.
       2) If minor wishes confidentiality to be maintained, remind parents of ground rules.

E. Checklist for disclosing confidential information to parent without legal custody of minor:

  1. Determine need for disclosure.
  2. Obtain consent from custodial parent, court, or guardian *ad litem*.
  3. Follow D above with regard to minor patient's interests.

F. Checklist for disclosures to third parties:

  1. Determine who has authority to consent.
  2. Obtain written consent from person with authority.
  3. If disclosure to benefit someone other than patient, if patient is adolescent, obtain consent of patient even when parent legally authorized to consent.

4. Limit disclosures to information necessary to serve interests in question.

G. Checklist for revealing information in judicial proceedings:

1. When request only (no subpoena):
   a. Request from party other than custodial parent:
      1) Refuse to make disclosure.
      2) Inform custodial parent.
   b. Request from custodial parent:
      1) Explain to parents potential harm to therapeutic relationship from testimony, suggesting alternative methods of obtaining same information.
2. When subpoenaed:
   a. Subpoena from third party for deposition:
      1) Determine who has right to exercise privilege in circumstances.
      2) Determine if appropriate consent is included or forthcoming.
      3) If no consent, inform issuing attorney that without consent or court order no patient information can be disclosed.
      4) If no consent but deposition not cancelled, attend, but limit disclosure as indicated.
      5) If consent, attempt to limit information to that necessary to serve relevant interests.
   b. Subpoena from third party for trial:
      1) Determine who has right to exercise privilege.
      2) Determine if there is consent from that person.
      3) If no consent, provide patient information at trial only after judge has considered and decided privilege issue.
   c. Subpoena from parents with legal custody:
      1) Contact parents, explaining potential harm to therapeutic relationship and suggesting alternative approaches.
      2) If parent persists, decide whether to comply with subpoena, move to quash or address judge about potential harm to treatment relationship and to request appointment of independent evaluator.
      3) If complying with subpoena, limit information disclosed to that necessary to extent possible.

VI. SUGGESTED READINGS

Gutheil, T. G. and Appelbaum, P. S. (1991), Clinical Handbook of Psychiatry and Law. Baltimore, MD: Williams & Wilkins.

Group for the Advancement of Psychiatry. (1990), A Casebook in Psychiatric Ethics (Report No. 129), New York, NY: Brunnel/Mazel.

Sheldon, M. and Sheldon, B. (1989), Confidentiality and the psychiatric treatment of children and adolescents. Rev Clin Psychiatry Law 1.

Committee on Confidentiality, American Psychiatric Association. (1987), Guidelines on confidentiality. Am J Psychiatry 144:1522–1526.

Gaylin, W., Macklin, R., ed. (1982), Who Speaks for the Child: The Problems of Proxy Consent. New York, NY: Plenum Press.

Dyer, A. R. (1988), Ethics and Psychiatry: Toward Professional Definition. Washington, D.C.: American Psychiatric Press, Inc.

6

Ethical Issues in Practice

ELISSA P. BENEDEK, M.D.

I. CASE EXAMPLES

A. Case Example 1

Susan, a 16-year-old adolescent, who has been in outpatient psychiatric treatment for a year and a half, comes into Dr. A's office distraught and visibly upset. Susan has been described as highly intellectual, calm, controlled, and without passion. She does not even bother to sit down in the doctor's office. She looks at Dr. A and says, "Dr. A, I think I might be pregnant, What should I do?"

B. Case Example 2

Johnny and his parents appear in the psychiatrist's office for a consultation. They are well-dressed, middle-class professionals. Mr. and Mrs. S are concerned about Johnny, their 14-year-old son. They describe him as "not listening" and "not obeying." They explain that Johnny listens to rock music all day, does not do his homework, and has been asking repeatedly for a driver's license. They believe they have a solution for Johnny's problem. Before the consultation they saw an ad on TV for New Waves Hospital, a private psychiatric facility located in their suburban environs which has a treatment program for "children who won't listen." They ask the doctor to arrange for Johnny's admission to the hospital.

C. Case Example 3

Dr. C listens to a radio talk show and hears long-time friend and colleague, Dr. R, responding to queries of a 16-year-old girl who complains of suicidal ideation, anorexia, sleeplessness, and pervading sadness. Dr. R suggests that this youngster take vitamins, exercise, and "call back if it doesn't work."

D. Case Example 4

Dr. S is confronted in the hallway by a hospital administrator who tells him that the psychiatric hospital is in financial jeopardy. Its beds are not being filled and "the doctors are going to have to do something or the hospital will not be able to keep the psychiatric ward open." The administrator tells the doctor, "You know you have a quota and if you fill it there is a bonus for you. If you don't fill it, you may not have a job next year."

II. INTRODUCTION

All of the clinical situations described above involve the potential for unethical behavior. A physician acts unethically when he or she *knowingly* and *intentionally* causes harm or acts in a way which increases the probability of causing harm toward another person or breaches his or her trusting relationship with his or her patient. There are many ways of acting unethically in clinical practice. Some unethical behaviors are clear: killing, causing pain, deprivation of freedom, deceiving, making a promise without justification. However, in daily practice, psychiatrists commonly carry out many of these actions toward patients. For example, they prescribe treatments which cause pain and many even cause risk of disability or death. They deprive patients of freedom by involuntarily committing the patient. Their treatments may disable patients. Psychiatrists are permitted these potentially unethical behaviors on two moral principles: (1) they do so with the patient's knowledge and consent, and (2) they do so to alleviate pain and suffering or to affect a cure of a patient's illness.

Making ethical judgments in a clinical situation is never easy, and frequently involves a complex series of decisions. Psychiatrists are bound by a series of ethical codes, and the forensic psychiatrist is bound by four ethical codes which are similar in some regard but dissimilar in others. These are the American Medical Association's Code of Medical Ethics, the American Psychiatric Association's Principle of Medical Ethics, the American Academy of Psychiatry and the Law's Ethical Guidelines, and the Principles of Practice of Child and Adolescent Psychiatry. During the practice of forensic psychiatry the clinician must be aware of all of these guidelines which are simply guidelines and not rules of behavior.

III. HISTORY OF MEDICAL ETHICS

These four sets of guidelines have their beginnings in prayers and incantations made long before the birth of Christ. These prayers sought inspiration and the granting of courage and determination from the deities or gods of a particular time and place in the care of the ill. The emphasis in these prayers was on honor, trust, and moral obligations. Most historians consider that medical ethics have their root in the Hippocratic Oath, which was probably written about 370 B.C. Moore (1978) suggests that the oath has two basis parts. The first is a sworn covenant for the physician to honor his teachers as a parent and to teach his teacher's son by the same covenant. The second part of the Hippocratic Oath is a series of rules (not guidelines) that are familiar to us today. Those rules include a discussion of such items as protecting patient confidentiality, avoiding sexual contact with patients, performing no surgery, and protecting the patient from harm. Although the Greek physicians of Hippocrates' time largely ignored the oath, except for the Pythagorean physicians who probably wrote it, this oath is the basis for contemporary concepts. Hebrew, Muslim, and Christian versions of the oath appeared. The major difference in these religious versions from the original Hippocratic Oath was the god or gods to whom one prayed. However, the Christian version did make a significant change to the sworn covenant. In the Christian version, the physician was obligated to teach whoever wished to learn medical practice, not only his teacher's sons.

In 1847, the fledgling American Medical Association adopted its first Code of Ethics. This Code highlighted the avoidance of cults, proper techniques of consultation, advertising, and advised physicians not to steal patients. This was a Code which emphasized etiquette and stemmed from the contemporary social situation in that in 1847 licensing of physicians had been discontinued, and quackery by mail-order physicians was rampant as was patient stealing. This Code was revised by the American Medical Association in 1903, 1912, 1947, 1957, and 1980.

In 1973, the American Psychiatric Association (APA) published the first edition of the Principles of Medical Ethics with annotations especially applicable to psychiatry. This Code is generally an elaboration of the American Medical Association Principles of Medical Ethics with Annotations. The Committee developing the Code was limited by the fact that the American Medical Association insisted that as physicians, psychiatrists were bound by the AMA Principles of Medical Ethics, and the APA could only add, not subtract, from those principles. The APA Committee was advised to look at real events rather than to focus on new or hypothetical cases. At that point in time, the APA simply annotated the AMA Code of Ethics. Subsequently, the Ethics Committee of the American Psychiatric Association received frequent requests for opinions with regard to handling ethical complaints and the ethicality of certain behavior and conduct. In 1973, the Ethics Committee began to provide answers to requests by members for consultation. Answers are provided by the chairperson of the Ethics Committee, who circulates the questions and possible answers to Committee members for their concurrence or for their different opinions. The Committee as a whole approves each opinion. They are then circulated to the Board of Trustees and received by the Board. The opinions are those of the APA Ethics Committee only. They do not represent official positions of the American Psychiatric Association. The Principles of Medical Ethics have been officially adopted by the American Psychiatric Association and are binding upon all members.

In 1980, the Council of the American Academy of Child Psychiatry adopted their current Code of Ethics. The Academy Code recognized that a Code of Ethics could not encompass all issues, that it was a dynamic entity, and that as such it was subject to growth, revision, and modification. The draft emphasized the fact that the principles were not laws but rather standards or guidelines and intended to guide the child and adolescent psychiatrist in the conduct of professional activities. The Code emphasized that the services of a child and adolescent psychiatrist were more often sought by a patient's parents or guardians than by children or adolescents themselves. They also recognized that agencies such as schools, community mental health agencies, and child protective services were more likely to use the services of the child psychiatrist than were individual children. With that recognition, they attempted to deal with some of the problems of dual or triple agency which will be discussed later in this chapter.

The Preamble to the Code also recognized the unique relationship between child and parent and the child's need for nuturing relationships and support of adults. Finally, the Code recognized that issues of consent and confidentiality in children needed to be viewed within the context of development and the overlapping of potentially conflicting rights of child or adolescent, parents, and society.

Subsequent to recognizing the unique nature of childhood and the child's relationship with parents and society, the Code articulated a series of 17 principles. These principles dealt with such issues as maximizing the development and potential of a child; the importance of parent and child participation in evaluation, treatment, and prevention; and recognizing the formal and legal responsibility for decision making in parents and the importance of participation by children. The Code also recognized that issues of confidentiality were different in children because of their relationship with parents and suggested that "regardless of the locus of the decision, the adolescent's psychiatrist will attempt to inform the child or adolescent of the need and intent to release information and will seek concurrence." It dealt with the special problems of children and balanced the benefits, risks, parental consent, and child assent to treatment. Finally, it dealt for the first time with issues of compensation and said quite clearly that the "professional opinions, judgments, and behaviors of child and adolescent psychiatrists shall not be influenced by the source of compensation." The Ethical Code of the Academy of Child Psychiatry is enforced using the same enforcement mechanism of the American Psychiatric Association, that is, a hearing by a district branch ethics committee, formal review of a decision by the APA Ethic's Committee, possible sanctions such as admonishment, reprimand, suspension, expulsion, and a right to appeal to the Ethic's Appeal Board. (These will be discussed in more depth.)

The American Academy of Psychiatry and the Law (AAPL) adopted ethical guidelines for the practice of forensic psychiatry in May of 1987 and revised those guidelines in October of 1989. The guidelines first defined forensic psychiatry as follows: "Forensic psychiatry is a subspecialty of psychiatry in which scientific and clinical expertise is applied to legal issues in legal context embracing civil, criminal, correctional, or legislative matters." The guidelines further specified that the forensic psychiatrist practices the subspecialty at the interface of two professions, each of which is concerned with human behavior and each of which has developed its own particular institutions, procedures, values, and vocabulary. As a consequence, the practice of forensic psychiatry entails inherent potentials for complications, conflicts, misunderstandings, and abuse. The guidelines elaborated on the

American Psychiatric Association's guidelines and dealt with issues of confidentiality, consent, objectivity, qualifications, and procedures with commentaries dictating the special problems in the forensic situation. With regard to enforcement, the American Academy of Psychiatry and the Law also does not adjudicate complaints of unethical conduct. These, too, are referred to the American Psychiatric Association. However, general questions with regard to ethical practice can be submitted to the Ethics Committee of the AAPL for consideration and review.

Finally, although psychiatrists clearly are not guided by legal ethics, it is important to at least be aware of the Canon of Ethics of attorneys. The sharpest contrast between the ethics of attorneys and that of mental health experts is the issue of objectivity. Attorneys are guided to work vigorously within the adversarial system representing *one* and only one side in a legal dispute to the best of their ability. On the other hand, forensic psychiatrists and psychologists are guided by their ethical principles to be objective, nonadversarial, and nonpartisan in presenting their clinical findings. Forensic mental health professionals often ask, "Do these people have any ethical standards and are there any constraints on the behaviors of attorneys?" However, attorneys are guided by ethical norms deriving from four basic sources: regulatory codes; professional standards; constitutional, evidentiary, and procedural laws; and personal values. Some of these are binding on the attorney, others merely advisory. Regulatory codes have been established in virtually every state. These codes are, for the most part, patterned after the ABA Model Code of Professional Responsibility adopted in 1969. These codes are significant in that they establish clear-cut boundaries for attorney behavior and if they are violated, the attorney is subject to disciplinary action. Sanctions for engaging in conduct proscribed by the code range from the most severe, disbarment, or the loss of one's license to practice law in a jurisdiction to relatively minor ones such as private admonition. In addition to enforceable rules of conduct, the ethical codes provide guiding principles for attorney behavior. While noncompliance with these principles will not ordinarily result in discipline, the guidelines do contribute to everyday legal ethics.

In addition to the regulatory codes, professional standards have been developed to guide the behavior of attorneys. The most significant of these, at least in the field of criminal justice, are the ABA Criminal Justice Standards developed in 1984. Particular chapters address the role of the prosecutor and the role of the defense attorney in criminal cases. There is a chapter dealing exclusively with issues of mental health consultation and the administration of criminal justice. The ABA standards also follow the two-part format of rules and guidelines. However, these are not enforceable.

Apart from ethical roles and professional standards, guidelines for attorney behavior can be found in the rules and procedures governing the trial of cases. These vary from state to state and in federal courts. There are rules of civil procedure which govern the conduct of civil trials and, for example, they may require attorneys to make good faith motions. Procedural rules are particularly important in defining the manner in which attorneys make use of experts. For example, if an attorney intends to call a mental health professional as an expert, she may be required by procedural rule to give notice of such intent well in advance of trial. In some states, after notice is given, procedural rules allow opposing counsel to have access to reports an expert may have prepared. Local rules of evidence define what an attorney *may ask* an expert to testify to (example, credibility). Finally, an attorney's personal moral values are always influential. For example, maybe the father charged with sexual abuse of his child articulates that it is a father's duty to teach a young child sexual behavior before he is sexually abused by a pedophile. The attorney's own sense of morality may compel her to withdraw from such a case, albeit there is a technical defense. She may feel that her own values will not allow proper representation of such a defendant.

IV. CLINICAL CONSIDERATIONS

A. Confidentiality

Confidentiality is essential and critical for psychiatric practice. Hippocrates addressed the issue of confidentiality: "Whatsoever things I see or hear concerning the life of man in any attendance on the sick or even apart therefrom which ought to not be voiced about I will keep silent thereon." The current status of confidentiality in the United States seems to be impaired because of third party payers, computer access, and patient access.

Psychiatrists and physicians are faced with balancing the welfare of their patients against the welfare of society—the public's right to know vs. the individual's right to privacy. Of all physicians, psychiatrists, as a part of their professional responsibility, come into possession of knowledge concerning a patient that may be embarrassing, destructive, or dangerous if revealed. Yet, this knowledge may shed light on a dangerous situation to other individuals or society. With regard to children in general, parents have the authority to make decisions and have access to information about their children. Children and adolescents should be informed about the limits of confidentiality both in the evaluation setting and in the therapeutic situation. It is critical that children understand that information they share with the therapist may be shared with parents or other third parties, particularly information about suicidality and homicidality and dangerous behavior. It is often advisable to suggest to the child that such information can be shared with the parent, in the presence of the child, if the child wishes with the exception of emergency situations. As teenagers approach maturity, the situation becomes more complicated and more difficult. Adolescents, too, should be informed about the necessity and limitations of confidentiality. In general, however, adolescent patients in treatment may have more confidentiality privileges as an adult except when there is risk to life of the adolescent or dangerousness to self or others. Confidentiality issues with an adolescent must be treated with care and sensitivity if there is to be a successful known outcome of treatment or if the treatment is to continue; a breach of confidentiality may end a treatment relationship.

It is rare for children or adolescents to ask for information from their records vis-à-vis the Freedom of Information Act. However, this does on occasion happen, and the psychiatrist is obligated to share such information with the patient. One acceptable way of doing this is sharing information from the chart with the patient in the patient's presence but not giving the child or adolescent the complete mental health records which clearly can be subject to misinterpretation. In addition, a chart may contain confidential material about a parent. If the psychiatrist evaluates the child or adolescent at the request of a third party such as a court or a child care agency, the psychiatrist again must inform the child or adolescent about the limits of confidentiality and the fact that information will be released to those requesting the information.

Maintaining confidentiality in multi-disciplinary settings and in training institutions poses special problems. Everyone, clerks, secretaries, aides, attendants, and trainees, should be informed of their professional responsibilities vis-à-vis confidentiality and the risks of discussing clinical material on elevators, in bathrooms, or at cocktail parties. A particularly vulnerable area is the use of audio-visual recordings of patients made in training institutions. Patient authorization and parental authorization for these should be obtained, and patients should be told they can rescind such authorization if they choose to do so. However, it is more advisable to use actors or actresses rather than real patients. It is particularly difficult to disguise information vis-à-vis a child as age and gender assume particular importance in the developing child.

With regards to AIDS, the APA has developed and disseminated a guideline on AIDS policy, confidentiality, and disclosure.

In summary, if a patient known to be infected with HIV refuses to agree to change his or her risky sexual behavior, or to notify the person or persons at risk and if the physician has good reason to believe that the patient has failed to or is unable to comply with this contract agreement, "it is ethically permissible for the physician to notify an *identifiable* person whom a physician believes to be in danger of contracting the virus." This policy may be in conflict with particular state laws or the AMA policy which focuses more on public health issues and encourages wider notification.

The forensic Code of Ethics, too, discusses issues of confidentiality and advises the psychiatrist to inform the client that he is not the evaluee's doctor. The Code advises the psychiatrist to indicate for whom he is conducting the evaluation and what he will do with the information obtained as a result of the examination. The Code also reminds the psychiatrist that although warning has been given, the client may believe he is being treated because of the intimacy of the clinical interview situation. This Code also suggests that the psychiatrist should clarify in initial screening conversation with a retaining attorney and prior to a formal agreement whether she will consider consultation with the opposing attorney if the psychiatrist decides not to accept the consultation. Practically, however, if a psychiatrist has been given information by an attorney representing a defendant or a plaintiff in a case, it is sensible, if not ethically prohibited, to decline participation in the case on an opposing side even if the psychiatrist decides not to accept the first consultation.

The Academy guidelines, too, deal with issues of confidentiality and address the need and right of parents to be informed. It also emphasizes the need to respect the confidences of parents and guardians with regard to the child.

All of the Codes/guidelines suggest when a clinical problem is particularly difficult it is imperative to seek consultation either from a colleague, from an institutional body (ethics board), or from an Ethics Committee of a professional organization describing the specific situation clearly and articulating the clinical ethical question.

B. Informed consent

1. SEXUAL ABUSE

All 51 jurisdictions in the United States require physicians to report suspected child abuse and sexual abuse. In most jurisdictions, reporting requirements override both confidentiality and privilege associated with the physician/patient relationship. Clinicians have argued that the child abuse reporting statues lead to both underreporting and overreporting of abuse and that reporting, while demonstrably beneficial to truly abused children, may lead to additional problems by condoning premature removal of a child or parent from the home and by interfering with the ability of abusing parents to deal with their family's problems and reintegrate their families. However, mandatory reporting exists in all the states. Physicians who do not report may be subject to criminal penalties, fines, and even imprisonment. However, only a few states mandate reporting of sexual involvement between psychiatrist and patient. The APA Principles of Medical Ethics with Annotations especially applicable to psychiatry are quite clear in specifying that sexual relations between psychiatrists and their patients are always unethical. No one knows for certain how common sexual exploitation of patient by therapist is, but studies suggest that five to seven percent of male psychiatrists are sexually involved in an erotic relationship and sexual exploitations with a patient. It would appear that sexual exploitation of child patients is less prevalent than that of adult females. However, cases involving male therapists and adolescent females, and homosexual exploitation have come to the attention of Ethics Committees. Generally, the exploitation begins with a confusion of boundaries leading to touching, fondling, and then frank sexual behavior. All studies dealing with this issue have recognized that sexual exploitation is ultimately harmful to the patient, leading to a lack of trust in any subsequent therapeutic relationship, an exacerbation of the initial clinical problems, and additional clinical problems such as substance abuse, depression, and even attempted suicide. There is no single profile of offending physician nor of exploited patient, and all patients seem to be at risk because of the nature of the therapeutic relationship, the intimacies involved in sharing confidential information, the power differential, and the trust that the patient places in the physician with the belief that the physician will "do no harm." Sanctions for this form of behavior generally are quite severe and include suspension and expulsion from professional societies. Civil and criminal sanctions also occur and, if convicted by a licensure board, a physician may permanently lose his license. This form of behavior is explicitly prohibited by the APA Code and implicitly prohibited by the Academy Code. The Academy Code in principle articulates the principle that the physician should avoid utilizing his or her unique relationship with the child . . . principally for his or her own gain or aggrandizement.

Although the Code of the American Academy of Psychiatry and Law does not deal with sexual abuse of patients per se, it does discuss issues of informed consent, honesty, and objectivity and, by inference, these principles can be used to sanction an offending psychiatrist.

2. CONSENT/ASSENT

Consent is one of the core values of the ethical practice of medicine and psychiatry. It reflects respect for the person. In particular forensic situations such as court-ordered evaluations, competency, involuntary commitment or custody, consent is not required. However, the psychiatrist is obligated to inform the client that an evaluation is legally mandated and that if the client refuses to participate in the evaluation, this fact would be included in any report, deposition, or testimony. With regard to consent in children, it is important to attempt to obtain the assent of the child for the evaluation. However, Principle Six of the Academy Code states that "a minor unemancipated child or adolescent may participate in evaluation, treatment, or prevention efforts without his or her full concurrence." The formal responsibility for decisions regarding such participation usually resides with the parents or legal guardians. While important in the clinical context, the agreement of the child or adolescent is not required. However, the child/adolescent psychiatrist should seek to develop with the child or adolescent being served as thorough an understanding of the professional judgments, opinions, and actions as is possible. This means that the nature of the proposed evaluation and its use should be discussed even with the very young child. An attempt should be made to ascertain that the child understands the purposes, risks, and benefits of the evaluation. The child may not fully grasp all the implications of the evaluation, much as the mentally ill patient may not grasp and appreciate all the implications of a proposed treatment. However, the clinician must attempt to inform and obtain assent.

C. Child custody

Psychiatrists are at great risk when conducting child custody evaluations if they do not know and understand ethical guidelines. A few clinical examples will serve. Occasionally the naive child psychiatrist may believe that a proper custody evaluation can be conducted simply by reviewing records and not necessarily interviewing parent or children. Such a record review can offer only limited information and may be difficult to justify ethically.

An additional concern exists as to whether one should conduct a child custody evaluation without having access to both parents. Unilateral evaluations are of limited value as one cannot make a comparison of parents and recommendation as to custody without having seen both parents. On the other hand, one can talk about a particular parent's parenting ability. Frequently, evaluators get trapped into assuming the position of both evaluator and treating physician in custody situations. It is difficult, if not impossible, to be objective when one is treating a parent and making recommendations about parental custody. In addition, parents in treatment may make disclosure which they would not have made had they known that custody was going to be an issue. Here, too, children must be informed that what they feel with regard to which parent they would prefer will be included in a report to the court, deposition, or testimony and may be seen by their parents as well as by the judge.

D. Termination of parental rights and adoption

In termination of parental rights situations, once again it is difficult if not impossible for the treating psychiatrist to serve as a forensic evaluator. Here, too, a parent may share information in therapy with regard to wishes and fantasies which will clearly be detrimental to their case if elaborated in legal proceedings. However, even more difficult is weighing the competing interests of a parent's mental health and a child's mental health. Termination clearly may affect a parent's mental health and may cause a parent on the verge of a depression to succumb to a serious illness. On the other hand, guiding principles of the Academy's ethical principles are that the child's best interests are always predominant. Ethical dilemmas also arise when clinicians deal with overburdened child protective agencies that do not seem to have time to actively pursue termination of parental rights when it seems to the clinician that it is in the best interest of the child.

E. Mental health and economics

There is a growing concern that economic changes in health care delivery may be exerting a negative impact on ethical psychiatric practice in that there is a new kind of intrusion of economics into the heart of psychiatry and the doctor/patient relationship. New reimbursement mechanisms seem to encourage violations of confidentiality. In addition, they also seem to encourage inadequate treatment of the patient (particularly managed care). New forms of revenue generation are emerging that pose potential conflicts of interest situations between doctors and patients. For example, physicians are offered financial incentives to admit to a given hospital or prepayment plans to select the least expensive (and perhaps least efficacious) form of treatment. Other issues center around physician's ownership of labs, facilities, and equipment. Questions arise as to whether owning expensive diagnostic equipment such as MRIs or a share in a hospital facility motivate a psychiatrist to overuse these diagnostic tools.

The for-profit sector has been accused of promoting ethical violations by physicians including skimming of well-insured patients and sending patients with no or little insurance to inadequate care facilities. Psychiatrists involved in these hospitals have also been condemned by colleagues. Excessive charges of patients or charging patients for services not rendered, or charging parents for services rendered to children when payment for dependents is not included in insurance plan, denial of access to care of indigent patients, and undue concern about profits are all possible violations. Finally, there is great concern about ethical problems in a period of diminishing resources for health care. When resources are not available for proper care, is improper care prescribed? This is particularly critical in the situation of the potentially suicidal patient who might be discharged prematurely. There are several consequences to the scarcity of resources. One is the problem of abandonment. Once a patient is the medical responsibility of a physician, he simply cannot be discharged when financial resources are depleted. It is difficult to find appropriate referral sources for chronically mentally ill patients who are indigent. The scarcity of resources may be producing a generation of demoralized professionals who feel defeated by a system and overwhelmed by fiscal constraints.

F. Education

Education with regard to ethics must begin at the time a student enters medical school. Pressures are rising for enhanced ethical knowledge in trainees. Some educators suggest that medical school admissions committees provide information about ethical duties in application forms. During preadmission interviews committees ask for explicit information about the tradition of medicine and the physician's ethical duties to society and patient. The rising epidemic of AIDS has brought to the forefront concern about the obligation to treat all patients, but recent scandals with ethical substrate such as fraudulent research, drinking alcohol on duty, drug abuse, and sexual activity with patients have made it eminently clear that students do not always learn about their ethical duties as they advance along the educational ladder to become physicians. Thus, many critics have suggested that ethical principles and codes should be explicitly slated to students before their admission to medical schools and they should be offered an opportunity to decide that they do not want to go into the profession of medicine if they cannot adhere to the code. In particular, the AIDS epidemic has created controversy over physician's ethical duty to treat patients when such care may pose health risks to them, their spouses, and their future children. However, even if students are not advised as to the AMA Ethical Code, it is clear that teaching in medical school and graduate medical education must include such Codes and clinical examples must explicate and elaborate on them. In addition, critics suggest that clinical ethics should be taught regularly at the bedside of patients. Clinical ethics should leave the calm environment of ethical discourse in the classroom for the urgency, uncertainties, and emotional environment of the bedside or a "patient" should not simply be an illustration of a principle but should be a discussion about a real person, and discussion should focus not simply on opinions about what ought to be done, but should include a commitment to do what ought to be done for a particular patient. Critics suggest that even if a physician uses a professional ethicist as a consultant, the physician must accept the responsibility of final decision-making and moral accountability.

G. Enforcement

Currently, ethical complaints against colleagues are investigated by District Branch Ethics Committees of the American Psychiatric Association after some preliminary screening or investigation of an ethical complaint by an ethics committee member. The complainant and defendant are invited to a hearing by the District Branch Ethics Committee. The purpose of the hearing is to give the defendant a full opportunity to respond to the specific charges of unethical conduct leveled by a complainant. The requirements of the hearing are spelled out and include fair notice to an accused member as to what he or she is alleged to have done. This requirement is usually satisfied by furnishing the member with a copy of a written complaint that sets forth the particular facts or circumstances underlying the charge of unethical conduct and the section of the Principle of Medical Ethics with Annotations that is violated. The member is allowed an opportunity to respond to the complaint in a live hearing. In theory, the member could make the presentation in a written form, but a meeting allows the accused member to provide more complete information and a more effective defense and the committee to elicit more information.

The complainant, too, may testify and may be subject to cross-examination. Such cross-examination may be done by a member of the Ethics Committee or an attorney and may be done by questioning the complainant or submitting written questions to him or her. Care must be taken to protect fragile patients in these difficult proceedings. It is critical to keep complete records of ethics proceedings; ideally a tape recording should be made of hearings. Subsequent to a determination by a District Branch and a recommended sanction, the matter is referred to the APA Committee on Ethics where the sanction may either be upheld or the matter referred back to the District Branch for further hearing and further and added testimony. If a member disagrees with either the proceedings or sanction, he or she may appeal to the Ethics Appeals Board of the American Psychiatric Association and may request a full hearing. Special rules guide the conduct and timeliness of that hearing.

It is important to note that a physician may be incompetent as a result of a physical, mental, or vocational disability, inadequate training, or practicing outside of his area of expertise. Incompetence does not necessarily mean unethical behavior, and an isolated mistake does not count as incompetence. A physician may also be impaired. A physician is impaired if he or she has a mental or neurological disorder which interferes on a significant number of occasions with ability to practice. A physician may also be impaired because of a physical disorder, for example, a blind surgeon. Incompetence, impairment, and unethical behavior are closely related concepts. An impaired physician is generally always incompetent or partially incompetent to carry out professional tasks. That is part of the meaning of impairment. Physicians can have mental or physical disorders which do not interfere with their ability to practice, but then we do not regard them as impaired. Physicians who are incompetent are usually impaired, but they may not be. For example, a psychiatrist may not be able to carry out a particular function which would not be expected of someone at his level of training, but he may attempt to do so. He is incompetent but not impaired. It is not necessarily unethical to be incompetent. For an action to be unethical, the psychiatrist must have known (or should have known) that this action was harmful or potentially harmful. If a psychiatrist were no longer competent to carry out some professional duties, he might be unaware of his lack of ability (a psychiatrist with a brain tumor or dementia). If he were ignorant about his disability, he would not be unethical. However, once a psychiatrist has been told about his disability, and if he is able to understand and remember what he has been told, if he continues to practice in the area of his disability, he is acting unethically.

V. CASE EXAMPLE EPILOGUES

A. Case Example 1

Prior to treatment, Susan has been informed that if she reveals material that might be dangerous to herself or dangerous to others, such material would be revealed to her parents or significant others with or without her permission. Susan, however, has said that she thinks she might be pregnant. It would be important first to explore realistic basis to Susan's concerns. Is she in fact pregnant? Has she consulted with an obstetrician? Secondly, it would be important to discover what Susan planned to do. Susan is 16, and if plans do not include dangerous behavior, the issues of confidentiality with regard to her treatment remain the same as those with regard to treating an adult. However, if Susan indicates that she is about to obtain a "back street abortion," or to marry her drug-dealing boyfriend, those behaviors might be dangerous. Thus, Susan was offered a choice. That is, the psychiatrist could share the information with Susan's parents with her parents and Susan together in the room, or separately.

B. Case Example 2

The physician is being asked to arrange for hospitalization which may be inappropriate prior to even evaluating the adolescent on an outpatient basis. Before any form of treatment a proper and complete evaluation is critical.

C. Case Example 3

The psychiatrist needs to decide whether Dr. R is impaired or unethical. Such a decision under the best of circumstances is difficult. In this situation, Dr. C decided to contact Dr. R, have lunch with her, and talk with Dr. R about her behavior before proceeding any further.

D. Case Example 4

It is clearly unethical to not place the needs of the patient first and paramount. Filling a hospital bed rather than providing for patient's needs is clearly unethical.

VI. ACTION GUIDELINES

A. Know the principles, guidelines, and ethical codes of your profession.
B. Be familiar with the opinions of ethics committees with regard to specific ethical problems.
C. Consult with colleagues when you are concerned about ethical standards and behavior.
D. Keep current with regard to changes in professional ethical guidelines.

VII. PITFALLS

A. *In accepting cases:* clinicians must be careful about their own biases in accepting forensic cases. These influence a clinician's objectivity and make it impossible to perform a reasonable forensic evaluation.
B. *In the evaluation:* issues of confidentiality and informed consent must always be discussed with children, their parents, and attorneys before beginning an evaluation, and it is imperative that the clinician evaluate whether the discussion results in appreciation of the information.
C. *In testimony:* the clinical evaluation and the application of data and testimony about it must be performed in a spirit of honesty and in striving for objectivity. The adversarial system places great strain to be biased and to distort opinions on the psychiatrist. The ethical forensic psychiatrist must strive to be objective.

VIII. SUGGESTED READINGS

American Academy of Child Psychiatry (1982), Principles of Practice of Child and Adolescent Psychiatry. Washington, D.C.: AACP.

American Academy of Psychiatry and Law (1984), Ethical Guidelines for the Practice of Forensic Psychiatry. Revised edition. Washington, D.C.: AAPL.

American Medical Association (1990), Current Opinions—the Council on Ethical and Judicial Affairs. Chicago, IL: American Medical Association.

American Psychiatric Association (1984), The Principles of Medical Ethics with Annotations Especially Applicable to Psychiatry. Washington, D.C.: American Psychiatric Association.

Bloor, R. D. and Weinstock, R. D. (1989), Conflict of interest between therapist/patient confidentiality and the duty to report sexual abuse of children. Behav Sci Law 5(2) 161–174.

Bouhoutsos, J., Holroyd, J., Lerman, H., et al. (1983), Sexual intimacy between psychotherapists and patients. Prof. Psychol: Res Pract 124(2) 185–196.

Fitch, W. P. L. P., Petrella, R. C., and Wallas, J. (1989), Legal ethics and the use of mental health professionals in criminal cases. Behav Sci Law 5(2) 105–117.

Gabbard, G. (1989), Sexual Exploitation and Professional Relationships. Washington, D.C.: American Psychiatric Press.

Gabbard, G. and Pope, K. (1988), Sexual intimacies after termination: clinical, ethical and legal aspects. Ind Pract, May 21–26.

Koocher, G. and Keith-Spiegel, P. (1990), Children, Ethics and the Law. Lincoln: University of Nebraska Press.

Rosner, R. and Weinstock, R. (eds.) (1990), Ethical Practice in Psychiatry and the Law. New York: Plenum Press.

Stone, A. The ethics of forensic psychiatry: A view from the ivory tower (1984), in: Stone, A.: Law, Psychiatry, and Morality. Washington, D.C.: American Psychiatric Press.

Weinstock, R. (1989), Perception of ethical problems by forensic psychiatrists. Bull Acad Psychiatry Law 17(2) 189–202.

SECTION TWO

CLINICAL ASSESSMENT

7

Child Custody Evaluations

STEPHEN P. HERMAN, M.D.

I. CASE EXAMPLES

A. Case Example 1

A court-appointed child psychiatrist was asked to evaluate the Slater family and to offer an opinion about custody of the 10-year-old son, Chad. At the start of the evaluation, Mrs. Slater's attorney informed the psychiatrist that Mr. Slater was "a chronically suicidal depressive" and on medication. Mrs. Slater told the psychiatrist that her husband had been hospitalized for depression and was in no condition to parent his son. She described with much detail her husband's depression of the year before, when he was unable to get out of bed for over 2 weeks. Mr. Slater confirmed that he had had two severe depressions in his life and had a family history of depression. He said that he had never made a suicide attempt and was routinely under a psychiatrist's care. He described his relationship with Chad as an excellent one and complained that his wife had had several affairs over the years and had not hidden them from her son.

In the joint interview with Chad and his father, the psychiatrist observed that they had a warm and comfortable relationship. They obviously were used to being together and enjoyed conversing and playing games. In the session alone with the psychiatrist, Chad told the doctor, "I know you said that you weren't going to ask me who I want to live with, but I want to tell you anyway. I really want to stay with my father. I'm not worried about him, and I know we'll be okay. My mother is angry all the time; I just don't want to live with her."

B. Case Example 2

In a custody case involving twin 7-year-old girls, their father contended that because of his wife's involvement in a religious cult, the children were being raised with a warped sense of values and would have difficulty relating to people outside the cult. He maintained an extensive, computerized file system documenting the way his wife was inadequately parenting his daughters. He told the psychiatrist about inappropriate medical care, poor nutrition, strange cult practices, and unusual ideas his wife had about education. "These children will never escape this cult," he told the expert, "unless I get custody."

C. Case Example 3

Two parents, both professionals, were disputing custody of their 8-year-old daughter and 6-year-old son. During the evaluation, each of the Dickinsons claimed that the other was not home enough. Frank Dickinson said that his wife's frequent business trips took her "out of the house more than she's in it." Alice Dickinson said that Frank's long hours at the office made him a stranger to his children. Yet, each admitted that the other loved the children very much and made special efforts to be with them as often as possible. Both parents had been involved with their children's schools, religious education, and afterschool activities. They knew their children's friends and their friend's parents. Mr. Dickinson had said at the start of the evaluation that he desired sole custody of the children; Alice thought that joint custody was workable for them.

The children told the court-appointed expert that they were very sad that the family was breaking up. They wanted to be able to live with each of their parents and to see them both regularly.

II. LEGAL ISSUES

A. Child custody

1. EVOLUTION OF JUDICIAL PRESUMPTIONS

Child custody disputes have always reflected societal views of the family and the specialized roles of mothers and fathers. In ancient Rome, children were considered property of their fathers. This absolute right of fathers carried over well into the eighteenth century in England and slowly began to change there and in the United States in the 1800s. Gradually, the state began to become more involved with families as the concept of parens patriae took hold. This theory held that government had the right to protect those of its citizens (especially children) not able to do so themselves. As social scientists began to observe that children were not simply small adults but developmentally unique, courts became more child-centered in their involvement with families.

The study of child development and psychoanalysis led to the legal presumption (a system of beliefs informing judicial opinion) of the tender years. This held that young children (from birth until about age 7 years) naturally belonged with their mother. Most custody disputes ended up this way, except in extraordinary circumstances. Sometimes, however, after the tender years were passed, courts reversed custody in favor of the father. In the second half of the twentieth century, as no-fault divorces became more common in this country, courts examined more closely the needs of the children involved in custody disputes and were less likely to concentrate on parental culpability. Thus, the tender years presumption gave way to the concept of the best interests of the child. Now courts began to examine custody disputes on a more individualized basis in order to determine the needs of each child. This is currently the guiding principle in resolving custody disputes, although for many judges, the tender years presumption dies slowly.

2. TYPES OF CUSTODY ARRANGEMENTS

Custody disputes arise when divorcing parents are not able to agree on a residential and parenting arrangement for their children, or when one parent uses the issue as a wedge against an unfavorable divorce outcome. Regardless of parental motivation, the possibilities for custody are sole custody or joint custody. In sole custody, one parent has the legal authorization to make all major decisions regarding the growth and development of the child. The noncustodial parent's rights are not terminated, but the decision-making powers are.

In a joint custody arrangement, the precise definition depends upon what the parties work out. It does not automatically mean that a child lives with each parent half of the time. It **does** mean, however, that both parents have the legal right and responsibility to share in their child's growth and development. Joint custody, heralded by some as a panacea for the ills of custody disputes, can be successful in certain circumstances if both parents are able to set aside their anger and frustration with each other, tolerate each other's different parenting style, and communicate frequently and comfortably with each other. However, such a post-divorce situation is unusual for parents and would probably not be possible for many. What seems to be most important psychologically for children of divorce is the ongoing relationship between the parents and between parents and children, rather than the legal custody arrangement.

3. VISITATION

Custody disputes often include determinations about visitation. Sometimes, in fact, the expert witness is evaluating a visitation dispute, rather than an argument over custody. Disorders of visitation arise when parents disagree about implementing a court-ordered visitation arrangement; when parents accuse each other of sabotaging a visitation schedule; when parents are unable to formulate a workable visitation arrangement; or when one parent maintains that the child is reluctant to visit the other parent. It has been argued that the sole custodial parent should control visitation arrangements in the interests of reducing the child's anxiety and avoiding further court interference in this family issue. However, courts **do** become involved in visitation disputes which are part of or separate from a custody dispute.

4. MEDIATION

Like joint custody, mediation has been heralded by some as an important alternative to the adversarial system. As most of the states adopted "no-fault" divorce laws by the 1980s, mediation's popularity grew. In several states, including California, Maine, and New Mexico, mediation is mandated by the court before custody litigation can begin. Maryland courts have also adopted this process except in cases in which a good-faith allegation of sexual or physical abuse has been made. Mediation programs may differ throughout the country in the professional backgrounds of the mediator(s), the number of sessions, the inclusion or exclusion of children from the process, and the presence or absence of lawyers. Thus, there is no single, clear-cut definition of mediation when applied to custody disputes.

Proponents cite the advantages of mediation: parents avoid litigation and the necessity for a court to direct their behavior; the process is more personalized, with more attention directed to the unique characteristics of the parents; parents take an active process in deciding their family's fate; and there is a greater likelihood of compliance afterward. Critics of mediation argue: there is too wide a variety of backgrounds and skills in mediators; there are no standards for what constitutes adequate mediation in custody disputes; failed mediation can lead to even more acrimony once the parties enter the judicial system; and mediation may lead to an imbalance of power which could favor men, who seem to mediate differently from women.

Mediation may work if couples are motivated to be child-centered in their custody negotiations and both parents are able to trust and work with the mediator or co-mediators. During or following the custody evaluation performed by the court-appointed expert, the process may evolve into mediation or may lead to the parents entering mediation with someone else. In this way the custody evaluation may serve a therapeutic purpose and may help the parents concentrate their energies toward a settlement and away from further litigation.

5. SPECIAL ISSUES

The child custody evaluation is often complicated by special issues presenting additional challenges to the expert witness. Many of these issues reflect current social dilemmas and raise ethical as well as clinical questions. These include: homosexual parenting and the impact of AIDS, grandparents' and stepparents' rights, mentally ill parents, parental kidnapping, allegations of sexual and physical abuse, and controversies in reproductive biology, such as surrogate parenting, oocyte donation, artificial insemination, and in vitro fertilization. The evaluating mental health professional faces the dual responsibilities of performing a competent and fair clinical evaluation and communicating to the court how the special issue affects the particular family.

For example, the expert evaluating a custody dispute in which one parent is homosexual will need to review the literature on children of homosexuals in order to best advise the court. The expert should know about the impact upon the child of parental kidnapping, if that has occurred. The expert should be aware of the legal and clinical ramifications of grandparents and stepparents seeking visitation rights or custody. In areas on the very frontier of reproductive biology, mental health professionals and legal experts alike will struggle and agonize over profoundly complex questions.

The evaluating clinician considers the special issue in terms of how it impacts upon the child and the parent-child relationship. The question then becomes not that a parent has a history of psychiatric illness, but, rather, what is the impact of the illness upon this particular child and the relationship with the child? In this way, the expert can put an issue in proper perspective and defuse what might otherwise be a false issue serving one side's legal strategy.

B. Role of the expert witness

Because custody disputes are complicated processes, the court-appointed mental health expert has an important role to play. Studies bear out that judges **are** influenced in their decisions by clinical evaluations, and many jurists rely on the expertise of psychiatrists and psychologists when deciding custody and visitation cases. Through the written report and testimony, the mental health professional provides important information to the judge. The expert witness may also assist the families by helping to make the clinical evaluation therapeutic. In the role of the child's advocate, the expert may be the first professional who is able to get the disputing parents on a more child-centered track. Sometimes, the child custody evaluation evolves into mediation or even arbitration, when both parents have come to trust the clinician and are motivated to reach an agreement themselves.

III. THE CLINICAL EVALUATION AND WRITTEN REPORT

A. Becoming involved

Therapists desiring to perform child custody evaluations may want to notify local courts (judges and family services clinics), attorneys, mental health colleagues, and agencies that they are willing to provide this service. Neophytes should make contact with an experienced colleague who can act as a mentor. Newcomers to this work should also read about their state's legislative and judicial history of handling child custody and visitation disputes. In some locales, it may be appropriate to contact judges directly; in others, there may be active family services clinics attached to courts or a chief clerk of the court that will assign such cases.

The initial call may come from the judge's law assistant, from an attorney for one side, or from a parent. The expert should know precisely what questions the judge is asking and whether, in fact, they can be properly answered. Sometimes, judges have unrealistic expectations of what a psychiatrist can do. The expert should inform lawyers and parents alike that he or she will perform a custody evaluation **only** if both sides agree that the expert will do an impartial, objective evaluation. Experts should avoid doing custody and/or visitation evaluations for just one side, seeing only part of the family. Judges (and lawyers alike) view such experts as "hired guns," whose credibility and objectivity become suspect. Mental health professionals should strive to avoid doing one-sided and incomplete evaluations. Occasionally, this rule may have to be modified if, for example, one party fails to cooperate or cannot be located. This situation should be clearly explained within the report.

Prior to the evaluation, the expert should explain the fee and request full payment. Some clinicians estimate the number of hours needed and charge by the hour; others have a flat rate. Up-front payment removes the fee as an issue during the evaluation and allows the expert to concentrate on the work. "Pay-as-you-go" arrangements are to be discouraged. They increase bookkeeping; payments may be skipped; and even a partial evaluation—halted by the expert because of non-payment—may result in the clinician having to testify anyway. Hourly rates range from $150 to $250 or more. Flat rates for custody evaluations (excluding court time) can be several thousand dollars. Some experts charge for their time reading court documents and speaking on the telephone; others include this in their fee. Payment is usually shared by both sides or the judge will order a payment plan based on each parent's financial situation.

B. Interviewing parents

The expert should offer both parents the opportunity to meet together with him or her for the first session. Sometimes, one or both parents decline this suggestion, saying that such a meeting would be too painful. The clinician should make it clear that refusing this initial meeting in no way prejudices that parent in the eyes of the clinician. But if such an opportunity is taken by both parents, the clinician has the chance to observe their interaction and to explore in a preliminary way whether or not there is any chance of a nonlitigated settlement. At the very least, the clinician can use the session to explain how the evaluation will be conducted and can assess the current level of animosity or cooperation between the parents.

Prior to the start of the session, the clinician should explain to parents that because of the forensic nature of this evaluation, they must waive the privilege of doctor-patient confidentiality. The expert should either have parents sign such a waiver or document in the chart that such an explanation has been given.

Each parent should be seen several times alone in sessions of 45 to 60 minutes. In the first session, the expert gives the parent a chance to speak about the background of the case, the marital problems, and desires regarding the arrangements for the children. In subsequent sessions, the clinician asks about the history of the parent-child relationship and seeks to know how well the parent knows the child, what the child's special needs might be, and what the parent's plans are for the child. One can expect that many parents will use these sessions to severely criticize the other parent and to "prove" to the expert that only he or she is the fit parent. The expert should allow this to a point, noting what each parent chooses to criticize in the other, but should also limit these critiques in order to cover other subjects.

The forensic psychiatrist is not a detective or a human polygraph. He or she is not the trier of fact. The object of these sessions with the parents is to get a sense of the parents and their relationship with the child—not to figure out who is telling the truth and who is lying. Parents in such a situation will try repeatedly to convince the clinician of one thing or another and will bring in "proof" to support their case. The clinician should remind parents what his or her function is. Sometimes, a parent will bring in a videotape or audiotape of a telephone conversation and ask that the expert watch or listen. In general, it is wise to decline such a request, unless both parents agree and request that the expert do so. Watching a video or listening to a recording (often made surreptitiously by one side) puts the psychiatrist in a difficult and uncomfortable position and threatens the impartiality of the evaluation.

The evaluation of the parents should include inquiring about their own family backgrounds and educational, social, and work histories.

The evaluation is **not** a formal psychiatric examination. The object is not to arrive at a psychiatric diagnosis but rather to assess parenting ability, the parent-child relationship, and the best interests of the child.

C. Interviewing children

Prior to the interview with the child, one or both parents may try to involve the expert in a controversy over which parent brings the child to the session. If just two sessions with a child are held, each of them can take a turn at bringing the child. Otherwise, they may ask the clinician to become involved in this aspect of the dispute. The expert should refrain and can suggest that the parents not struggle over this question. The parents may feel that the child will be influenced by whomever brings him to the session. The therapist should point out that in most cases the child already **is** influenced by the parents and that this will be factored in during the evaluation. Parents may also ask the therapist for advice about what to tell the child prior to the interview. The expert can turn the question around and ask the parent, "Well, what do you think you should say to Annie?" The parent's response may give additional information about how he or she relates to the child and appreciates the child's developmental abilities. Parents should be honest with the child about the purpose of the evaluation. Even a 3-year-old knows that parents are fighting about where he or she will live.

Although the parents should be seen for at least one session at the start of the custody evaluation, the child or children should be seen as early into the process as possible. Although custody disputes are supposed to be about chidren, the clinician may find himself caught up in the struggle between the parents and delayed in actually meeting the child. Children as young as 2½ or 3 years can be seen alone, assuming that they are able to separate from the parent. The therapist conducts the interview with the child as he would any evaluative session. He tries to develop a comfortable, anxiety-free relationship early on, through drawing, building blocks or other building toys, by playing a board game, an electronic game, and by talking. The expert is interested in how the child perceives the family conflict and what he thinks will or will not happen. The expert can explain to a child of 4, in many cases, what a judge is and how the doctor is meeting with the family to help the judge figure out where they are all going to live.

It is not necessary to ask a child his or her parental preference. Such a question puts added pressure on a child already dealing with enough. A child who volunteers such information, however, may do so because of having been prompted by a parent or because he or she has conviction about the preference. Either of these possibilities is more important for the evaluator than asking the child directly. The child's preference, when volunteered, should be noted and considered as part of the data collected. More weight may be given to preferences expressed by pre-teens than those of 4- or 5-year-olds. The expert will consider the developmental context, whether or not there is evidence of coercion, and the child's stated reasons for stating the preference. When siblings are involved, each should be seen alone and also with each other. A child may be more inclined to speak about the home situation when supported by the presence of a brother or sister.

1. INTERVIEWING PARENT AND CHILD

It is important to hold one or two interviews jointly with each parent and the child (or children). This joint session should be unstructured and should occur following the child's visit to the office. Thus, he or she will be familiar with the furniture, toys, games, etc., and can direct the play and/or discussion with the parent. The evaluator should not be an active participant in this session but, rather, should observe parent and child behavior. The expert should factor in parental anxiety at seemingly being "graded" during this interview and should stress that this is a time for parent and child to "be together" in any way they wish. The therapist observes the interaction, the ease with which parent and child are together, how they play a game or work on a drawing, what they talk about, and the level of anxiety or conflict.

The therapist might want to conduct this session in the parent's home. A home visit—even though it is planned and, therefore, not a surprise drop-in— nevertheless affords a view of the family in its own surroundings. There may be much material gained in such a visit that would otherwise be missed if the evaluation is conducted solely at the office.

D. Interviewing others

Occasionally, the expert may wish to interview others who play an important role in the proceedings. For example, a divorcing father may already be living with someone he intends to marry. Such a potential stepparent for the child should be interviewed. Sometimes a nanny, babysitter, or grandparent who has known the child a long time may provide useful information. In general, the expert should seek the agreement of both parents before involving others in the custody evaluation.

E. The written report

The expert communicates to the judge, a family services court clinic, or the attorneys through the written report. This report should be succinct, in plain language without undefined psychiatric jargon, long enough to provide a complete picture, and short enough to maintain the professional interest of those who read it. The report can be written in letter form, addressed to the judge, the clerk of the court, or another appropriate individual, depending upon the locale. The expert should determine in advance who the primary recipient will be. The report should begin with a summary of the questions it will address and include a listing of people seen and the times spent interviewing them, and a summary of any documents read by the expert. It should contain summaries of the interviews with the family members. Using direct quotes from parents and children is helpful and conveys the tone of the interview. A separate section, perhaps labelled "Conclusions and Recommendations," should contain the expert's formulation of this case along with specific recommendations regarding custody and general suggestions about visitation, if that is part of the evaluation.

The written report should not contain language that is inflammatory or bespeaks bias or value judgments by the expert. For example, it would not be helpful to say, "Mr. Jones is a rigid man who is self-centered and unable to cooperate." Instead, the report could include, "Mr. Jones seems to find it difficult to compromise on a number of issues and cannot always see the other person's point of view." Psychiatric diagnoses are not necessary; this evaluation is of parenting—not mental status. The report should be written with the expectation that at some point the parent might be reading it. It should be carefully proofread.

F. Testimony

A complete and conclusive written report, accurately reflecting the clinical interviews, may stand on its own and help lead to a settlement. Occasionally, however, one side may request that the expert appear in court to testify about the report. The side with which the expert seemed to agree may want the clinician to expand on the conclusions and indicate to the judge how he reached his conclusions. This direct testimony will be friendly and respectful and will attempt to bring out the therapist's "superb" qualifications as well as the conclusions. The cross-examination, on the other hand, is a process by which the clinician's report will be challenged and criticized. The cross-examining attorney will attempt to point out inconsistencies and deficits in the report and will suggest that the expert did not have all the information at hand at the time of the evaluation.

The expert must be polite and professional during testimony and must remember that he or she is not on trial. Answers should be short and directly to the point and should not be expanded upon, unless requested by the attorney or the judge. If the expert does not understand a question or feels that a question cannot be answered as posed, he should so state.

The expert witness has a right to be paid for courtroom time. Fees vary with locale but may be $1000 or more for part of a day in court. The expert should ask for the fee prior to the testimony and should not hesitate to answer any fee-related questions when on the witness stand.

IV. PITFALLS

A. In accepting cases

An expert may be under intense pressure from an attorney to evaluate a child and one parent—the attorney's client—involved in a custody dispute. The attorney may state that the expert will not be asked to offer an opinion as to custody—just to evaluate the parent-child relationship. The expert should avoid such one-sided participation, as already mentioned in Part III. Such a limited evaluation puts added stress on the child and does little to enhance the professional reputation of the expert. It is just not possible to compare two parents if only one has been seen.

The treating therapist should not assume the additional role of forensic expert. Nor should a court-appointed impartial expert become involved in treatment. Wearing two hats in this manner may violate confidentiality, impedes both the forensic and treatment processes, and will cause great discomfort to patient and expert alike.

The forensic expert should avoid situations suggestive of a conflict of interest or instances in which his or her impartiality may be challenged.

B. In the evaluation

Parents often feel that they have not had enough time to explain their point of view to the expert witness. It is important to give them an opportunity to be heard and not be unduly strict about limiting their time. On the other hand, the clinician should explain that the evaluation cannot be prolonged indefinitely. The expert should not refuse to read documents given by a parent, even if he or she feels the papers will have little relevance. It is important for parents to feel that they have been heard and that they are being evaluated by an impartial person. The biggest pitfall, alluded to earlier, is the danger of the expert trying to decide which parent is lying and which is telling the truth and confusing his role with that of the judge.

C. In the report

A major pitfall in preparing the written report is failure to have the conclusions follow from the data presented. The reader should appreciate a flow in the material and a cogent formulation at the end. The conclusions and recommendations should emerge in a rational way and should not take the reader by surprise. The report should contain enough process from the interviews so that the judge can appreciate that the expert did solicit enough information.

D. In the testimony

A common pitfall is not being prepared for court. The expert should review the written report as well as handwritten notes prior to testimony. In most situations, he should meet beforehand with one or both attorneys to go over the planned testimony. Although it is permissible to bring notes along when on the witness stand, it is important for the expert to convey the impression of having taken the work seriously and of having given the evaluation and report considerable thought.

V. CASE EXAMPLE EPILOGUES

A. Case Example 1

The child psychiatrist reviewed the issue of depression with Mr. Slater. The man assured him that he was in regular treatment with a psychiatrist and was complying with his antidepressant medication regimen. He invited the expert to call the psychiatrist, who did confirm that Mr. Slater was under his care and was taking his medication regularly. The expert learned that although Mr. Slater had suffered two episodes of depression, he was in every other respect an excellent father who had a warm, loving relationship with his son. At the time of the custody evaluation, Mr. Slater displayed no signs or symptoms of depression.

Further evaluation revealed that Mrs. Slater was extremely angry with her husband. She accused him of being "a mental case" and a danger to Chad. She said that she was even thinking of asking the court to prevent overnight visits with Mr. Slater for fear that he might make a suicide attempt with Chad present.

The child psychiatrist was struck by how forcefully Mrs. Slater was attempting to portray her husband as an ill man. The expert also learned of some other false accusations by Mrs. Slater. He met with both parents at the end of the evaluation and offered them the opportunity to try mediation with him. Mr. Slater readily accepted, saying that he would prefer to reach some kind of shared custody agreement with his wife. "We both love Chad very much," he said. "It would be a shame to have to drag out this litigation."

Unfortunately, Mrs. Slater refused the offer of mediation. The evaluating child psychiatrist went on to recommend that Mr. Slater have custody of Chad, and the judge agreed with the recommendation.

B. Case Example 2

The psychiatrist observed a close relationship between the daughters and their mother. He learned that the "cult" was a philosophical organization which the mother had joined but was not a residential group. The mother had friends both within and outside the organization and made sure that her daughters had friends from a variety of families. The children spoke excitedly about their school, their friends, and their life with their mother. They recognized that their parents were fighting over their custody and said that they loved their father. However, they expressed concern that, "Daddy is against anything Mommy wants to do with us. He wants to put us in a different school and move away. We're happy where we are."

The expert was particularly concerned about the father's computerized data bank of information gathered to prove his wife's unfitness. He did in fact review all of the data given him but was more concerned with the father's mission to prove maternal unfitness than with anything included in the "facts" provided by the father. The psychiatrist recommended that the mother be given custody.

C. Case Example 3

Following the child custody evaluation, the impartial expert realized that it was extremely difficult to recommend custody to one parent or the other. Both Mr. and Mrs. Dickinson were devoted to their children, psychologically minded, and upset about the ligitation. When the psychiatrist suggested they try for a mediated settlement, they readily agreed. He met with them for six sessions following the completed custody evaluation. Although the Dickinsons were often angry and frustrated with each other during the mediation, the clinician helped them to remain child-centered and suggested a number of compromises. They were able to reach a joint custody agreement involving a living arrangement for the children, their future educational needs, summer vacations, and holidays. They were even able to work out a number of financial matters. Out of this mediation they drafted a complete agreement which was submitted to the court and which ended their litigation.

VI. ACTION GUIDE

A. Getting involved

1. Agree to be a court-appointed expert only, or someone agreed to by both sides. In most cases it is not advisable to participate in one-sided custody or visitation evaluations.
2. Make sure the questions posed by the court are understood and reasonable for a mental health professional to answer.
3. Make fee requirements clear and request payment in full prior to the evaluation.

B. Doing the evaluation

1. Explain to all parties how the evaluation will be conducted.
2. Consider the evaluation a profile of parenting—not a psychiatric report.
3. Be sure that all important people in the children's lives are seen and for enough time.

C. Writing the report

1. Remember that the report is a communication with a non-mental health professional.
2. Clearly indicate who was seen, when, and for how long. Include all important data from interviews.
3. Check that conclusions and recommendations flow naturally and logically from the data that are presented.
4. Proofread carefully.

D. Testifying in court

1. Be prepared!
2. Be professional, courteous, respectful, and avoid arrogance.
3. Do not hesitate to indicate if a question is unclear or cannot be answered as posed.

VII. SUGGESTED READINGS

American Psychiatric Association (1988), Child Custody Consultation: A Report of the Task Force on Clinical Assessment in Child Psychiatry. Washington, D.C.: APA.

American Psychiatric Association (1992), Disclosure of Psychiatric Treatment Records in Child Custody Disputes. A report of a task force of the American Psychiatric Association. Washington, D.C.: APA.

Ash, P. and Guyer, M. (1984), Court Implementation of Mental Health Professionals' Recommendations in Contested Child Custody and Visitation Cases. Bull. Am. Acad. Psych. and the Law 12:137–147.

Ash, P. and Guyer, M. (1986), Relitigation after Contested Custody and Visitation Evaluations. Bull. Am. Acad. Psych. and the Law 14:323–330.

Atwell, A., et al. (1984), Effects of Joint Custody on Children. Bull. Am. Acad. Psych. and the Law 12:149–157.

Benedek, E. and Schetky, D. (1985), Custody and Visitation: Problems and Perspectives. Psych. Clin. N.A. 8:857–873.

Bozett, F., ed. (1987), Gay and Lesbian Parents. New York: Praeger.

Curran, W. (1985), The Vulnerability of Court-Appointed Impartial Experts in Child-Custody Cases. NEJM 312:1168–1170.

Derdeyn, A. (1976), Child Custody Contests in Historical Perspective. Am. J. Psychiatry 133:1369–1376.

Derdeyn, A. and Scott, E. (1984), Joint Custody: a Critical Analysis and Appraisal. Am. J. Orthopsych. 54:199–209.

Emery, R. and Wyer, M. (1987), Child Custody Mediation and Litigation: an Experimental Evaluation of the Experience of Parents. J. Consult. Clinc. Psych. 55:179–186.

Goldstein, J., Solnit, A., and Freud, A. (1973), Beyond the Best Interests of the Child. New York: Free Press.

Goldzband, M. (1983), Current Trends Affecting Family Law and Child Custody. Psychiatric Clin. N.A. 6:683–694.

Herman, S. (1990), Special Issues in Child Custody Disputes. J. Am. Acad. Child Adolesc. Psychiatry 29(6) 969–974.

Herman, S. and Levy, A. (1989), Does Peer Review Have a Place in Child Custody Evaluations? Children Today 18:15–18.

Johnston, J. and Campbell, L. (1988), Impasses of Divorce. New York: Free Press.

Kleber, D. et al. (1986), The Impact of Parental Homosexuality in Child Custody Cases: A Review of the Literature. Bull Am. Acad. Psych. and the Law 14:81–87.

Levy, A. (1982), Disorders of Visitation in Child Custody Cases. J. Psych. and Law (Winter) 471–489.

Miller, T. and Veltkamp, L. (1987), Disputed Child Custody: Strategies and Issues in Mediation. Bull. Am. Acad. Psych. and the Law 15:45–56.

Nicholson, E. B. and Bulkley, J. (1988), Sexual Abuse Allegations in Custody and Visitation Cases. Chicago: ABA.

Schetky, D. and Haller, L. (1983), Parental Kidnapping. J. Am. Acad. Child Psychiatry 22:279–285.

Steinman, S. (1981), The Experience of Children in a Joint-Custody Arrangement: A Report of a Study. Am. J. Orthopsych. 51:403–414.

Steinman, S., et al. (1985), A Study of Parents Who Sought Joint Custody Following Divorce: Who Reaches Agreement and Sustains Joint Custody and Who Returns to Court. J. Am. Acad. Child. Psych. 24:554–562.

Tibbits-Kleber, A., et al. (1987), Joint Custody: A Comprehensive Review. Bull. Am. Acad. Psych. and the Law 15:27–43.

Weithorn, L., ed. (1987), Psychology and Child Custody Determinations. Lincoln: University of Nebraska Press.

8

Clinical Indicators of Child Abuse

CATHERINE DeANGELIS, M.D., M.P.H.

I. CASE EXAMPLES

A. Case Example 1

An 8-month-old male infant is brought to the pediatric emergency room by ambulance. His mother reported that he'd fallen from a bed onto a carpeted floor but appeared to be fine except for some crying. She'd put him into his crib for a nap and returned about 15 minutes later to find him seizing. She'd called the ambulance, and he continued to seize all during the 10 minute ride to the hospital. The seizing stopped with the administration of intravenous medication.

According to the mother, there was no history of any pre- or perinatal problems and he'd been "perfectly healthy" up to today. The entire physical examination is within normal limits except for the presence of retinal hemorrhages bilaterally. The physicians send the child for a computed tomogram (CT) of the skull and a radiological series of all long bones and the skull.

B. Case Example 2

The mother of a 3-year-old girl asks you to evaluate the child because she has told the mother that, "Daddy touched my hinnie with his peenie." The parents recently were divorced after a very stormy fight in court about custody and visiting rights regarding their only child. The child allegedly told the mother about a month after the incident which occurred during a weekend visit with the father.

The child's regular physician suggested the referral to you because the father had called him and warned him that the mother ". . . was trying to make trouble with ridiculous allegations." The physician know both parents well and didn't want to get involved in the issue. Also, he didn't feel sufficiently qualified to make such a medical judgment.

You make an appointment to evaluate the child the next day. When you interview the child, using anatomically correct dolls, she tells and shows you how her daddy touched his penis to her vaginal area. She denies having been hurt, and the mother denies seeing any discharge or blood on the child's panties. The physical examination of the genital area reveals an intact hymenal ring with a vaginal opening of 3 mm. There are no scars, tears, or other abnormalities of the genital or anal region.

C. Case Example 3

A 2-year-old boy is brought to you by his mother because of vomiting and poor weight gain "since birth." The family recently moved, and the child's past medical record reveals intermittent episodes of severe vomiting and chronic diarrhea since the child was several months old. The child has had at least three thorough medical evaluations including hospitalization at two major medical centers. No specific diagnosis has been made, and the mother has devoted most of her time to feeding the child special (and varied) diets, including nasogastric feedings. In fact, the child's previous physician stated in the record that the child would probably have not survived were it not for the mother's dedication and diligence with him.

The child is irritable and difficult to examine because he clings to his mother. His height, weight, and head circumference are at 50% for a 12-month-old. However, the rest of his physical examination is normal. His developmental milestones are normal.

II. LEGAL ISSUES

A. Definition of abuse

While the specific legal definitions of child abuse are established by the individual states, most base their definition on The Child Abuse Prevention and Treatment Act of 1974 (PL 93–247). That Act defines child neglect and abuse as ". . . the physical and mental injuring, sexual abuse, negligent treatment or maltreatment of a child under the age of 18 by a person who is responsible for the child's welfare under circumstances which indicate that the child's health and welfare is harmed or threatened thereby . . ." Because state definitions, interpretations, and enforcements differ, the professional who deals with child abuse must become familiar with the specific law within the state where he practices.

B. Reporting

In all 50 states physicians and others who work with children professionally are required to report cases of suspected child abuse to child protective agencies. The legal requirement to report supercedes all claims to confidentiality. Those who report and/or are involved in the evaluations and investigations are granted immunity from any civil action provided their report is reasonable and made in good faith. A precedent exists for civil liability for failure to report suspected abuse.

Reporting laws vary widely regarding the specific abusive acts to be reported, the amount of suspicion required, and the time frame in which a report must be made. In general, the major requirement is that there is a clinically sound reason for suspicion and that the report is made within a time frame adequate to protect the child from potential further abuse.

C. Expert testimony

Health professionals, and especially those who report suspected child abuse, are frequently required to testify in court. While this is time consuming and often unpleasant, it is necessary to provide fair legal treatment to the child and to the suspected abuser. Because testimony is often given some time after the child has been evaluated, careful notation in the medical record is of vital importance (See VI. Action Guide). Sound advice for providing expert testimony can be found in

Wissow, 1989, pp 209–217. It also is an excellent resource on child abuse in general.

D. The child's testimony

While the abused child's testimony in court may provide the most important evidence, the act of testifying can be very traumatic to the child. Traditionally child witnesses were treated no differently than adults in courts, but in the past few years the legal system has attempted to minimize the anxiety and trauma to the child by using videotaping, eliminating reporters and audiences from the courtroom, and by permitting a psychiatrist to veto sensitive questions addressed to the child (Baum, 1987 and Landwirth, 1987).

The abused child, especially one who has been sexually abused, can be further harmed by publications of the event. Because some children have been harmed in this way, The American Academy of Pediatrics has recommended that all states adopt laws forbidding public disclosure of the identities of abused children in the mass media unless ordered by a judge (Krugman, 1988).

III. CLINICAL ISSUES

A. Physical indications of abuse

Child abuse and neglect occurs in children of all ages and from all socio-economic classes. A wide range of indicators may suggest abuse, but many children who have been victimized present with non-specific complaints such as failure to thrive; "doctor shopping"; multiple emergency room visits for apparently trivial complaints; a complaint or history that is incompatible with physical findings; chronic complaints such as abdominal pain, headaches, and recurrent vaginal discharge; or unexplained or poorly explained trauma.

The following physical, potential indicators of abuse should arouse the suspicions of the health professional:

1. *Bruises and welts* including those on any infant and especially those on the face, the posterior side of a child's body, in non-bony areas, and in unusual patterns that might reflect the type of instrument used; bruises in various stages of healing; unexplained bruises and welts; bilaterally symmetrical bruises; human bite marks; and clustered bruises indicating repeated contact with a hand or instruments.
2. *Burns* including immersion burns indicating dunking in a hot liquid (i.e., a sharp line of demarcation on the skin), cigarette burns, rope burns that indicate confinement, dry burns indicating that a child has been forced to sit upon a hot surface or has had a hot implement applied to the skin, and unexplained burns.
3. *Lacerations* of the lip, eye, or portion of an infant's face (e.g., tears in the gum tissue which may have been caused by force feeding); any laceration or abrasion to the external genitalia; and unexplained lacerations and abrasions.
4. *Skeletal injuries* including epiphyseal fracture, periosteal elevation, and metaphyseal or corner fractures of long bones possibly caused by twisting or

pulling; linear skull fractures in infants; and unexplained fractures or multiple fractures in various stages of healing.

5. *Head injuries* including absence of hair and/or hemorrhaging beneath the scalp due to vigorous hair pulling, subdural hematomas due to shaking or hitting, retinal hemorrhages or detachments due to shaking, jaw and nasal fractures, and unexplained head injuries.

6. *Internal injuries* including duodenal or jejunal hematomas or rupture of the inferior vena cava due to kicking or hitting, peritonitis due to a ruptured organ, pancreatitis and pancreatic pseudocysts, and unexplained internal injuries.

7. *Genital and rectal injuries* including scars, clefts, abrasions of the hymen, fourchette, or anus; increased vascularity of the tissue; skin tags outside the midline of the anus; enlarged anal or vaginal orifices (the introital diameter is generally considered to measure up to 5 mm in prepubertal children; however, this can vary with positioning and age and should not be used as the only indicator); attenuation of the hymen, i.e., a small rim rather than a sharp or rounded border; genital ulcers or warts; and vaginal discharge in a prepubertal girl. Table 8.1 shows the various organisms normally found in the vaginal area and those indicating abuse.

When any of the above abnormalities are found, the clinician must be sure they had not been caused by something other than abuse. For example, the child might have sustained perineal injuries from falling on a hard object or straddling hobby horses. Injuring the anal region can result from severe constipation. Also, iatrogenic injury can occur when a foreign object is removed from a child's vaginal orifice by a physician. Some professionals believe that the mere presence of any foreign object in the vagina of a child, including when it is placed there by the child, is indication of sexual abuse because someone taught the child to do so. Others believe this is normal exploratory behavior since no one teaches children to put foreign objects into other orifices, including the ears and nose. When any doubt exists, consultation with an experienced professional should be sought.

B. Behavioral indicators of child abuse

The following behaviors that can be associated with abuse should arouse the suspicions of the health professional. The child is different or difficult at birth, physically or mentally handicapped, developmentally delayed, cries very little or excessively during treatment or examination, is unusually fearful or docile, distrustful, guarded and shows no expectation of being comforted, does not look to parents for reassurance, wary of physical contact, unusually upset when other children cry, on the alert for danger and continually sizes up the environment, uses avoidance and denial to get out of anxiety producing situations, attempts to meet parents' needs by role reversal and superficial relationships with adults, has a low frustration tolerance, manifests behavioral extremes such as hyperactivity, aggressiveness, or withdrawal, is unusually fearful of parents, afraid to go home, reports injury by parent, is seen as different or bad by parents, and seems less afraid than other children when admitted to hospital and settles in quickly. Sexualization or eroticization behavior by the child can also be an indication of previous sexual abuse (Frederich, 1988).

TABLE 8.1   VAGINAL FLORA

Nonpathogenic Flora
   Bacteroides
   Diphtheroids
   E. coli
   Group B streptococcus
   Group D streptococcus
   Klebsiella species
   Lactobacilli species
   Peptostreptococcus
   Proteus species
   Pseudomonas species
   Staphylococcus aureus
   Staphylococcus epidermidis

Infectious: Not Sexually Transmitted
   Bacterial
      Gram negatives (UTI)
      Group A beta-hemolytic streptococcus
      H. influenzae
      Shigella
      S. pneumoniae
   Parasitic
      Enterobius vermicularis
   Viral
      Adenovirus
      Echovirus
      Molluscum contagiosum (pox virus)
      Varicella-Zoster
   Yeast
      Candida albicans

Infectious: Sexually Transmitted
   Bacterial
      Chlamydia trachomatis
      N. gonorrheae
   Protozoa
      Trichomonas vaginalis
   Viral
      Herpes simplex
      Papilloma virus

Suspicious
      Gardnerella vaginalis
      Mycoplasma hominis
      Ureaplasma

C. Indicators of neglect

The following potential indicators of neglect should arouse the suspicion of the health professional. The child is not up-to-date for immunizations and health care; is constantly fatigued; frequently runs away from home; has developmental delay; appears rejected, withdrawn, apathetic; is overly compliant or passive; is overly hostile, aggressive, unsocialized; or does not expect comfort from parent. Other indicators include consistent hunger; poor hygiene; inappropriate dress; lack of supervision especially in dangerous activities or for long periods of time; unattended physical problems or medical needs including dental care; abandonment; failure to thrive; prostitution; alcohol or drug abuse behaviors; and injuries or ingestion as a result of poor supervision. The child has caretaking responsibilities beyond expectations for age, displays role reversal, refuses to return home, states there is no caretaker, begs or steals food, is habitually truant or late to school, is inappropriately dressed for weather, or is not enrolled in school.

D. Characteristics of abusive and neglectful parents

The following characteristics that can be associated with abuse and neglect should alert the health professional. They can be used as indicators for parents who might need additional support or education to prevent an abuse from occurring.

The parent displays poor coping skills; is experiencing unusual stress or marital discord; considers excessive physical methods as legitimate forms of punishment; is isolated and has difficulty trusting others; has a poor support system; has unrealistic expectations and/or rigid expectations of the child; sees child as bad or demanding; has low self-esteem; looks to child for nurturance; has temper outbursts; is impulsive; shows loss of control or fear of loss of control; uses alcohol or drugs; does not involve self with child's care; can not think of good qualities in child; seldom touches or looks at the child; has a psychiatric disorder or chronic illness but no social support system; leaves the child unsupervised in potentially dangerous situations; consistently fails to keep the child's medical appointments; and consistently ignores child's crying or reacts with aggression. Finally, be alert to the parent who was repeatedly beaten or severely deprived as a child and was unable to depend on any adult to meet physical or emotional needs, those with a past record of serious mental illness or repeated difficulty with the law, or a parent previously suspected of physical abuse.

E. Munchausen syndrome by proxy

Munchausen syndrome by proxy (Meadow, 1977) is a condition in which one person, usually a parent, persistently fabricates signs or symptoms for another, usually a child. It is a form of child abuse because the child is exposed to potentially dangerous drugs and numerous and unnecessary traumatic physical evaluations in the search for a diagnosis. Examples of this problem include giving a child syrup of ipecac to force vomiting or cathartics to induce diarrhea, deliberately suffocating an infant to induce apnea, and feeding blood to an infant and smearing it on his face to simulate bleeding. Some victims have died.

The psychodynamics in this situation seems to be quite different from those operative in the more typical child abuse case. The parent, usually the mother, is almost always described as a model parent who has a substantial knowledge of clinical medicine, and the diagnosis is invariably delayed. She or he seems to thrive on the attention and support given by health professionals who receive reciprocal positive feedback from the payment. The physician must be alert to this possibility when a child recurrently presents with symptoms that defy diagnosis.

IV. PITFALLS

A. General

While the actual prevalence of child abuse is not known, over the past 20 years or so officially recognized cases have risen from several thousand to over a million annually. This represents about 2% of American children (Russell, 1984). It is difficult, if not impossible, to determine if all appropriate cases are being reported. There is some feeling that they are not. On the other hand, only about two-thirds of sexual abuse cases are substantiated (Green, 1986).

No one, and especially no professional who works with children, would want a child to be continually exposed to an environment where he will be abused. On the other hand, it is equally wrong for an innocent person to be accused and possibly incarcerated because of false accusations. These issues, involving an area where it is often clinically impossible to determine with a reasonable degree of certainty whether abuse actually did occur, can lead to under- or overreporting.

B. Denial and underreporting

The two major reasons for underreporting are failure to recognize abuse (especially sexual) and denial in the face of overt clinical signs. Even though pediatricians and mental health professionals often are called upon to assess the likelihood that sexual abuse has occurred, many have a surprisingly limited knowlege about the medical and social aspects of this problem (Ladson, 1987). In an effort to alleviate this problem, child abuse currently is being better and more frequently addressed in residency training and continuing education programs for physicians. Training in child abuse, per se, is included in the Accreditation Council on Graduate Medical Education special requirements for pediatric training programs that went into effect January 1, 1990.

Even when child abuse is clinically apparent, it is unpleasant to become involved in the legal actions that often ensue. Appearing for deposition or in court is time consuming and an alien environment to most health professionals. The health professional sometimes can overidentify with upper middle class families and give them more than a fair benefit of doubt. Also, the accusation might alienate a parent. It can be easier to "look the other way" and attribute bruises or peculiar behavior to other etiologies. It is simply wrong, not to mention illegal, to do that.

C. Overreporting

Children with injuries resulting from normal activity and those with bleeding disorders can be mistakenly determined to have been abused. Carelessness in performing a history, physical examination, and appropriate diagnostic tests can lead to false accusation.

There is a growing concern that some health professionals have developed a so-called "cottage industry" by serving as expert witnesses in sexual abuse cases. This can be a lucrative practice and lends itself to abuse or at least allegations of abuse of the medical and legal systems. Often, these alleged abuses occur when parents are involved in embittered divorce and custody cases. The estimated frequency of fictitious sexual abuse claims in such cases ranges from 8% to 55% (Paradise, 1988). It is difficult to believe that any health professional would deliberately aid in a false accusation, especially of such magnitude. The best way to eliminate such individuals from the profession, if they do exist, is for other professionals to gain expertise in the area. Most of the time, unethical professionals are not countered by ethical professionals. If all health professionals who deal with children were knowledgeable in the area of sexual abuse, they could eliminate unethical practices.

A major legal problem (but a medical blessing) is that physical wounds from sexual abuse can heal over time (Cantwell, 1987 and Muram, 1989). If several months or so have expired between examinations, the later normal physical examination might be irrelevant. Therefore when doubt exists it is imperative for the child to be examined by a second professional as soon as possible after "abnormal" findings are found by the first.

V. CASE EXAMPLE EPILOGUES

A. Case Example 1

Nonaccidental head trauma must be considered in any infant with a sudden onset of seizures with no previous history. In fact the diagnosis of shaken (or shaken impact) baby must be entertained in any child under 1 year who has signs of unexplained brain injury and/or altered consciousness with no overt signs of trauma. Infants and small children rarely sustain accidental brain injury of sufficient severity to result in seizures or loss of consciousness. Minor falls, as described in this case, rarely result in brain damage even when accompanied by significant linear skull fractures. Retinal hemorrhages are found in the majority of children who have been shaken.

Upon further interview by the physicians and a social worker, the mother admitted having become very angry with the infant who wouldn't stop crying. She had shaken the baby in her crib but hadn't realized she'd been seriously injured until she began to seize. The child was admitted to the hospital, and a report was made to Protective Services.

B. Case Example 2

You tell the mother that there are no physical findings consistent with sexual abuse but that the lack of such findings do not eliminate the possibility that sexual abuse occurred. Fondling or other non-penetrating sexual acts usually leave no physical findings. Also, since more than a month has passed since the alleged incident, healing of abnormalities might have occurred. Because of the child's testimony, the mother decides to pursue the case legally and you agree to present your findings. Because the mother reported the problem to the police the next day, you do not make a separate report to Protective Service. The case is still pending.

C. Case Example 3

The child vomits while you are examining him, and (mostly on a whim) you send off the vomitus for a toxicology screen. Somewhat to your surprise, the laboratory technician calls and tells you that she has identified syrup of ipecac in the vomitus.

After you confront her with the laboratory test results, the mother admits that she has been administering syrup of ipecac and laxatives intermittently to the child. You arrange for the mother to be evaluated by a psychiatrist and for her to have the child's maternal grandmother help the mother care for him.

VI. ACTION GUIDE

A. History

1. GENERAL

a. Take a careful history while remaining calm and non-judgmental. The goal is to assure the child's safety and not to extract a confession from the parent. Use direct quotes whenever possible, and refrain from making inferences about what a child or parent says. Be compassionate and open when talking with the victim of abuse, and reassure him that the abuse is not his fault.
b. If possible, interview the child and parent(s) separately. However, a child should not be forced to be separated from his parent(s).
c. Ascertain and document the child's usual caretaker, alternate caretaker(s), family structure and stresses, daily routine, usual eating and sleeping patterns (including nightmares), level of activity, and recent changes in these areas. Determine whether the child displays acting-out behaviors, crying/clinging, the support system available to the parent(s), the quality of the parent's interaction with the child and with you, and the child's usual source of health care and her immunization status.

B. Interviewing different age groups

1. PRESCHOOLER

Do not ask leading questions; ask neutral questions such as, "How did you get hurt?" If the child gives an answer, record it as a quote. The child may be too frightened to talk, but picture-drawing is enjoyed by children and may elucidate the needed information. Ask the child what he has drawn and label the drawing(s) with his own words in quote. Save it as part of the medical record. If sexual abuse is suspected, use of anatomically correct dolls may depict what the child cannot or will not communicate.

2. OLDER CHILD OR ADOLESCENT

Ask how the injury occurred, why he thinks he has chronic pains, and how his symptoms started and progressed. Ask him about his life at home, at school, and with friends. Encourage him to talk and don't interrupt. If a child admits to being abused, ask him if he will tell you who did so. Record his answers as quotes, and note any non-verbal cues (crying, bowing of the head, etc.). Children are frequently afraid to provide the name of the abuser because they fear the consequences. Respect this fear, and do not harass a child for the identity of the abuser. Be a good listener, and don't write while the child is talking if your writing seems to upset him.

C. Assessment and documentation of presenting complaints

1. TRAUMA

If the child presents with trauma, ascertain and document when the episode occurred, who saw it, how the injury occurred (e.g., for closed head trauma, what did the child's head hit, how high was the fall, etc.), and history of previous trauma/hospitalization (verify the parent's history by the medical record if possible).

2. SUSPECTED ABUSE REFERRAL

If the child presents as suspected abuse, ascertain and document why abuse is suspected and who suspects it; who the suspected abuser is and why he is suspected; when and where the suspected abuse occurred; length of time during which the suspected abuse has occurred; and precipitating factors for abuse.

3. FAILURE TO THRIVE

If the child presents with failure to thrive, chronic complaints, or psychosomatic complaints, ascertain and document the history of the presenting complaint; presence of related symptoms; parent's and child's reactions to these complaints; precipitating factors that trigger the complaints; and stresses in the family/school/social life of the child.

4. GENITOURINARY

If the child presents with genitourinary complaints, ascertain and document the onset, progression, and character of symptoms; parent's and child's reactions to these symptoms; history of other contributing factors (e.g., if vaginitis is suspected, history of masturbation, tight clothing, bubble bath usage, new soaps, etc., should also be elicited); and whether anyone else in the household has genitourinary complaints.

D. Physical exam

1. GENERAL

When abuse is suspected, a complete physical exam including the genital and anal areas should be performed and documented carefully.

2. APPEARANCE AND BEHAVIOR

Note the child's general appearance (hygiene, state of nutrition); his behavior (fear vs. bravado); and his rapport with the parent and you.

3. DOCUMENTATION OF POSITIVE FINDINGS

Note and record positive physical findings. If feasible, take photographs of suspicious skin findings or mark suspicious areas on the human drawings (Fig. 8.1). Photographs are preferred and should be marked with the child's name, date, and body part. Full pictures of a young child may also be helpful.

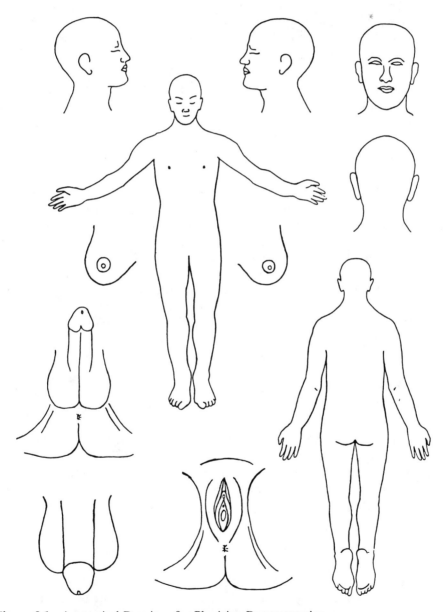

Figure 8.1 Anatomical Drawings for Physician Documentation

4. CLOSED HEAD TRAUMA (CHT)

When evaluating CHT, perform a complete neurological exam. Check the skull and scalp for bruises and lacerations and the rest of the body for evidence of trauma. A fundoscopic exam must be performed because retinal hemorrhages are frequently seen with shaking injuries but not with benign CHT.

5. SUSPECTED LONGSTANDING SEXUAL ABUSE

When longstanding sexual abuse is suspected, a complete genital and rectal exam is performed. The appearance of the genitalia (rashes, lesions, swellings, lacerations, hymenal ring integrity, anal sphincter tone, etc.) must be noted. Also, check the child's pharynx carefully for evidence of inflammation or trauma.

6. DOCUMENTATIOIN OF NEGATIVE FINDINGS

Document pertinent negative findings. If abuse is suspected the lack of any bruises, cuts/burns on the skin is an important pertinent negative and should be noted.

E. Diagnostic tests

1. LABORATORY

Be reasonable. If the patient says that the child bleeds (or bruises) easily, a hematocrit, platelet count, and clotting studies are advisable. If the child has a genitourinary complaint, the urine should be examined microscopically for cells and organisms. If the complaint is sexual abuse, gonococcal cultures should be taken of the throat, rectum, vagina/cervix, or male urethra; a test for syphilis, a wet prep for Trichomonal and Chlamydia cultures, and pregnancy test (if applicable) should be obtained. If the sexual abuse occurred within the past 48 hours the vaginal canal, head, and pubic hair and skin are examined carefully for the presence of semen (sperm and/or acid phosphatase). Document what tests were ordered and what results are already available.

2. RADIOLOGY

Order a trauma series and/or computerized tomography tests judiciously. Generally, they are most useful in infants and toddlers and are less useful in older children and teenagers. The only exception to the latter is in severely mentally retarded children who cannot provide information about pain or past injuries. A trauma series is generally advisable for children 3 years and under for whom abuse or severe neglect is suspected. Obtain radiological tests of injured parts as dictated by the physical exam.

F. Assessment

After the history, physical exam, and pertinent laboratory or radiological studies are obtained, the chart should be completed and an assessment noted. Enumerate the historical, physical, and diagnostic studies that are pertinent. Avoid assessments that categorically indicate abuse unless you are certain. Otherwise, the term "suspected" should be used.

G. Disposition and plan

The plan should include acute management of the child's injuries, reporting of the episode to Protective Services, explaining to the parent why the episode must be reported, planning for the child's disposition, and long-term follow-up.

1. Treat the child's injuries.
2. Report the family to Protective Services and/or to an interceding group such as Social Services (if such is available).
3. Inform the parent that a report of *suspected* abuse is being made. Tell them that it is the law and that the protection of the child is the primary concern. Be sympathetic and compassionate but firm. Do not "make deals" with the parent. Avoid taking sides if the family members attempt to blame each other.
4. Disposition can be a complex issue which must be decided carefully. The major concern is the child's immediate safety. The physician and others involved (Social Services, Protective Services, etc.) should jointly review disposition alternatives and come to a consensus based on their assessments and identification of appropriate resources available for disposition. Disposition alternatives include the return of the child to his home, placement of the child with relatives, placement of the child in an emergency shelter care, foster home, or admission to the hospital, if necessary.

VII. SUGGESTED READINGS

A. LEGAL CONSIDERATIONS

Baum, E., Grodin, M. A., Alpert, J. J., and Glantz, L. (1987), Child sexual abuse, criminal justice, and the pediatrician. Pediatrics 79:437–439.

Green, A. H. (1986), True and false allegations of sexual abuse in child custody disputes. J Am Acad Child Psychiatry 25:449–456.

Krugman, R. D., Chadwick, D. L., Helfer, R. E., McHugh, M. T., and Whitworth, J. M. (1988), Public disclosure of private information about victims of abuse. Pediatrics 82:387.

Landwirth, J. (1987), Children as witnesses in child sexual abuse trials. Pediatrics 80:585–589.

Myers, J. E. B. and Peters, W. D. (1987), Child Abuse Reporting Legislation in the 1980's. Denver: The American Humane Association.

Paradise, J. E., Rostain, A. L., and Nathanson, M. (1988), Substantiation of sexual abuse charges when parents dispute custody or visitation. Pediatrics 81:835–839.

Paul, D. M. (1986), What really happened to Baby Jane? The medical aspects of the investigation of alleged sexual abuse in children. Med Sci Law 26:85–102.

Runyan, D. K., Everson, M. D., Edelsohn, G. A., Hunter, W. M., and Coulter, M. L. (1988), Impact of legal intervention on sexually abused children. J Pediatr 13:647–653.

B. ASSESSMENTS AND MANAGEMENT

Cantwell, H. B. (1987), Update on vaginal inspection as it relates to child sexual abuse in girls under thirteen. Child Abuse Negl 11:545–546.

Chadwick, D. L., Berkowitz, C. D., Kerns, D., McCann, J., Reinhart, M.A., and Strickland, S. (1989), Color Atlas of Child Sexual Abuse. Chicago: Yearbook Medical Publishers.

DuBowitz, H. (1989), Prevention of child maltreatment: What is known. Pediatrics 83:570–577.

Ellerstein, N. S. (1979), The manifestations of child abuse and neglect. Am J Dis Child 133:906–909.

Enos, W. F., Conrath, T. B., and Byer, J. (1986), Forensic evaluation of the sexually abused child. Pediatrics 78:385–398.

Erickson, M. R. and Egeland, B. (1987), A developmental view of psychological consequences of maltreatment. School Psychol Rev 16:156–168.

Finkel, M. (1988), The medical evaluation of child sexual abuse. In: Schetky, D. H. and Greene, A. H.: Child Sexual Abuse: A Handbook for Health Care and Legal Professionals. New York: Brunner-Mazel.

Frederich, W. (1988), Behavior problems in sexually abused children. In: Wyatt, G. E. and Powell, G. J. (eds.): Lasting Effects of Child Sexual Abuse. Beverly Hills, CA: Sage Publications.

Hegger, A. and Emans, S. J. (1990), Introital diameter as the criterion for sexual abuse. Pediatrics 85:222–223.

Ladson, S., Johnson, C. F., and Doty, R. E., (1987), Do physicians recognize sexual abuse? Am J Dis Child 141:411–415.

Meadow, R. (1987), Munchausen syndrome by proxy: The hinterland of child abuse. Lancet 2:343–345.

Muram, D. (1989), Child sexual abuse: relationship between sexual acts and genital findings. Child Abuse Negl 13:211–216.

Troy, M. and Sroufe, L. A. (1987), Victimization among preschoolers: role of attachment relationship history. J Am Acad Child Psychiatry 26:166–172.

U.S. Dept. of Health and Human Services, Office of Human Development Services (1988), Study findings: National Study of the Incidence and Severity of Child Abuse and Neglect. Washington, D.C.: U.S. Government Printing Office.

Waller, A. E., Baker, S. P., and Szocka, A. (1989), Childhood injury deaths: national analysis and geographic variations. Am J Public Health 79:310–315.

C. GENERAL

Finkelhor, D. (ed.) (1986), A Source Book on Child Sexual Abuse. Beverly Hills, CA: Sage Publications.

Kessler, D. B., and New, M. I. (eds.) (1989), Child abuse and neglect. Pediatr Ann 18:467–513.

Russel, A. B. and Trainor, C. M. (1984), Trends in Child Abuse and Neglect: A National Perspective. Denver: The American Humane Association.

Wissow, L. S. (1990), Child Advocacy for the Clinician. An Approach to Child Abuse and Neglect. Baltimore: Williams & Wilkins.

9

Interviewing Children for Suspected Sexual Abuse

KATHLEEN M. QUINN, M.D., AND SUE WHITE, PH.D.

I. CASE EXAMPLES

A. Case Example 1

A 5-year-old girl and her 3-year-old sister had attended a local daycare center for a time when they had first moved to town. After 6 months the mother removed them due to concerns that the head teacher used physical punishment described by the older girl as hitting her on the face. Shortly thereafter the mother was called by another mother who stated that there were also concerns that sexual abuse had occurred at the center. The 5-year-old and 3-year-old were interviewed together by the local department of human services and police. The first two interviews were unstructured and included the protective worker sitting on the floor with the children whispering questions and answers. Puppet play was used in an attempt to understand the girls' vocabulary concerning body parts.

B. Case Example 2

A couple who have been divorced for several years were engaged in a visitation battle in domestic relations court over their children, aged 9 and 7. The mother had restricted visitation in the past, due to her ex-husband's history of physical abuse towards herself and the children and his alcoholism. Now sober and in AA, the father insisted upon visitation. The court awarded a limited visitation plan beginning with a half day a week and a gradual increase to alternating full weekends. Three months into the resumption of the visitation the mother and the 9-year-old girl alleged the child had been approached sexually by her father. The 7-year-old boy made no allegation. A report was made by the mother to the local department of human services. A motion to terminate visitation was filed by the mother's attorney in domestic relations court.

C. Case Example 3

A 3-year-old boy alleged his teenaged stepbrother had touched his bottom. The child was not yet toilet trained, and the intake worker taking the complaint found that the stepbrother assisted the 3-year-old in the bathroom. The mother who reported the allegation stated that the 3-year-old had immature language skills.

Sexual abuse allegations have emerged as the fastest growing type of abuse complaint. Effective investigation, validation, intervention, and treatment all depend upon a working knowledge of both the clinical and legal issues surrounding abuse. This chapter will describe the major issues surrounding investigation of sexual abuse.

II. LEGAL ISSUES

A. What Is Child Sexual Abuse?

Child sexual abuse is a sexual act imposed upon a child. Further definition of what constitutes sexual abuse has resulted in differing definitions among mental health, legal, and social professionals as well as researchers. Finkelhor (1979) has described three possible standards to define abuse—the consent standard, the report of the victim, and the community standard. The consent standard establishes that an act is abusive if a child does not consent to it. Finkelhor rejected using the consent standard, concluding that children cannot give informed consent to participate in a sexual act with an adult. Another method would be to consider someone abused if they reported feeling victimized. Victimization, Finkelhor concludes, can occur whether or not the victim feels victimized. Young children may not appreciate their victimization. The power and knowledge differences between adults and children imply that sexual acts between adult and child are abuse. The community standard includes consideration of the age difference between the victim and perpetrator, their relationship, and legal definitions which are seen as a reflection of public policy. As Finkelhor concludes, such a standard is objective and easy to use.

B. The Laws

Legal definitions of child sexual abuse are found in child sex offense, incest, and child protection statutes (Bulkley, 1985). Sexual activity with children by adults is a crime in every state. Both the age of the child and of the perpetrator as well as their relationship often determines the nature of the offense and resulting penalties. Consenting intercourse may be specifically prohibited if the adult is a parent or legal guardian or someone acting in a position of authority over a child, such as a foster parent, teacher, or household member.

Numerous inconsistencies exist in the laws across states. The lower age at which children can consent to sexual activity ranges from 11 to 17 years. Penalties for perpetrators range from minimum sentences to life imprisonment or death. In addition, the definition of prohibited acts vary widely.

Most states have incest laws. These incest laws limit the criminal act of incest to sexual intercourse. These laws were primarily written to prevent the biological risks to the resulting offspring. More recently, many states have revised their laws to protect the integrity of the family by forbidding sexual relationships between adoptive parents or stepparents and their children.

Two types of civil statutes, mandatory reporting laws, and juvenile or family court jurisdiction acts exist for the protection of abused and neglected children. More than 20 state statutes now specifically include sexual abuse. However, statutory definitions in every state can be interpreted to include sexual abuse. Legal action may be brought against both the actively abusive parent as well as a complicitous spouse.

All 50 states have mandatory reporting acts which require certain professionals working or caring for children to report suspected abuse or neglect to public child protective agencies and/or the police. The purpose of reporting laws has been to establish a comprehensive public policy mechanism for child protection designed to encourage reports of abuse to protect children and to designate one agency to handle abuse and to offer services to children and families. In most states a mental health professional or other named professional can be charged with a violation of criminal law for failure to report known or suspected cases of child abuse. Failure to report may also make the professional liable for civil damages in a malpractice case. All state statutes provide the mandated reporter with immunity from suit for negligence or defamation if a suspected case of abuse is reported in good faith.

Although reports of abuse have increased dramatically in recent years due to both increased public awareness and the reporting acts, child abuse, including sexual abuse, is still significantly underreported. Despite protections and possible sanctions, many professionals fail to report suspected abuse. However, sexual abuse appears more likely to be reported than other forms of abuse and maltreatment (Burgdorf, 1981). Mandated reporters must follow their child protection laws to avoid both criminal and civil liability. Professionals encountering cases raising issues concerning abuse should consult with knowledgeable colleagues and/or legal counsel to determine their responsibility for reporting. Mandated reporting of abuse is a well-recognized exception to confidentiality. In addition to professionals caring for children, almost half the states require "any person" to report suspected abuse or neglect.

C. Legal Interventions

If a child is found to be abused (or neglected) the state has two routes of intervention: 1) criminal prosecution against the perpetrator, or 2) child protection intervention and civil action in juvenile or family court in order to protect the child when the parent or caretaker is the abuser. Either or both interventions may take place. In the cases of parental abuse or neglect a child protection investigation is initiated although the case may not proceed to juvenile court. Sexual abuse of a child more frequently results in a criminal prosecution than does physical abuse or neglect unless the child is severely injured or dies. Thus in child sexual abuse cases involving a parent, two legal proceedings may occur.

In the criminal justice system the burden of proof is high. The state must prove that the accused is guilty beyond a reasonable doubt. The rights to a fair trial and to be proven guilty only by reliable evidence is a fundamental concept of our criminal system. Therefore, there is a strict adherence to rules of evidence in criminal court, particularly the rule against admitting an individual's out-of-court assertion to prove the truth of the allegation (the hearsay rule). Significant problems occur in proving sexual abuse in criminal proceedings, including the lack of eyewitnesses and the lack of medical evidence. The child may not be competent to be a witness, or the child may be viewed as not credible due to limited cognitive or verbal skills. Advocates of using the criminal justice system argue that child abuse is a crime, that unlike the juvenile court, the criminal justice system exercises control over the offender while providing full due process and other constitutional safeguards to protect the offender's rights. Since the late 1970s and 1980s a number of states have reformed laws and procedures aimed at reducing the trauma children experience in the criminal justice system and to modify restrictions on the admissibility of evidence at trial.

The juvenile court system has certain advantages and disadvantages over the criminal justice system. The juvenile court may rapidly protect the child by removing the child. The court has greater access to both services and treatment for family and children and can offer long-term monitoring. More informal evidence and procedural requirements, lack of a jury or a public trial may make the court proceeding less traumatic to the child and make abuse easier to prove. A guardian *ad litem* representing the child's best interest may be appointed.

The disadvantages of child protection intervention include a lack of direct control over the offender, resulting in the removal of children from their own homes, often placing them in foster homes for excessive amounts of time. Other disadvantages include a lack of specialized treatment for sexually abusive families by protective service agencies. Critics have also pointed to the risk of unwarranted invasion of privacy and the lack of due process and other legal safeguards in juvenile court.

Although states maintain broad authority to intervene within families under child protection laws, recent federal and state reforms have been adopted to limit state interventions and to prevent unnecessary and overly long placements of children. The federal Adoption Assistance and Child Welfare Act (1980) initiated many of these reforms.

D. Procedural Reforms in the Courtroom

Many clinicians involved with child victims believe the children are often further victimized by their involvement with the legal system. Although few sexually abused children testify in open court (Rogers, 1982) much attention has been paid to reforms in trial procedures because of their potential impact both on victims and on the rights of defendants. The major areas of reform have included 1) testimonial alternatives and 2) special hearsay exceptions.

1. ALTERNATIVE TESTIMONIAL APPROACHES

At least 34 states have laws permitting the child's testimony to be videotaped before the trial. Twenty-seven states allow the child's testimony to be taken by closed-circuit television outside the courtroom and shown for the jury and defendant to see. Although many states have adopted these reforms, some have been criticized as unconstitutional. The most frequently raised constitutional issue involves the Sixth Amendment's confrontation clause. The confrontation clause has generally been interpreted to require the prosecution to produce a witness whose prior testimony is offered into evidence and to show that the previous statements appear reliable. The confrontation clause has three purposes: 1) to ensure the witness provides testimony under oath; 2) to require the witness to submit to cross-examination; and 3) to permit the jury to observe the witness as a means to assess credibility. Two major issues are raised by the use of alternative testimonial methods: 1) Must the child physically confront the defendant?, and 2) Must there be a finding that the child is unable to tolerate normal courtroom procedure before an alternate method such as closed-circuit television is used?

A recent Supreme Court case (*Coy v. Iowa*, 56 USLW 4931 no. 86-6757) has established some guidelines concerning testimonial innovations in child abuse cases. The case involved an unusual Iowa statute that permitted two girls to testify behind a one-way screen in front of the defendant without a showing for need. The conviction was struck down on the Sixth Amendment right to confrontation grounds. The majority found that "face to face" was an essential element of confrontation. However, it was left open as to whether or not any exception to physical confrontation would be recognized. After *Coy*, question of the constitutionality of numerous state statutes remains unanswered. However, nearly every state appellate court that has ruled on the constitutionality of its closed circuit and videotaped prior testimony statutes has taken the position that face-to-face confrontation is preferred but may be overridden by competing interests such as the child's well-being.

Although videotaping has been vigorously debated, in actuality it is seldom used in states where it is permitted. Many of the statutes are cumbersome to put into practice. Many prosecutors consider a deposition more stressful than courtroom testimony for several reasons. Depositions take place in small rooms putting the child and defendant in close proximity. In addition, the judge may not be present to monitor the proceedings and the behavior of the participants. Often victim advocates are not permitted in the room to support the child. Finally, if a finding of emotional trauma is required the child must undergo mental health exams. Thus many prosecutors believe that a child who can withstand the investigation process leading up to a deposition or preliminary hearing can succeed at trial as well.

2. SPECIAL HEARSAY EXCEPTIONS

Hearsay is defined as "a statement, other than one made by the declarant while testifying at the trial or hearing, offered into evidence to prove the truth asserted" (Federal Rule of Evidence 801). An example relevant to sexual abuse might include the teacher of the alleged victim who was told by the child that her stepfather was abusing her. If the teacher is permitted to testify about these statements and the child does not testify, the stepfather has lost his ability to confront his accuser (the child) through cross-examination.

There has always been a recognition of the need for some exceptions to the general rule of excluding hearsay. The Supreme Court has held in *Ohio v. Roberts* (448 U.S. 56, 1980) that out-of-court statements do not deny the defendant the right to confrontation guaranteed in the Sixth Amendment if two requirements are met—1) if the witness is unavailable and 2) if the statements are judged to be sufficiently reliable. Each request for the admission of hearsay evidence must be determined on an individual basis by the trial judge using these two criteria. A child is most often found to be "unavailable" because he/she is incompetent to be a witness; is too distressed to testify; would be emotionally harmed by testifying; or "freezes" on the stand.

The three major hearsay exceptions currently used in sexual abuse trials are 1) "excited utterances" or *res gestae*; 2) statements made to a physician during diagnosis and treatment; and 3) residual hearsay, an exemption permitting such evidence when it can be shown to be reliable. An excited utterance is a "spontaneous declaration made by a person immediately after an event and before the mind has an opportunity to conjure a falsehood" (*Black's Law Dictionary*, 1979:1173). The time span permitted between the events and the statements has usually been several hours, but in some jurisdictions it has been as long as 24 hours.

An area of legal reform has been the expansion of traditional hearsay exceptions. At least 27 states have enacted special hearsay exceptions allowing a person to testify about a child victim's out-of-court statements concerning abuse. Most special exception statutes conform to the requirements of *Ohio v. Roberts* to ensure that the confrontation clause is not violated. Several appellate court decisions have upheld the constitutionality of the special exception statutes written in this manner. A recent case, *United States v. Inadi* (89 L.Ed. 2d. 390, 1986), has also left open the possibility that the prosecution may not need to call an available child to testify as a condition to the admission of his or her earlier out-of-court statements as hearsay.

III. CLINICAL ISSUES

A. General concepts

1. VALIDATION OF COMPLAINTS

When faced with an allegation of sexual abuse, the clinician is presented with a number of problems in attempting to validate the complaint. First, few of the cases have any physical corroboration (DeJong, 1986; DeJong et al., 1983). The estimated percentages of those which have physical signs vary widely. Sexually transmitted diseases (STD) have been reported in anywhere from 2%–12% of victims (Cupoli and Sewell, 1988; DeJong, 1986; DeJong et al., 1983; Grant, 1984; Shamroy, 1980; White et al., 1983). The range of female victims which has been noted to have positive physical trauma is between 25% and 33% (Cupoli and Sewell, 1988; DeJong et al., 1983; Ellerstein and Canavan, 1980; Tilelli et al., 1980), while documented trauma in male victims has been reported in 34%–68% of the cases (Ellerstein and Canavan, 1980; Reinhart, 1987; Spencer and Dunklee, 1986).

A second problem in the validation of sexual abuse complaints is that of retractions, whether they be allegations of abuse which are later denied or initial denials which are subsequently reversed. Most clinicians have been faced with both types of situations and have had to make a decision regarding which statement of the two appeared to be most valid. Those children who initially make an allegation which is later denied are often felt to be sensing the negative impact their statement is having upon their own lives and that of their families. The children who initially deny an allegation (usually brought by an adult) and later support the allegation may be described as initially being fearful of the interviewer, of what they perceive they may be doing to their families, and/or of some actual threat made to them by the perpetrator. In some cases the children may be seen as simply echoing the adult's allegation.

Third, in attempting to validate an allegation of sexual abuse, the clinical investigator may be confronted with the problem of interviewing children of special populations who present unique problems. These special populations may include those with sensory losses (e.g., deafness), mental disabilities (e.g., retardation), and/ or communication problems (e.g., language disabilities). These children often require interviewing techniques which the average clinician does not possess.

Fourth, the alleged victim may not appreciate the abusive nature of the alleged events. Victims of sexual abuse have been reported from under 6 months of age (Cupoli and Sewell, 1988; Ellerstein and Canavan, 1980; Farber et al., 1984) to their late teens. It is estimated that from 15%–47% of all documented victims are under 5 years of age (Conte and Berliner, 1981a; DeJong et al., 1983; Mrazek et al., 1983; Shamroy, 1980). These children do not understand that they are indeed victims of abuse.

Fifth, behavioral problems cited as the basis for sexual abuse allegations frequently overlap with other sources of a child's problems. A child's experience with divorce, adjustment problems at home and/or at school, and other situational factors, such as medical problems, may give rise to behavioral and emotional indicators which mimic symptoms arising from abuse. The clinician must be very careful in using behavioral indicators as support for sexual abuse allegations. The only consistently reported behavior in clinical as well as controlled research is that of sexual acting out (Cavaiola and Schiff, 1988; Kolko et al., 1988; Runtz and Briere, 1986), especially in children under 7 years (Friedrich and Reams, 1987; Gale et al., 1988; White et al., 1988a).

Sixth in the list of validation problems is that the alleged perpetrator is often well-known and loved by the child. Younger victims are felt to be more likely abused by members of their intimate social network (Finkelhor, 1979). Of those victims who presented with masked symptoms, the alleged perpetrator was more likely to be the father (Hunter et al., 1985). After family members, the next highest frequency of offenders for females is found among family friends. Percentages range from 23% (DeJong et al., 1983) to 50% (Shamroy, 1980). Sexual abuse by strangers has averaged only between 8% and 25% (Conte and Berliner, 1981b; Grant, 1984; Mrazek et al., 1983; Russell, 1983; Shamroy, 1980).

All of these factors make investigating an allegation of abuse a difficult problem and one which deserves the highest degree of care to detail in order to provide the clinical and judicial systems with the best set of data.

2. BASIC CONCEPTS OF INVESTIGATORY INTERVIEWING

Independence. The primary goal of investigatory interviewing is to document the chronology, context, and consistency of an allegation. The data gathered should be as uncontaminated as possible for use by the mental health and judicial systems. *Contamination* occurs when the source of the child's memory of the alleged event becomes distorted or falsified by factors inside or outside the interview. In order to achieve this goal of uncontaminated data, the interviewer must adhere to two specific concepts: external and internal independence. *External independence* is the evaluator's objective stance of not allying himself/herself with any particular individual involved in the investigation of the allegation (White et al., 1988b). In other words, the evaluator must deal with all individuals on an equal basis, whether they be the alleged victim's mother, father, a parent's lawyer, the prosecutor, or the protective services worker. Care must be taken not to ally oneself with one particular side of the allegation.

Internal independence is the evaluator's internal ability not to be biased relative to the allegation (White et al., 1988b). In practical terms, internal independence is the interviewer's ability not to lead or otherwise influence the data that the child brings to the evaluation. The task of the investigator is to gather the child's information in unaltered form. The internally independent interviewer does not add to or change the child's information by his/her manner of interacting or questioning.

3. MODELS OF INVESTIGATION

Debate continues regarding the interviewer's initial lack of knowledge of the allegation itself. If an interviewer consistently interviews children without knowing the allegation, he/she will come to be believed when he/she testifies that any and all information provided to the court came from the child. While not totally eliminating the possibility of the child being led by the interviewer, the chances are decreased. Disadvantages include the interviewer's being restricted from reviewing the child's background data prior to the interviews, thus forcing the interviewer to work harder to understand the child's developmental status and to obtain the child's story. The interviewer must realize that any information he/she may get from the child may be incomplete, as children tend to make more errors of omission than of commission (Goodman and Aman, 1990). If an evaluator has prior information, he/she is better able to understand the context of the child's complaints but must guard against leading or coercing the child to disclose information consistent with what the evaluator knows of the complaint.

One model of the investigation of child abuse is a two-person abuse team. On such a team one person is the designated *intake* professional and one is the *child interviewer*. In such a system, the intake person is responsible for all the contacts with adults, for securing the background documents, for gathering intake information, and for conducting the initial history sessions. After this person feels there is adequate evidence that a sexual abuse evaluation is in order, he/she then arranges for the child interviewer to see the child. Until this time, the child interviewer knows nothing of the case and then only learns about the child's name, birthdate, and any special qualities the child may have (e.g., language impediment). After the child's interviews, the child interviewer may elect to interview the parental figures on his/her own in spite of having the information from the intake interviewer.

A second model is for one person to be responsible for all the duties of investigation. This is the most common model in current use. Because of the higher probability of losing one's independence in such a one-person system, the clinician must be especially careful to keep all parties on an equal footing and not to contaminate the child's interviews by his/her having prior knowledge of the allegation.

a. Interviewer characteristics

Anyone with adequate child interviewing training and experience may be qualified to interview a child relative to a sexual abuse allegation, including child psychiatrists, child psychologists, clinical social workers, protective services workers, police, pediatricians, or family practitioners. Regardless of the discipline, the interviewer should have certain qualities and characteristics.

(1) The interviewer needs to be able to manage parents in a positive manner. The parents who bring a child for a sexual abuse allegation are frequently quite anxious. Unless properly handled, the parent may become more distraught and transmit this anxiety to the child. Then the child's information may become distorted because of his/her perception of the parent's anxiety and/or he/she may not be able to disclose as he/she might have. By addressing a number of issues in advance, the clinician can frequently ease the anxiety of the parent. These issues include preparation of the parent and child as to *what* will be happening to the child, as well as by *whom*, *where*, and *why* the child will be interviewed alone (to decrease probability of contamination and increase chances of data being utilized by the judicial system). The parent should also be prepared, prior to bringing the child, that the interviewer will not provide immediate feedback unless there is a need for immediate protection of the child. It should be explained that if the parent receives immediate feedback between the child's interviews, there might be an issue of parental contamination raised in subsequent events (i.e., court hearing) regardless of whether or not it actually happened. If these issues were posed in such a way as to help the parent understand that the precautions are really of long-term benefit to the child, he/she is usually less anxious, because he/she knows what to expect and is more helpful in assisting the clinician gain the child's cooperation.

(2) The interviewer must be comfortable in interacting with children of various ages and developmental levels.

(3) The interviewer must have at least a basic knowledge of child development principles. He/she should know what to expect of average children within differing age brackets. Misjudging the child's cognitive or language level may lead the interviewer to pose questions and interactions on an inappropriate developmental level, resulting in ineffective communication with the child.

(4) The interviewer must be skillful in managing a wide range of children's behaviors. Behaviors to be managed in order to obtain the best level of response from the child include shyness, anxiety, tears, manipulation, aggression, and/or temper tantrums.

(5) The interviewer must also be knowledgeable about child sexual abuse dynamics and child witness issues. These fields are changing very rapidly, and the interviewer must remain current regarding the most recent information as it affects his/her interviewing techniques and interpretation of the child's responses.

b. Role confusions

Interviewers must be careful to avoid role confusions. The interviewer must remember that he/she is the professional interviewer, not a therapist or child advocate for any particular case. Techniques of investigation must not be mixed with those of therapy during an assessment of child sexual abuse. In some states, it is a violation of the mental health professional's code of ethics to do both within one case. There needs to be a sharp demarcation between evaluation and therapy. For example, the interviewer must be careful not to provide an emotional interpretation of the events revealed by the child. Comments such as, "I'm sorry this awful thing happened to you . . ." may make the child feel better and may make the interviewer feel he/she is building a stronger relationship with the child. In reality, however, such comments are potentially contaminating in that they are mixing investigation with therapy by providing a value judgment concerning the report of the child's experiences.

A second role confusion often exhibited by interviewers is mixing investigation with inappropriate advocacy. Statements to the referrant such as, "I'm sure she'll tell me what happened . . ." demonstrate a lack of independence on the part of the interviewer. Promising to the child that "nothing like this will ever happen again" is an empty promise in that the interviewer has no way of providing total protection to the child once he/she leaves the office. In addition, telling a child after a disclosure that "things will be better now" is likewise a potentially empty promise because the child who experiences the court proceedings may find that things do not get better for a long time. In fact, for the child himself, things may actually get worse.

A third role confusion to avoid is being the judge or jury. Interviewers must remember that the judge or jury makes the ultimate decision regarding the legal issues. It is not the interviewer's role to decide that Uncle Joe is guilty. The interviewer can have opinions and can provide data from the interview to support these opinions, but it is not the interviewer's responsibility to indicate guilt or innocence in a court of law.

B. Stages of Investigatory Interviewing

1. INTAKE

a. Triaging the initial contact

One of the most important contacts an evaluator in child sexual abuse allegations has is the initial one in which he/she is first approached about evaluating an alleged victim. An evaluator may become acquainted with an allegation of sexual abuse in several ways. First, he/she may be a legally mandated evaluator in that he/she must investigate any and all allegations. Such a role is taken by protective services workers and/or police. There is usually no choice as to *if* the allegation is investigated; the choice is *how, when, where*, etc.

For the nonlegally mandated evaluators, the decision whether or not to investigate is voluntary. He/she may refer the complainant to those legally mandated to investigate the evaluation or may decide to evaluate the allegation himself/herself. Mental health professionals in clinic settings, private practice, and/or hospital settings are frequently faced with this decision. The referrals to these individuals may arise in one of several ways. First, the complainant may be a parent (usually a mother) who requests the clinician to evaluate her child because of her own suspicion of abuse. Second, the complaint may become known to the clinician through an attorney representing one side of a custody dispute. Third, the clinician may be asked by a court to provide an independent evaluation. Fourth, the legally mandated agencies (e.g., protective services) may ask the clinician for his/her special expertise in the evaluation of a case already known to that agency.

b. Intake questions

A number of questions need to be answered to assist the evaluator in deciding whether or not to take the referral. One of the primary issues to be clarified relates to the marital status of the child's parents. Information about separation, divorce, court actions, visitation, and custody arrangements must be an integral part of the initial intake procedure. The clinician must ascertain what each party is seeking and if there are other family members (e.g., grandparents) who are trying to be included. This data are helpful in establishing the context of the complaint. It also provides questions for further exploration such as the pattern of the child's visitations and the reasons for any interruption or symptoms related to contact with the visiting parent.

A second area of intake investigation on the clinician's part is the assessment of any previous evaluation(s) the child has experienced. Unless directly asked, many parents do not volunteer that the child has had an evaluation prior to the one presently being sought. The clinician must be careful not to become one of a number of evaluators who have agreed to see the child without knowing that others have preceded him/her. The degree of contamination in such cases can be extremely high. Thus as a part of the intake procedure, the clinician should routinely ask about any previous evaluations the child has had regarding the issue at hand. The clinician should be especially cautious in determining the circumstances of any previous evaluations. Information to be gathered includes the location of the previous evaluation, who was present, who the evaluator was, and his/her training, techniques utilized, number of sessions, type of documentation, who received feedback, and any contamination and/or inadequacies present. It is the wise clinician who does not accept the referral until he/she has been thoroughly convinced that any previous evaluation was inadequate *and* that he/she can provide information which will be helpful in sorting out the allegation.

c. Clarification of issues

Upon receiving any telephone call or formal contact requesting the clinician to evaluate any young child, the present-day clinician must be cautious to ascertain whether or not an evaluation concerning sexual abuse is being requested. There are numerous ways complainants gain the clinician's agreement to see the child for an abuse evaluation when the clinician believes he/she is seeing the child for, among other things, a behavioral evaluation, an emotional status exam, a school adjustment issue, reaction to divorce, and so forth. Direct inquiry should be made as to whether or not there are any concerns of unsafe or abusive acts by others.

In all cases of mental health evaluation, the clinician should make sure that the referrant knows the *clinician's areas of competence.* For instance, someone who specializes in adolescent and adult evaluations should not allow himself/herself to be pressured into evaluating a young child. Or, the child clinician who has expertise in evaluating parenting skills, but not in chemical dependency, should not agree to provide the referrant an evaluation on how the father's alcoholism affects his propensity to perpetrate the alleged abuse.

The clinician should have the attorney clarify any legal issues in the case being referred. This permits the clinician to decide if he/she has competence in the relevant area. The clinician may also wish to request a copy of relevant statute or case law to clarify the focus of the evaluation (for example, in a case of parental termination).

Lastly, the clinician should clarify his/her posture regarding his/her willingness to testify on the ultimate legal issue. Each state has its own guidelines regarding to which opinions an expert witness may testify. In addition, some clinicians may favor leaving the ultimate decision to the legally mandated factfinder (judge or jury).

d. Clinician's requirements

If the clinician accepts the referral, some practical elements should be discussed with the referrant. The clinician should emphasize his/her stance regarding independence and should attempt to become court-appointed if at all possible. In the absence of court appointment, the clinician should obtain a written agreement between the parents and their attorneys regarding the independent status of the clinician.

Another practical issue is the clinician's time constraints. If he/she is being asked to provide an evaluation of sexual abuse in the midst of a custody dispute, he/she must find out if there is a court hearing already scheduled. If there is, the clinician must ascertain if there is adequate time to complete the evaluation. The estimated time must include the availability of the child and parents, the time to gather other documents, and the time to write the report.

e. Document gathering

In addition to a copy of any evaluation previously done on the alleged victim, other sources of information must be gathered as quickly as possible. These documents include any mental health evaluation of the child or either parent, school records and teacher reports, medical examinations, police reports, and, if applicable, copies of court filings. Of course a legal custodian must sign for the release of the child's records, and each adult must sign for his/her own materials. If the parents had been seen for marital counselling, both must sign for the release of such materials. Without these materials, the results of the evaluation may not be considered complete in assessing all possible sources of the allegation.

2. DOCUMENTATION

a. Why?

Documentation of the clinician's contacts and interviews needs to be meticulously kept in order to show the chronology of the investigation and how the disclosure, if any, emerged through the various stages of the evaluation. Documentation should preserve the initial complaint to professionals. Documentation of the child's statements facilitates the clinician's presentation of the data in court and helps to counter any attacks concerning contamination. Good documentation should demonstrate the clinician's attention to maintaining independence.

b. What?

Documentation should be made regarding any and all contacts with anyone in the case, including telephone calls, from the initial call to the end. The file should contain a collection of any failed and/or cancelled appointments and the reason for such. All interviews, whether with the child, parent, or others (including attorneys), should be documented. The total time of each contact should also be noted.

c. Methods

The most usual means of documentation is that of written notes, preferably taken contemporaneously with the event. The clinician who trusts his/her memory to keep the details of such important interviews until a later time for transcribing or dictating is not acknowledging the very real possibility that important details are lost, that quotes are mistakenly remembered, and that a child's concomitant behaviors are frequently underemphasized and not reported.

A second means of documentation is through audiotaping. While helpful in reconstructing the events, audiotaping omits a major portion of data: the behavioral reactions of each participant in the interview. As humans, we transmit important messages through nonverbal communication, and this information is not captured on audiotape.

The best means of documentation is videotaping the entire interview. By capturing the behavioral reactions of both the child and interviewer, others will know what occurred during the interview and what is the degree of contamination. The interviewer's skills are shown. If the clinician's skills were adequate and there is little to no contamination, the chances of the child's being subjected to multiple investigations are decreased.

Problems with videotaping the interview include the highlighting of any interviewer errors. In addition, parts of the videotapes may be used out of context or inconsistencies of the child's revelations may be highlighted during a court hearing. In such instances, it would be the clinician's job to explain the proper context and/or why the child appeared to be inconsistent in his/her report. In addition, the videotape process may prove distracting for the child as well as for the interviewer.

Regardless of these disadvantages, however, videotaping is still considered the best means of interview documentation.

3. INTERVIEWS

For parents who are separated or divorced, some clinicians prefer to offer the parents separate interviews. Others, however, contend that more information is gathered in interviews in which both parents are present, regardless of their marital status. When both parents are present they often keep each other honest.

The parental interviews should be carefully scheduled so that there is relative balance in number and timing. If the parents are being seen separately, the interviews should occur so that all of one parent's interviews are not done prior to those of the other parent. Whether or not the child is seen before or after the parents' interviews depends upon the model of investigation the clinician has developed. In a two-person system, the child is usually seen after the parents. In a one-person system, the child is sometimes seen very early in the process in order to minimize the interviewer's use of information from the parent to interview the child.

The child is always seen alone. While there are some who suggest that children may be interviewed with a supportive adult present (Boat and Everson, 1986; MacFarlane and Krebs, 1986; Sgroi et al., 1982), others are adamantly opposed

(Friedeman and Morgan, 1985; White et al., 1988b) because of the problem with parental contamination. Even with the most understanding and supportive parent, there are factors which may contaminate the child's disclosure. The child may feel he/she must satisfy the perceived expectations of the parents and/or not hurt their feelings by revealing the experience. Children may also feel they will get into trouble if sensitive information is revealed in front of the parent because the parent has always lectured them on not letting anyone touch their private parts. When the reasons for interviewing the child alone are explained to parents, the overwhelming majority become supportive of such independent interviews.

When custody and visitation are at issue in addition to a sexual abuse complaint the child should be seen for additional appointments in order to observe the child's interaction with each parent. The clinician performing this set of interviews should be the one doing the custody/visitation assessment. The purpose of this set of interviews is not to further determine the credibility of the allegation but rather to observe the quality of the overall relationship between the child and each parent. These data are often helpful in recommending the nature and frequency of any contact between the child and the alleged perpetrator. Much resistance should be anticipated in attempting to set up such appointments.

a. Parent interviews

Psychosocial issues. There are a number of psychosocial issues which must be clarified either in the intake or during the parental interviews. Especially in cases involving divorce and/or visitation/custody, a chronology of escalating allegations should be documented to ascertain if previous attempts by the complainant have not been successful in changing the visitation/custody arrangements. The possible utility of the allegation as perceived by the complainant and child should be assessed, especially as it relates to custody and visitation changes. The complainant's potential for deceptive motives should be addressed, including the possibility of that person's having a major mental illness which may lead him/her to distort reality. The clinician should also be aware of any person involved in the case who repeatedly sexualizes relationships.

The child's baseline sexual behavior and sexual knowledge as well as the presence of overstimulation should be assessed. A listing of those individuals who come in contact with the child should be made. A good history of the child's symptoms should be made, including the date of initial appearance, any increases or decreases in symptom severity, and the coexistence of other stresses which have occurred. The clinician should also investigate the child's fears or alienation, which might be fueling the allegation.

Family history. From each parent, a thorough family history is necessary. This history should include a review of each parent's family of origin, the parents' dating, marriage, divorce, and remarriage history, a review of each child's history in the family, the presence of significant others, history of abuse or neglect of any member (adult or child), and an evaluation of significant mental and/or physical health problems of all family members. Efforts to obtain a conception of the family's daily living patterns, their traditions concerning privacy and nudity, their approach to sexuality and sex education, and the child's exposure to sexually explicit materials and activities need to be made.

Child's history. Information from each parent should be gathered regarding his/her memory of the child's own history, including prenatal, birth, developmental, medical, caregiving, school, significant separations, and present living circumstances. Significant behavioral or emotional problems should be investigated also.

b. Child interviews

Number of interviews. The child is to be interviewed two to three times. If only one interview is conducted, there is a problem of trying to judge consistency of the complaint as well as allowing the child time to feel comfortable enough to reveal sensitive secrets. Over three interviews increases the chances of the child's feeling coerced into elaborating the story and/or the degree of contamination of the child's story by the interviewer.

Environment and materials. The interview environment needs to be in a quiet private place, away from telephones and beepers. The room should have toys appropriate for the child's age and developmental level. For the preschool child, this includes, among other items, markers and paper, play telephones (2), doll house, and trucks and cars. There should not be an overabundance of toys which may distract the child, causing the interviewer to have a more difficult time in getting the child to pay attention to the abuse interview.

The use of anatomical dolls continues but also is debated on a number of fronts. For a review of the doll debate, see White and Santilli (1988) and White (1988). For suggestions on the use of the dolls, see White (1991).

Anatomical dolls continue to be utilized, and the primary topic of debate is whether or not the presentation of dolls sets the stage for the child to give a false disclosure and/or to encourage the child to exhibit sexualized behaviors (Yates and Terr, 1988a,b). Even though the research data on anatomical dolls are rather sparse, those studies which have been published in refereed journals indicate that for nonreferred children (and assumed to be nonabused), the dolls do *not* encourage false reporting or sexualized play (Glaser and Collins, 1989; Sivan et al., 1988). Several studies have also found that children who had been referred for a sexual abuse evaluation and/or who had been diagnosed as being abused presented more sexualized play with the dolls than their nonreferred counterparts (August and Foreman, 1989; Jampole and Weber, 1987; White et al., 1986).

In addition to the clinical arguments concerning doll usage, the appellate courts have consistently ruled doll usage to be appropriate in the preparation of a witness by a prosecuting attorney (*State v. Eggert*, 358 N.W. 2d, 1984), as anatomically "correct" (*Commonwealth v. Reid*, 511 N.E. 2d 331, 1987; *Cleaveland v. State*, 490 N.E. 2d 1140, 1986), and as props during a victim's court testimony (*Kehinde v. Commonwealth*, 338 S.E. 2d 356, 1986; *People v. Rich*, 520 N.Y.S. 2d 911, 1987). Some jurisdictions have indicated that the dolls should be considered a psychological test (*In re Amber B. v. Ron B.*, 236 Cal. Rptr. 623, 1987), while others have totally rejected the test argument (*Rinesmith v. Williams*, 376 N.W. 2d 139, 1985). More importantly, however, are the conclusions several courts have reached which indicated that dolls were coupled with inappropriate interviewing techniques to produce contaminated evidence for the courts (*In re J. H.*, 505 N.E. 2d 1360, 1987; *In the matter of X v. Syme*, 714 P. 2d 13, 1986). Appellate decisions involving doll interviews fulfilling the criteria for various hearsay exceptions can be found on both sides, supportive or rejecting. For a review of the doll picture, see White and Santilli (1988) and White (1988).

Materials which are felt to be inappropriate for use in a clinical evaluation of sexual abuse include materials which have been designed to promote sexual education and/or abuse prevention, puppets, media materials (e.g., newspapers, TV footage), or lineups of suspected perpetrators.

Freeplay. There are two major parts of a child sexual abuse interview: freeplay and the structured interview. The freeplay portion is designed to achieve several goals: first, to allow the child *and* interviewer to become comfortable in the room and with each other; second, to establish a positive rapport between the two; third, to allow the interviewer to informally assess the child's developmental levels.

The developmental abilities to be assessed include the child's suggestibility, ability to deceive, cognitive style and level, and language and speech abilities. It should be remembered that children's memory, as adults', is basically divided into two types: free recall and recognition. When a child is able to reveal information through free recall by open-ended nonleading questions, there is more likelihood that the information is coming from the child's own memory unless there is proof of prior contamination factors. To get to a child's recognition memory, leading cues must be provided.

In assessing a child's ability to deceive or distort, the clinician must assess if the child appears to be pursuing a goal by lying (e.g., change of custody or visitation), if the child echoes the adult's report, and/or if the child's presentation is consistent with a mental disorder which could compromise a child's capacity to perceive reality.

The level of sexual knowledge must be part of a sexual abuse assessment. Efforts must be made to match that expected for that child with what is known about his/her cultural and class background. Even though it is known that preschoolers and early latency age children have little explicit sexual knowledge and that children's major information about sexual matters concerns pregnancy and birth (Bernstein and Cowan, 1975; Goldman and Goldman, 1982), each child's understanding must be individually assessed relative to his/her own culture and background because of widely differing levels of knowledge.

Structured interview. After the freeplay portion of the interview, a structured interview should be administered. There are several available methods for interviewing (Conerly, 1986; MacFarland and Krebs, 1986; Sgroi et al., 1982), utilizing various materials and degrees of structure (Boat and Everson, 1986; Friedman and Morgan, 1985; White et al., 1987). It is the authors' recommendation that a structured interview be completed with each child for a number of reasons. First, the structured interview can specifically address the child's level of sexual knowledge, especially if dolls or anatomical drawings are employed on a systematic basis. Second, all children will be receiving the same basic interview technique, and their responses can be compared. Third, charges that the interviewer is contaminating the child's story by using leading questions can be better defended if the interviewer has a structured and consistent manner of interviewing children.

4. CREDIBILITY OF ALLEGATIONS OF SEXUAL ABUSE

The investigating clinician should document and discuss factors which argue for or against the validity of the allegation. The strongest validation criteria are based upon documenting explicit sexual experiences with a progression of sexual acts over time described by the child. The interviewer should look for sexual experiences beyond the child's expected knowledge or experience, a description told from the child's viewpoint and vocabulary, and an emotional response consistent with the nature of the abuse. The assessment of a sexual abuse complaint should also include possible motivations for the issuance of a false sexual abuse complaint by either the child or the adult (Quinn, 1988).

Several clinical factors should not be used to assess the credibility of a child's complaint. For example, so-called behavioral indicators often lack specificity for sexual abuse as the stressor. The only consistently reported behavior in clinical as well as controlled research is that of sexual acting out, especially in children under age 7 (Friedrich and Reams, 1987). The child's feelings towards an alleged perpetrator are also not specific validation criteria. A child often wants the relationship maintained but the abuse to stop. On the other hand, children may become alienated from a parent for many reasons other than abuse.

False sexual abuse allegations remain rare. The most likely explanation for a false allegation is either misperception or distortion by the child or parent bringing a complaint or a conscious lie by a parent to deceive regarding the complaint. Particular concern has recently been focused on leading or coercive investigatory techniques which may result in a false assessment of a complaint (Quinn, 1988). The techniques described in this chapter should assist investigators in avoiding such pitfalls.

5. EVALUATION RESULTS

In analyzing the data available, the clinician must look at a large number of factors which may have influenced the child's report of the allegation. Figure 9.1 (Data Influences: Quinn et al., 1989) summarizes these factors. The clinician has the responsibility to assess each area and report the effects of each in the final report. Failure to do so provides the judicial system with an incomplete report. Clinicians and other professionals in the field must recognize that the interview process itself can distort the child's data and/or allow for the incorporation of foreign data into the child's report. It is critical that interviewers do their best not to allow such intrusions to occur.

C. Pitfalls of Investigation

After an evaluation has been completed, each interviewer should review his/ her own work for evidence of contamination as well as evidence of how other factors may have altered the child's responses between the initial disclosure and

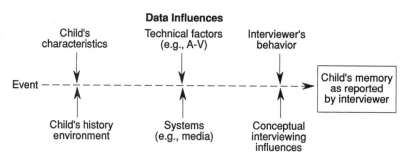

Figure 9.1

the present time. In the following discussion, a number of pitfalls are described which should be examined for their presence as well as for their effect on disclosures of sexual abuse.

1. AGENDA

An agenda is "the conscious or unconscious effort on the part of the interviewer to have the child describe, confirm, or verify the interviewer's assumptions concerning the allegation" (White and Quinn, 1988:270). While it is apparent that everyone has some purpose when interviewing a child, those individuals who do not recognize that they do and make no provisions for decreasing an agenda's influence on the child's interview are making a serious mistake. Such individuals often use specific techniques, such as leading or coercion, to obtain the information they are determined to confirm.

2. LEADING

Leading is "the introduction of specific material [into the interview] which the child has not previously revealed to that interviewer" (White et al., 1988b). Leading material is frequently introduced through yes-no questions (e.g., "Didn't he put his hand in your pants?") and/or multiple choice questions (e.g., "Was it Joe, Harry, or Sam who did that to you?"). When the child shakes his/her head or responds with one of these names, the interviewer with an agenda is satisfied: the child has confirmed the information provided by someone else. In reality, however, the interviewer does not really know what the child's response meant, because the child did not provide additional information spontaneously. The person with a strong agenda will then report to the judicial system and/or parent that the child actually "told" him/her something. This is an extremely inappropriate conclusion to make.

3. DISCONFIRMATION

Disconfirmation occurs when the interviewer refuses to accept a child's answer and then institutes one of several techniques to influence the child in a new direction (White and Quinn, 1988) Everyone has disconfirmed a child at some time. When we ask our children, "Do you want to go to bed now?" we're really saying, "You are going to bed whether you want to or not." When the child responds, "No, not yet," we disconfirm his/her answer by saying, "Well, yes, you are." This is an example of disconfirmation followed by coercion. In an abuse interview, the person with a strong agenda will frequently tell the child he/she is wrong or will ignore a child's answer unless it is consistent with the interviewer's preconceived idea of the abuse.

4. COERCION

When an interviewer uses his/her position of authority in an attempt to pressure the child to answer in a manner consistent with expectations of that interviewer, coercion is being used. There are many ways coercion is exhibited, including questioning about the child's knowledge of truth, reinforcement with tangible items, repetitive questioning, and actual threats. Although numerous clinicians inquire about a child's truthfulness through several means (e.g., "You know what truth is, now, don't you?"; "If I say this dress is red, am I telling the truth?";

"Now today, we're going to tell the truth, aren't we?"; and "If you don't tell me the truth, I'm not going to let you see your mommy again."). Regardless of how a child responds to any of these statements, there is no guarantee that the child either knows what truth means or that he/she intends to always speak the truth to the interviewer. Truth-lie questioning really belongs to the area of competency qualification for being a witness. Only within the jurisdiction of judicial proceedings does the factfinder (judge or jury) have the obligation to listen and make a judgment regarding the child's understanding of truth and determination to speak it. This becomes part of the child's credibility. When truth-lie paradigms are used in interviewing, it is essentially a coercive technique.

Other coercive techniques include offering a child food, drink, or a tangible present during contacts with the interviewer. While such reinforcements may or may not be influential in getting the child to answer in a certain direction, they are best left to others to give in order to maintain the appearance of interviewer neutrality.

Still another technique of coercion is that of repetitive questioning. When we do not like the answers children give, we often question them again and again until they produce the desired response. For instance, "Who spilled this milk?" will often receive a "Not me." response. Knowing full well who spilled the milk, the parent will repeat the question until the culprit finally confesses. Investigatory interviewers also have been known to use this technique. For example, upon receiving no response to "Jenny, who touched you?", the interviewer rephrases it, "Jenny, I know somebody did. Now who touched you?". Repetition of such questions signals to the child that she is not giving the answer the interviewer wants to confirm his/her agenda.

The most serious form of coercion is that of threatening the child with a potentially serious consequence if he/she does not cooperate. A common threat is, "You cannot see your mother again until you tell me who hurt you." Such a threat is inappropriate in investigatory interviewing.

5. Interviewer's behaviors

An interviewer must be aware that his/her physical and verbal behaviors may alter a child's response to questions. A clinician can alert a child to the fact that he/she has just given a "good" answer by the clinician becoming more positive by touch and/or voice. Similarly, a clinician can tell a child nonverbally when he/she is not providing the "proper" answers. Table 9.1 (Quinn et al., 1989) illustrates the many ways such interview influences arise.

TABLE 9.1   INTERVIEWER'S BEHAVIORAL INFLUENCES

	Communication of Emotions	*Inappropriate Patterns*	*Discontinuity*
VOICE	Overly solicitous Inapprop. reward Harsh, cold tone	Inappropriate level	Tone change
PHYSICAL	Controlling Caressing Interfering/grabbing	Body posture Anatomy ID	Position changes

Reprinted with permission from Bull Am Acad Psychiatry Law, Vol. 17, No. 1, 1989.

6. TECHNICAL FACTORS

While videotaping is the best way to document an interview with a child, there are potentially contaminating factors. If the equipment is set up in the same room with the child, it may become too distracting and/or anxiety provoking for the child. In addition, the child may wish to continually see how he/she looks on the TV monitor. Third, unless warned specifically, the child may think that he/she will appear on the 6 o'clock news tonight. The child needs to be informed regarding the future use of the videotape. Fourth, some interviewers have emphasized the use of videotape by continually telling the child to speak into the microphone or to be sure and sit on the "X" so the TV can see the child.

7. SYSTEMS FACTORS

Systems contamination is a result of the factors outside the interviewer's control which may directly affect the data reflected in the interview. Such factors may arise from the media, peers, school officials, neighbors, etc. While the interviewer cannot control such factors, he/she can review the effect he/she thinks they had on the child's disclosures and can discuss this impact in the interview report.

8. PARENTAL FACTORS

When a parent interrogates a child relative to suspicion of abuse through leading and/or coercive techniques, the child's memory for the events may become distorted. This is parental contamination. The clinician should guide the parent into not interviewing the child; however, frequently the damage is done prior to the child's coming into contact with the professionals. Still the clinician can caution the parent about the reasons not to repeatedly interview the child.

IV: CASE EXAMPLE EPILOGUES

A. Case Example 1

Several months after the first set of interviews the investigators became concerned that their techniques would be criticized. They redid the interviews, this time separating the children and using an interview protocol which contained a series of questions surveying the child's knowledge of body parts and screening for abuse. The children were much less forthcoming at the time of the second set of interviews, denying all sexual abuse. Due to the inconsistencies between the interviews and the poor techniques used initially, the prosecutor decided not to include these children in the pending lawsuit against the daycare. Repetitive nightmares and traumatic play suggested that the children had been abused in some way.

B. Case Example 2

The social worker for the department of human services initially worked up the case by interviewing the girl in her mother's home and made no attempt to interview the father. However, a psychiatrist associated with the domestic relations court consulted with the worker and recommended an interview of the child at a neutral site, the social worker's office, and contact with the father. A series of two interviews with the girl revealed a consistent history of fondling and nudity within the father's home. The disclosure was noted to be in age-appropriate language with unique details such as who said what to whom. The social worker, after her initial skepticism that this might be a false allegation, concluded that the abuse was substantiated. The case was scheduled to be heard in domestic relations court to determine what, if any, contact between the father and daughter would be permitted.

C. Case Example 3

The intake worker, upon hearing this history, decided that additional expertise would be required on this case. She called the local hospital-affiliated sex abuse team and asked to speak to the coordinator. The two professionals decided that a senior member of the sexual abuse team with experience in early childhood development and special-needs children would interview the child while the social service personnel watched behind a one-way mirror. The two interviews which were conducted over the next several days appeared to indicate that the 3-year-old was describing hygienic touching as opposed to abuse. The family readily decided to change their handling of the 3-year-old's toileting. No other over-stimulating or inappropriate experiences were detailed during the evaluation. The 3-year-old was also referred for a speech and language assessment.

V. ACTION GUIDE

A. General principles

1. *Document* the chronology, context, and consistency of complaint.
2. *Establish* principles of independence.
   a. *External independence*: not allying oneself with any particular individual involved in investigation.
   b. *Internal independence*: not allowing oneself to be biased relative to the allegations.
3. *Gather* uncontaminated data for the court system.
4. *Establish* evaluation roles.
   a. *Intake worker* who obtains allegation information, makes contacts with appropriate individuals, gathers documents, explains procedures.
   b. *Child interviewer* whose primary task is to interview the child in the least contaminating manner possible.

B. Interviewer requirements

1. *Be skilled* in managing parental behaviors, emotions, reactions.
2. *Be comfortable* interacting with children.
3. *Have knowledge* of basic child development principles.
4. *Be skillful* in managing a wide range of children's behaviors.
5. *Remain current* with regard to child witness and child sexual abuse literature.
6. *Maintain reliability* and expertise in a disciplined interviewing format.

C. Avoiding role confusions

1. *Maintain* evaluation stance rather than engage in therapeutic procedures.
2. *Avoid* emotional interpretation of events to child.
3. *Remember* who is trier of fact (judge/jury).
4. *Maintain* independence by avoiding inappropriate advocacy.

D. Triaging intake

1. *Determine* whether evaluation by clinician is mandatory or voluntary. If possible, get court-appointed status.
2. *Determine* ability to perform requested evaluation; *learn* the legal issues at stake.
3. *Assess* amount of time available for necessary procedures and availability for any court procedures.
4. *Inform* participants of financial considerations.
5. *Assess* divorce, custody, visitation arrangements.
6. *Obtain* pertinent court information.
7. *Assess* quality of any previous evaluations, including who did it, kind of training, techniques utilized, availability of written report, who received feedback, contaminatory influences.
8. *Determine* levels of documentation to be utilized (e.g., audiotaping, videotaping, written report, etc.).

E. Interviews

1. *Arrange* for parental interviews, separate and balanced, if desire to see each parent separately.
2. *Obtain* psychosocial, family, and child histories from each parent.
3. *Make* appointments for child interviews, informing parent of need to see child alone.
4. *Prepare* child interview room with minimum number of toys and desired evaluation materials.
5. *Establish* freeplay period for child, with goals of (a) making child comfortable and relaxing interviewer, (b) rapport building, (c) informal developmental assessment of memory, suggestibility, capacity to lie, cognitive style, and level of sexual knowledge.
6. *Guide* child through structured interview.

F. Ancillary services

1. *Arrange for* psychological testing, if indicated.
2. *Refer* for medical exam if not already done.

G. Assessment of contamination

1. *Assess* degree of one's agenda relative to use of (a) leading, (b) disconfirmation, and/or (c) coercive techniques.
2. *Review* interviews for effect of interviewer's behaviors which may have affected child's responses.

3. *Judge* technical, system, and/or parental factors which may have influenced child (videotaping, intensive questioning, etc.).

H. Report writing

1. *Complete* report, including (a) referral information, (b) time, place, and participants of each contact, (c) background information, (d) behavioral observations, (e) type of procedures utilized in evaluation, (f) information gathered from interview, (g) testing report if done, (h) impressions, (i) diagnosis, and (j) recommendations.
2. *Include* degree of factors which may have affected child's responses in past as well as present evaluations.

VI. SUGGESTED READINGS

August, R. and Forman, B. (1989), A comparison of sexually abused and nonsexually abused children's behavioral responses to anatomically correct dolls. Child Psychiatry Hum Dev 20:39–47.

Bernstein, A. C. and Cowan, P. A. (1975), Children's concepts of how people get babies. Child Dev 46:77–91.

Black's Law Dictionary (1979), 5th ed. St. Paul, Minnesota: West Publishing Co.

Boat, B. and Everson, M. (1986), Using Anatomical Dolls: Guidelines For Interviewing Young Children in Sexual Abuse Investigations. Chapel Hill, N.C.: University of North Carolina.

Bulkley, J. (1985), Child Sexual Abuse and the Law. 5th ed. Washington, D.C.: American Bar Association.

Burgdorf, K. (1981), Results of the National Incidence Study. Washington, D.C.: National Center on Child Abuse and Neglect.

Cavaiola, A. A. and Schiff, M. (1988), Behavior sequelae of physical and/or sexual abuse in adolescents. Child Abuse Negl 12:181–188.

Conerly, S. (1986), Assessment of suspected child sexual abuse. In: MacFarlane, K. and Waterman, J. (eds.): Sexual Abuse of Young Children: Evaluation and Treatment. New York: Guilford: 30–51.

Conte, J. R. and Berliner, L. (1981a), Prosecution of the offender in cases of sexual assault against children. Victimology 6:102–109.

Conte, J. R. and Berliner, L. (1981b), Sexual abuse of children: implications for practice. Soc Casework: J Contemp Soc Work 62:601–606.

Cupoli, J. M. and Sewell, P. M. (1988), One thousand fifty-nine children with a chief complaint of sexual abuse. Child Abuse Negl 12:151–162.

DeJong, A. R. (1986), Sexually transmitted diseases in sexually abused children. Sex Transm Dis 13:123–126.

DeJong, A. R., Hervada, A., and Emmett, G. (1983), Epidemiological variations in childhood sexual abuse. Child Abuse Negl 7:155–162.

Ellerstein, N. and Canavan, J. W. (1980), Sexual abuse of boys. J Dis Child 134:255–257.

Farber, E. D., Showers, J., Johnson, C. F., Joseph, J. A., and Oshins, L. (1984), The sexual abuse of children: a comparison of male and female victims. J Clin Child Psychol 13:294–297.

Finkelhor, D. (1979), Sexually victimized children. New York: Free Press.

Friedemann, V. and Morgan, M. (1985), Interviewing Sexual Abuse Victims Using Anatomical Dolls: The Professional's Guidebook. Eugene, Oregon: Shamrock Press.

Friedrich, W. N. and Reams, R. A. (1987), Course of psychological symptoms in sexually abused young children. Psychotherapy 24:160–170.

Gale, J., Thompson, R. J., Moran, T. and Sack, W. H. (1988), Sexual abuse in young children: its clinical presentation and characteristic patterns. Child Abuse Negl 12:163–170.

Glaser, D. and Collins, C. (1989), The response of young, non-sexually abused children to anatomically correct dolls. J Child Psychol Psychiatry 30:547–560.

Goldman, R. and Goldman, J. (1982), Children's Sexual Thinking: A Comparative Study of Children Aged 5 to 15 in Australia, North America, Britain and Sweden. London: Routledge & Kegan Paul.

Goodman, G. and Aman, C. (1990). Children's use of anatomically correct dolls to report an event. Child Dev 61:1859–1871.

Grant, L. J. (1984), Assessment of child sexual abuse: eighteen months' experience at the Child Protection Center. Am J Obstet Gynecol 148:617–620.

Hunter, R. S., Kilstrom, N. and Loda, F. (1985), Sexually abused children: identifying masked presentations in a medical setting. Child Abuse Negl 9:17–25.

Jampole, L. and Weber, M. (1987), An assessment of the behavior of sexually abused and nonsexually abused children with anatomically correct dolls. Child Abuse Negl 11:187–192.

Kolko, D. J., Moser, J. T. and Weldy, S. R. (1988), Behavioral/emotional indicators of sexual abuse in child psychiatric inpatients: a controlled comparison with physical abuse. Child Abuse Negl 12:529–541.

MacFarlane, K. and Krebs, S. (1986), Techniques of interviewing and evidence gathering. In: MacFarlane, K. and Waterman, J. (eds.): Sexual Abuse of Young Children: Evaluation and Treatment. New York: Guilford: 67–100.

Monoghan, J. (ed.). (1980), Who Is the Client? Washington, D.C.: American Psychological Association.

Mrazek, P. J., Lynch, M. A. and Bentovim, A. (1983), Sexual abuse of children in the United Kingdom. Child Abuse Negl 7:147–153.

Quinn, K. M. (1988), The credibility of children's allegations of sexual abuse. Behav Sci Law 6:181–200.

Quinn, K. M., White, S. and Santilli, G. (1989), Influences of an interview's behaviors in child sexual abuse investigations. Bull Am Acad Psychiatry Law 17:45–52.

Reinhart, M. A. (1987), Sexually abused boys. Child Abuse Negl 11:229–235.

Rogers, C. (1982), Child sexual abuse and the courts: preliminary findings. J Soc Work Hum Sexual 1:145–153.

Runtz, M. and Briere, J. (1986), Adolescent "acting out" and childhood history of sexual abuse victims. J Interpers Viol 1:326–334.

Russell, D. E. H. (1983), The incidence and prevalence of intrafamilial and extrafamilial sexual abuse of female children. Child Abuse Negl 7:133–146.

Sgroi, S. M., Porter, F. S. and Blick, L. C. (1982), Validation of child sexual abuse. In: Sgroi, S. M. (ed.) Handbook of Clinical Intervention in Child Sexual Abuse. Lexington, MA: Heath: 39–80.

Shamroy, J. (1980), A perspective on childhood sexual abuse. Soc Work 25:128–131.

Sivan, A., Schor, D. P., Koeppl, G. K. and Noble, L. D. (1988), Interaction of normal children with anatomical dolls. Child Abuse Negl 12:295–304.

Spencer, M. J. and Dunklee, P. (1986), Sexual abuse of boys. Pediatrics 78:133–138.

Tilelli, J. A., Turek, D. and Jaffe, A. C. (1980), Sexual abuse of children: clinical findings and implications for management. N Engl J Med 302:319–323.

White, S. (1991). Using Anatomically Detailed Dolls in Interviewing Preschoolers. In: Schafer, C., Gitlin, K., and Sandgrund, A. (ed.): Play Diagnosis and Assessment. New York: John Wiley.

White, S. (1988), Should investigatory use of anatomical dolls be defined by the courts? J Interpers Viol 3:471–475.

White, S., Halpin, B., Strom, G. A. and Santilli, G. (1988a), Behavioral comparisons of young sexually abused, neglected, and nonreferred children. J Clin Child Psychol 17:53–61.

White, S. and Quinn, K. M. (1988), Investigatory independence in child sexual abuse evaluations: conceptual considerations. Bull Am Acad Psychiatry Law 16:269–273.

White, S. and Santilli, G. (1988), A review of clinical practices and research data on anatomical dolls. J Interpers Viol 3:430–422.

White, S., Santilli, G. and Quinn, K. M. (1988b), Child evaluator's roles in child sexual abuse assessments. In: Nicholson, E. B. and Bulkley, J. (eds.): Sexual Abuse Allegations in Custody and Visitation Cases. Washington, D.C.: American Bar Association National Legal Resource Center for Child Advocacy and Protection: 94–105.

White, S., Strom, G., Santilli, G. and Halpin, B. (1986), Interviewing young children with anatomically correct dolls. Child Abuse Negl 10:519–529.

White, S., Strom, G., Santilli, G. and Quinn, K. M. (1987), Clinical guidelines for interviewing young children with anatomically correct dolls. Cleveland, Ohio: Case Western Reserve University School of Medicine. Unpublished manuscript.

White, S. T., Loda, F. A., Ingram, D. L. and Pearson, A. (1983), Sexually transmitted diseases in sexually abused children. Pediatrics 72:16–21.

Yates, A. and Terr, L. (1988a), Debate forum: Anatomically correct dolls: should they be used as a basis for expert testimony? Am Acad Child Adolesc Psychiatry 27:254–257.

Yates, A. and Terr, L. (1988b), Debate forum: Issue continued: Anatomically correct dolls: should they be used as a basis for expert testimony? J Am Acad Child Adoles Psychiatry 27:387–388.

10

Intervention in Child Abuse

ELI H. NEWBERGER, M.D.

I. CLINICAL EXAMPLES

A. Case Example 1

A 3-week-old white boy is brought to the hospital emergency room by his mother. She informs the nurse and the physician that within the half hour, the baby awakened in the middle of the night as he always does. It was his father's turn to go into the baby's room and to give him a bottle. The mother reports that she was half awake and that she heard what she thought was a slap. She went into the child's room and saw a developing area of bruising on the face. She said she was frightened and brought the child promptly to the hospital.

The medical staff conducts an examination which indicates that the child is neurologically intact and has a single area of bruising. They admit the child to the hospital for observation and for protection.

The following morning, there is conflict with regard to the management of the case. The assigned private physician indicates that he would prefer to not call the case one of child abuse and to make a mandated report, as law requires. He reports that he has known the child's father, a physician, for many years and would prefer to call the case an "accident" in order not to take action which might stigmatize the man and possibly harm his career.

After much discussion, there is agreement to consult with a social worker knowledgeable about child protection issues. She interviews both parents and finds that the child's father appears to harbor angry feelings against his son, associated in some measure with a profound sense of his wife's abandoning her attentions to him after the child was born. She strongly recommends case reporting and further psychiatric, diagnostic, and therapeutic work with the family.

B. Case Example 2

A 10-month-old black girl is brought to the emergency room with symptoms of severe malnutrition. The mother reports that the child has not been feeding well but gives no further history. On examination, the physical hygiene is poor; the weight and length are well below the third percentiles of the normal distributions; there are moderate knee and elbow contractures; and the child can neither roll over, sit unsupported, nor vocalize in response to the examiner. The child is admitted to the hospital. Without any specific diagnostic or therapeutic interventions, she begins promptly to regain weight and to recoup her lost developmental milestones.

Discussion of the management of the case focuses on whether to initiate actions to separate the child's custody from her mother. A social work consultation is obtained, and further history is gathered.

The mother moved to this city approximately 18 months prior to the admission with two preschool children and a fantasy of making life better for her family and for her ailing, elderly parents in the rural South. She found work, and things went well for a while. She became involved with a man, however, by whom she became pregnant, and he abandoned her shortly before the birth of this child.

She found herself isolated, without kin or friends, and dependent on the program, Aid to Families with Dependent Children (AFDC). She had to pay 70% of her AFDC stipend for rent.

It was noted that she spoke with little modulation in her affect. She complained of her teeth and of her back aching her constantly. There was concern that she might have a propensity to somatize rather than to express in words her deep feelings of sadness. She did, however, appear to love this infant deeply and to comprehend the tasks of giving her care.

A referral to an internist led to the diagnosis of the mother's chronic urinary tract infection, and a referral to a dentist disclosed she had markedly carious teeth. The mother formed strong relationships with social service, nursing, and medical staff.

C. Case Example 3

Three girls, aged 2½, 4, and 9 years, were referred by the Family Service Office of the Probate Court for evaluation of the 4-year-old's disclosure of having been sexually victimized by her father, who was seeking the children's custody. Interview of the mother yielded a history of a tumultuous and violent marital relationship beginning in late adolescence when the parents were members of a circle of friends who abused drugs together. The mother had been psychiatrically hospitalized for depression. She reported that she had been sexually abused in her own childhood and that her own mother had denied her victimization. The maternal grandmother was associated with the children's father in a fundamentalist church and shared his view that the mother, because of her preoccupation with her own victimization and her psychiatric instability, was responsible for the children's disclosures.

The initial clinical interview suggested a severe depression on the mother's part and a sense of futility with regard to her capacity to retain the custody of her children.

Interview of the father suggested that he was earnest in his effort to seek custody of the children. He argued vociferously that he had been falsely accused and that the allegations of sexual abuse were attributable entirely to his wife's preoccupation with her victimization and its psychiatric impact. He admitted that he had been violent toward her, but he insisted that she had provoked his rage.

The children were interviewed with appropriate examination techniques, including the use of anatomically detailed dolls. On the fourth interview, the 4-year-old clearly disclosed that her father had, on several occasions, inserted his fingers into her vagina. Subsequently, all three children disclosed sexual abuse by their father.

At the custody hearing at the Probate Court, the father's attorney relentlessly grilled all of the professionals who were involved in the assessment, examining one witness for 36 hours. He challenged the entire system of diagnosis and treatment for victims of child sexual abuse and suggested that the professionals colluded with one another and with the mother against his client. The judge appeared to be sympathetic to his argument.

II. LEGAL ISSUES

A. Child abuse case reporting

As noted in Chapter 8, all states have laws which require all professionals who have responsibility for the care of children to report situations in which they suspect or believe that a child is a victim of abuse. These statutes define child abuse and neglect broadly. The agencies to which the reports are mandated to be made are generally state departments of social services or of welfare. In some jurisdictions, there is an obligation to make reports directly to the police or to a prosecutor's office as well.

In mental health settings, a child abuse case report can be conceived and has been described as a therapeutic intervention. It indicates unequivocally the professional's concern for the safety of the child and his or her interest to fulfill the legal obligation to assure that the child is protected. It is appropriate to inform the parents of the making of the report and to prepare them for the anticipated subsequent interventions, explaining that the objective of the action is to protect the child, not to punish the parents, and to assure that whatever may have happened will not recur. If one takes the time to listen responsively to the parents' responses, including their expressions of anger, one can help lay the groundwork for successful future interventions. It is important also to indicate one's concern to continue to follow the child and family and to assure that they receive needed help and appropriate intervention.

B. Liability for failure to report

The statutes contain in them civil, and in some states, criminal, penalties for failing to report child abuse. Additionally, there is now an extensive body of case law which defines a professional liability risk for not reporting. Malpractice awards in the hundreds of thousands of dollars have been made in response to the argument that the failure to report is an intervening cause of a child's subsequent injury.

C. Custody initiatives

1. COMPLAINTS ON A CHILD'S BEHALF

If a child is believed to be in danger in her or his home, a family or juvenile court can be approached and asked to transfer the child's legal and physical custody to the state. These complaints can be initiated by any professional person, although they are generally made by child protection agencies. They frequently culminate in a child being placed in one or another form of substitute care (in a foster home, a group home, or an institutional setting), and they very often begin a protracted process of investigations, hearings, and interim placements until some future time when the child's family is perceived to be able to provide appropriate protection and care, or when a child may become eligible for adoption.

2. CUSTODY CONFLICTS IN THE FACT OF DIVORCE

Many child victims of physical, and especially sexual, abuse are identified in the context of legal conflicts over their custody. These cases are burdensome for the divorce courts, and professional consultation is often sought to establish the validity of the allegations or disclosures, to assess the psychological status of children, and to make recommendations for custody and for visitation.

D. Criminal prosecution

Since the late 1970s, there has been an increasing trend toward treating offenses within the family in the criminal justice system. In many jurisdictions, child abuse case reports to social welfare agencies are now transmitted directly to the prosecutors' offices if they meet certain definitional criteria, such as severe child physical abuse or substantiated child sexual abuse.

The cases pose special challenges to these prosecutors, who alone in the system have discretion with regard to the principal professional choices concerning whether charges should be filed (in contrast to mandated child abuse case reporters, who, at least according to law, have no alternative but to report). Prosecuting attorneys, who are elected officials, may be particularly oriented to obtaining convictions, as opposed to protecting children and supporting their mental health. They may aggressively gather all data, including medical and psychiatric data, which could help them to meet the high standard of proof ("beyond all reasonable doubt") in the criminal court.

It is well always to keep in mind that when a severe case of child abuse is seen in consultation, some contact with the criminal justice system may follow. Mental health professionals should be prepared for the unique ethical challenges which these contacts impose, especially with regard to confidentiality and informed consent. One's own lawyer may be needed to provide guidance with regard to the use of one's data and to giving testimony in a case, as well as how best to handle inquiries from prosecutors for expert witness service. (In this connection, when one is asked to testify as an expert, it is entirely appropriate to be paid for consultation and the giving of testimony, at prevailing rates.)

Mental health professionals' services are increasingly in demand, e.g., for evaluations and for making the case for adapting the courtroom appropriately to the needs of children. The United States Supreme Court has overturned state legislation making such courtroom adaptations part of the regular routine in cases of child victimization. The Court gave priority to the Constitutional guarantee to confront one's accuser. It left open the possibility of the prosecutor's demonstrating in a particular case possible harm to a child who might have to face an assailant. Upon such demonstration, adaption may be allowed.

In many jurisdictions, enlightened prosecutors have established excellent programs to support witnesses through the often difficult ordeal of giving testimony in these cases. These victim-witness specialists may help also in getting their clients access to helpful interventions and services, including psychotherapy and shelter, and in keeping offenders away from them. They can turn into a personally validating and psychologically beneficial process a victim's participation in a criminal prosecution.

III. CLINICAL ISSUES

A. The context of intervention

Effective clinical work on child abuse is best oriented to the child and family in their life setting, taking cognizance of cultural and social values, especially with regard to sex, violence, power, and the status of women. It is essential to understand the context of one's work.

1. THE CHANGING AMERICAN FAMILY

There are now in excess of a million divorces each year. On average, each divorce includes at least one child. Most children remain in the care of their mothers. Their economic and social status declines precipitously. Much of the developmental attrition associated with divorce is believed to be connected to its accompanying economic adversities.

2. THE FEMINIZATION OF POVERTY

Most divorcing fathers do not pay the amount of child support which they agree or are ordered to pay. Indeed, many judges believe that women can and should quickly go into the workforce and provide for themselves and their children. Because women's wages, however, are less than men's, only very rarely can mothers sustain their and their children's living standards. There have been substantial cutbacks in governmental support programs for child care, housing, nutrition, and welfare during the 1970s and 1980s, a period in which housing costs have outstripped inflation. Additionally, during the 1980s, the relatively flat minimum wage became increasingly less sufficient to bring a family over the federal poverty line.

In 1990, a parent's minimum wage employment is sufficient only to bring a family to a level 30% below this income level.

The convergent impacts of these events have been characterized as the "feminization of poverty." They are associated with dramatic increases in the participation of mothers in the workforce and with patchwork child care arrangements which may render children who are given care by boyfriends, step-parents, and unlicensed family daycare facilities vulnerable to physical and sexual abuse. Many of the most serious cases of sexual and physical abuse now seen in practice are inflicted by caregivers while their mothers are at work.

3. CONFUSION IN THE SOCIETY ABOUT VIOLENCE AND SEX

The average American child witnesses the killing of over 13,000 persons on television during the period between the ages of 5 and 15 years. Violence and coercion are favored in many contexts as appropriate ways to settle human conflicts. Advertisers take advantage of the heightened arousal from exposure to sexually stimulating visual metaphors, mostly featuring female models, to draw attention to advertisements, and to attach excitement to commercial products. Television and the movies take advantage of sex to draw viewers and to sell goods. Sex and sexuality are lively elements in the debate on the control of abortion. Women and children are the particular objects of this clamor, which concerns who controls their bodies and their lives. Their disempowerment, most experts in the family violence field believe, is connected to their special vulnerability as victims of violence and sexual exploitation.

Unfortunately, many professionals, in the face of this fascination and confusion in the larger society, treat with denial their patients' disclosures of symptomatic manifestations of violent or sexual exploitation. Because these cases stimulate vexing emotions and conflicts, it is sometimes easier to push out of conscious acknowledgement the possibility of victimization.

4. CONVERGENCE OF THE FORMS OF FAMILY VIOLENCE

There is increasing evidence of overlap among the forms of family violence. Children who are victims of physical abuse are likely to have victimized mothers. With regard to child sexual abuse as well, current thinking suggests that these offenses are better understood as distortions in power relationships in the family than as disorders of adult sexual expression. In many of these cases, because of the similar power dynamics, mothers are also battered.

Unfortunately, however, health, mental health, and social service professionals and their institutions are not well equipped to contend with the spectrum of family violence. Agencies which treat child abuse may be unable to address the needs of battered women, for example. Psychotherapists for adults may neglect the needs of children. Courts may focus on the custody of children and ignore the status of their mothers.

Because this is a rapidly evolving area of practice, where in the face of shortened resources and a slow dissemination of newer knowledge, service responses are not always timely and well informed, professionals who see these cases need to be knowledgeable and aggressive in their contacts with the human service systems.

B. The philosophy of helpful intervention

Since the "rediscovery" of child abuse in the 1960s, an ambivalent response has developed in the United States. The humane imperative of research and practice in the 1960s and 1970s—the notion that help can be made available to families whose children are not adequately protected in their homes—has to some extent given way in the 1980s to a notion that criminal sanctions are more effective individual and social deterrents. The emphasis in this section is on the conceptual underpinnings of mental health work.

1. ECOLOGICAL APPROACHES TO SERVICE DELIVERY

Families in which abuse occurs have been described as suffering from a variety of stresses in their life contexts in addition to individual psychological disturbances. Addressing the many sources of distress, from marital discord to social isolation to substance abuse, requires a multifaceted and systems-oriented approach. Inadequate resources often constrain what services can be provided. But the philosophical foundation is: where possible, to strengthen family life. This is also the underpinning of the modern "family preservation movement."

A conceptual watchword of this movement is "ecological." The notion is that family life is embedded in the realities, cultural values, and idiosyncratic qualities of a community, and that services to children cannot be defined as separate from families and their environments. This idea has particular relevance to the prevailing state of the official child protection agencies, which are to a great extent still rooted in the limited knowledge about child abuse which prevailed in the 1960s.

At this time, it was widely believed that child abuse was principally an artifact or consequence of parental psychopathology. The expanding literature on parental and family characteristics in the 1970s, however, drew attention to the relative rarity of definable psychological disturbances in parents and the frequency of family stresses, social isolation, marital conflict, and problematic issues of child health, temperament, and development.

Child protection agencies, however, in part because of the constricted understanding of child abuse but, equally importantly, because of diminished resources, generally offer counseling approaches based on a psychotherapeutic model of "treatment." When for whatever reasons these do not result in the desired changes, many take or threaten action to separate children from their parents' care.

It is important to establish a good diagnostic base in each case, identifying strengths in parents and families, as well as deficits. Often it is necessary aggressively to assert a child's and family's needs in order to assure that appropriate services are given to them. These services will be described below.

2. THE FAMILY SUPPORT MOVEMENT

The movement is a recent phenomenon, beginning in the early 1980s growing from the perception that social support is associated with improved maternal-infant attachment and better adjustment of children following divorce. It takes cognizance of the merit of such comprehensive programs as Project Head Start and the sense, especially in the course of the program cutbacks in the 1970s and 80s, that social service programs simply could not meet the needs of families. Family functioning is understood as being inextricable from the realities (and adversities) of the family's life setting. Many of the support programs are grass roots efforts, offering home visitors who provide friendly and warm connections to knowledgeable professionals, linkage between parents, and education about children and child rearing.

The focus is on sustaining strengths in families rather than on compensating for their faults, and the programs particularly are concerned to correct the perceived focus of many social welfare programs on family deficits which are often biased, its proponents assert, against poor people and cultural and ethnic minorities. These programs are also concerned to prevent family breakup, that is to say, to assure that where possible family members stay together, even in the face of a history of violence. The programs are not available everywhere, but they provide an important orientation point with regard to services to abused children in the latter part of the 20th century and will almost certainly influence the evolution of social and psychiatric services.

3. The child welfare tradition

a. Child protection services

These are the principal services to abused children and their families. In the statutes which establish these programs, the agencies are mandated to protect children in their homes where possible, and to undertake efforts to remove them from parental care if not. Social workers working within child protection service agencies, which are generally located within county or state departments of social services or welfare, have suffered from inadequate funding and consequent worker overload, inadequate training and supervision, and staff turnover. In several states, however, substantial improvements have been made in these programs, generally after strenuous advocacy efforts. In these jurisdictions, child protection agencies may offer publicly funded child care services, homemaker services, psychotherapeutic interventions, excellent liaison with medical and nursing services, and, in a few states, multidisciplinary diagnostic and treatment teams. Unfortunately, these initiatives are rare, and the prevailing standard of social work in the child protection world appears to be low.

b. Social control agenda

Historically, the families served by these agencies have been poor, and the agencies' functions included larger social control mandates. (These are not, obviously, the focus of this chapter, however, but it is important to know about them. They are treated in one of the suggested readings: Linda Gordon's *Heroes of Their Own Lives*.) The social control functions include obliging women to remain subservient to their husbands, to stay home with their children, and to limit their educational and employment opportunities. Also, the agencies have been concerned historically to regulate the lives of poor people by threatening them with the loss of their children if their behavior does not measure up to society's expectations with regard, for example, to self-sufficiency, personal deportment, and work.

C. Specific interventions

1. SOCIAL CASEWORK

This is the core service in child protection. Social workers assess a child's and family's needs with a focus on a child's protection. They offer, obtain, and coordinate counseling and other services. With parents, they develop, and in some jurisdictions sign, service plans with defined objectives for improvement of family functioning. They may initiate proceeds for the removal of a child if change does not take place.

"Case management," the coordination of services of other providers, is a concept which is increasingly supplanting the notion of casework, or direct service provision, in the face of the high volume of child abuse referrals and the shortage of protective service resources.

2. PSYCHOTHERAPY

Among the valuable psychotherapy interventions are individual and group treatment of adults and children, as well as couples and family treatment. The latter two forms of therapy are believed by many to be inappropriate in situations where a woman may have been abused, and it has been recommended that prior to making a referral for couples or family treatment one be certain that a woman is not a victim of abuse.

Psychotherapy for children should be considered in all cases of abuse, in order to address the important child developmental and psychiatric impacts of the victimization experience. There is now a wide professional consensus on its special significance for child sexual abuse victims, nearly all of whom will bear psychological scars in the absence of treatment.

3. HEALTH SERVICES

a. Pediatric continuing care

All children should have regular medial care; victims of child abuse suffer more than usual burdens of acute and chronic illness. These children's medical needs are often neglected, however, especially if they may be placed outside their parents' care.

A systematic effort should be made in each case to assure that a child is given a full physical examination and that the child's health needs are documented and addressed.

b. Public health nursing

A nurse may visit frequently and regularly to assure that specific child health and nutritional problems are attended to and that there is good liaison with medical services. Public health nurses also provide information on child development, a sympathetic ear, an orientation to the strengths of individuals and relationships, and prompt access to help when it is needed. Their work has been shown clearly to have been effective in the prevention of child abuse.

c. Adult medical and dental care

For many parents, chronic medical and dental problems can affect their capacities to protect and nurture their children. When these problems are addressed, and, hopefully, ameliorated, children's well-being may improve.

4. FAMILY-FOCUSED INTERVENTIONS

a. Homemaker services

These paraprofessionals help with the organization of daily living activities and serve as models for giving appropriate care to children. They may significantly ease the burdens of parents who may be impaired themselves or who may not be able to contend with a child who may be handicapped or ill.

b. Homebuilders

This relatively new family intervention assigns a very small number of families to a homebuilder, who may be a social worker or someone without a formal professional background. That individual may spend the majority of his or her employment hours with one family. Homebuilders get to know the individuals in great depth, forming a deep relationship in a short interval of service, and engage with the family in all the tasks of family life, including giving care to children, going shopping, helping people get access to essential resources, services, and supports, and, importantly, working to change behavior that would result in the breakup of the family if it were to continue. The period of the intervention is generally under two months, and the preliminary evaluations of these programs suggest an impressive effectiveness for well-selected cases.

Parent aide programs have grown from an initial effort to provide "lay therapy" parallel to social workers' interventions to a national paraprofessional and sometimes volunteer program. The results appear to be favorable and cost-effective with the focus on family strengths versus pathology and on keeping the family together.

c. Child care services

Child care can be seen as a form of family service. It provides for the child an opportunity to socialize with peers and to change patterns of behavior which may be distressing to parents. For parents, it may provide the chance to work, linkages to other parents and to professionals knowledgeable about children's development, and in the case of comprehensive programs such as Project Head Start, access to nutritional food, child health, and counseling services.

5. ALCOHOL AND SUBSTANCE ABUSE TREATMENT

When child abuse occurs in the face of alcohol and substance abuse, specific treatment can make the difference in a family's capacity to give care to children. In the absence of these services, children of substance-abusing parents may be vulnerable to being placed outside the home. The services are typically in short supply, and they are often not congenial to the needs of parents. (Few, for example, offer child care while adults participate in their programs.)

6. SUBSTITUTE CARE: FOSTER HOME AND INSTITUTIONAL PLACEMENTS

When families are perceived not to be able to care for and protect their children sufficiently well, arrangements are made to place them outside their parental homes. This can be done on either a "voluntary" or a court-mandated basis.

In best practice, substitute care is conceived as a form of family service. Too frequently, however, it is conceived as a form of punishment. It is well to be alert to the risks of substitute care, which include a higher than usual risk of exposure to sexual abuse.

Approximately a third of children entering substitute care have physical or psychological handicaps, and relatively few are given treatment for these in the overburdened child welfare system. It is thus important at the outset of a substitute care plan to assure that a child's needs are well-delineated and that appropriate services are brought into place.

Documentation of these service needs on a "medical passport" has been implemented in states such as California, Massachusetts, and North Carolina. By virtue of their status as residents in substitute care, children are eligible for Medicaid. This means that the foster parents have some insurance for specialized services to these children. It is important to encourage foster parents to utilize them. Medicaid programs in some states are able to pay for long-term child psychotherapy.

Longitudinal studies of children in foster home care suggest a substantial developmental attrition to children in care, attributed in part to the relatively long average length of stay (3–5 years) and the relatively frequent disruptions in the care settings (the average child is placed in several homes, and many children are placed in more foster homes and institutions than they can remember, culminating in what has been characterized as an institutional psychopathy which may severely compromise their capacities to form and sustain intimate relationships, including those with their own children, in later life).

"Permanency planning" has become the watchword of a movement beginning in the 1980s to restrict the inappropriate use of long-term foster care. Here, regular reviews are mandated of the child's status, in accord with the requirements of Public Law 96-272, and if progress is not being made with regard to the family of origin's capacity to give care to the child, prompt action may be taken to terminate the parental rights and to place the child in adoptive care. Conversely, efforts can be made to invest home-based services to preserve the families and to obviate the need for long substitute placements. These, however, require resources which are frequently lacking in today's child welfare programs.

Residential treatment settings are often needed for children with substantial psychological burdens associated with child abuse. The quality of these programs varies tremendously. Some integrate therapeutic and educational efforts with family interventions with a long-term perspective to enhance the functioning of the child and the child's relationship with his or her kin. Others may offer no more than a roof over a child's head, and some, unfortunately, have been disclosed to be settings in which children are vulnerable to further abuses.

Tragically, many children leave substitute care to become homeless. The developmental problems associated with what is quaintly characterized as "aging out" of the child welfare system have begun to receive serious public scrutiny.

In the absence of a committed parent to assure a child's care and support, children are often cut adrift when they enter substitute care. For this reason many professionals advise that until more uniform standards are articulated and the overall quality of the system is improved, it should be avoided where possible.

7. PARENTS ANONYMOUS

This national self-help movement began in the early 1970s. There are now thousands of chapters across the United States. Toll-free telephone numbers are available in many states for parents who sense they are on the verge of doing something harmful to their child. They may call, talk with someone, and come to a meeting. The program is similar in outline to so-called "12-step" programs, but it varies substantially from place to place. Evaluations of the program suggest that it is of enormous value for selected individuals, and it also appears to be salutary to their children. Parents who participate in Parents Anonymous often report feeling empowered and validated by sharing the experience of coming to terms with the adversities of giving parental care. Most programs have professional sponsors, and some have formalized linkages to established service agencies.

8. CRIMINAL JUSTICE SYSTEM INTERVENTIONS

a. Testimony as an intervention

Testimony in a criminal trial against an offender has been documented to have useful psychological effects in several studies. For some children, however, it can be a threatening and traumatic experience. (See Chapter 16.) For this reason, it is well to discuss a child's possible participation in a criminal case with a prosecutor and to offer guidance (or intervention) with regard to the possible use of the child as a witness in a court proceeding.

b. Victim witness services

Victim witness services are available in many prosecutors' offices. Here, specialized personnel, some but not all of whom have human services training, tend particularly to the victim's needs in the course of the prosecution, explaining the court process, accompanying the victim to all proceedings, making available access to certain specialized services including psychotherapy and victim's compensation funds, where they are available, and serving generally as an ombudsman for the victim in the criminal system. These programs appear to have been successful in reducing the occasional adverse impacts on child and women victims who give testimony in court proceedings.

c. Offender treatment

Under the aegis of the criminal justice system, many offenders are brought into treatment. Increasingly, adolescents are given treatment in this setting when they have committed sexual offenses against children. Often the threat of incarceration is needed to compel participation, and there are encouraging data which suggest positive outcomes, dispelling the popular myth that there is no useful treatment for sex offenders.

d. Incarceration

Offenders against children generally spend less time in jail than offenders against adults. Incarceration offers only a short amount of protection for children from the perpetrators of violent and sexual offenses. Only rarely, unfortunately, are specific therapeutic services related to offending behaviors against children available in the course of an imprisonment.

9. BATTERED WOMEN'S SERVICES

Because of the increasing understanding of the connections among the forms of family violence and the high prevalence of battered women in recent studies of child abuse, it is well to be informed about the battered women's service network in one's community.

This is largely a self-help and severely underfunded movement which started when battered women's problems came into public view in the late 1970s. There is a vivid sense of counterculture in many of these programs, and mental health professionals may experience a lively sense of mistrust.

This is often especially the case for professionals who are concerned about the possible abuse of children, since many of the people who work in the battered women's service movement have been burned by the tender ministrations (and the aforementioned "social control functions") of the child protection system, which is widely perceived as being unsympathetic to the needs of battered women. An adroit focus on the *mother's* protective needs may stimulate an interested response, however, as one endeavors to provide protection to a child.

Asking a woman about her own safety is often the only way to get information about her possible abuse. Action taken to protect her may be an important component of building a trusting relationship with her and addressing her child's needs effectively.

IV. PITFALLS

A. Class and culture biases

1. REPORTING

Studies of child abuse case reporting demonstrate a clear bias which favors poor and minority children for identification and reporting as child abuse victims. This perpetuates the widespread myth that child abuse is restricted to homes which are different from where the majority lives. When making judgments about the capacity of parents to give care to children, prejudices may often impose themselves. Professionals need to be alert to the possibility of making prejudicial value judgments, and the actions of practice should be considered thoughtfully in relation to the family's social and cultural status. Interdisciplinary decision making, with professional representation from various cultural groups, has been demonstrated to lead to more effective and less biased practice.

2. SUBSTITUTE CARE

There is a well-documented increased risk for poor and minority children being separated from family and placed in foster home or institutional care.

3. PSYCHIATRIC SERVICES

Minority children also appear from recent research to be less likely to receive psychiatric services after the diagnosis of child sexual victimization.

4. CRIMINAL PROCESS

The criminal justice system principally deals with poor individuals, and there is a far greater proportion of minorities in prisons than their distribution in the population would appear to suggest.

B. To punish or to help?

In the course of the 1980s, a perceptible shift away from therapeutic services toward punitive interventions for family offenses took place. Therapeutic resources are in increasingly short supply. The promise of help in the child abuse reporting statutes may be an empty promise. This situation presents vexing contradictions to child mental health professionals. One may wonder whether a legally mandated intervention may do more harm than good. In general, practice is best when it abides by the statutory requirements and struggles to make the system work for individual children and families. Mandatory reporting has also been documented to help the psychotherapy process for certain children and families.

C. Countertransference

These cases stimulate in all of us feelings of anxiety, sadness, revulsion, and rage (see Chapter 15). Actively processing with our colleagues the personal impact the cases may exert, creatively displacing angry feelings in the direction of the struggle to improve the service system, and rounding out one's professional life with less burdensome clinical work have been identified as valuable pathways toward professional sanity in the victimization field. It is well always to be alert to how these cases may affect oneself, lest the actions of practice not be driven by the force of emotion. The risk of burnout for those immersed in this area of practice is great.

D. Turf struggles

At a time of too many cases and too few resources, there are divisive strivings among the professions to control pieces of a shrinking pie. Issues of control in child protection cases can be paramount for social welfare agencies and prosecutors, in particular. It is well to be aware of their sensitivities to the higher social status of mental health professionals, always to be respectful and gracious in one's dealings with them, and to choose carefully to fight the battles which really make a difference for a child.

V. CASE EXAMPLE EPILOGUES

A. Case Example 1

After much discussion, a child abuse case report was filed as law required. A coordinated program of services was brought into place. These included adult psychiatric services and social services oriented toward the protection of the child. The child was not reinjured.

B. Case Example 2

At a five-year follow-up interval, the child was functioning appropriately for her age on physical examination and psychological study. The mother had another infant who was thriving. At no time was it necessary for any of the children to leave the care of their mother.

C. Case Example 3

All three children required psychiatric hospitalization for symptoms attributable to their victimizations, to their mother's severe depression, and to the custody conflict. In a protective setting, all three children disclosed multiple sexual victimizations by their father. Their mother was successful in her bid to retain their custody. The father, armed with new counsel, intends to appeal the judge's decision.

VI. ACTION GUIDE

A. Priority to Understanding Rather than to Punishment

1. Conduct thorough and thoughtful diagnostic studies of all victims.
2. Focus on building relationships with their parents.

B. Focus on the Welfare and Protection of the Child

1. Hospitalize the child if necessary for physical protection.
2. Take adroit action, where indicated, to assure that the systems to protect children are brought effectively into play. Report all cases where there is reasonable cause to believe the child is being abused or neglected. Cooperate in court initiatives on the child's behalf and to assure that whoever offended against the child will not do so again. Assure that all the interventions which may have possible adverse effects are monitored, and intervene where necessary to prevent adverse developmental consequences to the child.
3. Sustain contact with the child and the family.

C. Advocate for helpful services for individual children and for the improvement of services for child victims more generally.

D. Deal maturely and graciously with all professionals. Choose one's battles carefully.

E. Document professional work systematically.

VII. SUGGESTED READINGS

PHILOSOPHY AND TECHNIQUE OF INTERVENTION:

Bentovim, A., Elton, A., Hildebrand, J., Tranter, M., and Vizard, E. (eds.) (1988), Child Sexual Abuse within the Family: Assessment and Treatment. London: Wright.

Daro, D. (1988), Confronting Child Abuse: Research for Effective Program Design. New York: The Free Press.

Gordon, C. (1988), Heroes of Their Own Lives: The Politics and History of Family Violence. New York: Viking.

Newberger, E. H. (1990), Child abuse. In: Rosenberg, M. (ed.) Violence: A Public Health Approach. New York: Oxford University Press.

Watson, H. and Levine, M. (1989), Psychotherapy and mandated reporting of child abuse. Am J Orthopsychiatry 59:246–256.

Zigler, E. and Black, K. B. (1989), America's family support movement: strengths and limitations. Am J Orthopsychiatry 59:6–19.

IMPACTS OF CHILD ABUSE:

Bass, L. and Davis, L. (1988), The Courage to Heal: A Sourcebook for the Survivors of Incest. New York: Harper and Rowe.

Lynch, N. A. and Roberts, J. (1982), Consequences of Child Abuse. New York: Academic Press.

Oates, K. (1986), Child Abuse and Neglect: What Happens Eventually? New York: Brunner/Mazel.

Schetky, D. H. (1985), Role Models for Violence. In: Schetky, D. H. and Benedek, E. P., Emerging Issues in Child Psychiatry and The Law. New York: Brunner/Mazel, Inc.

Wyatt, G. and Powell, G. J. (eds.) (1988), Lasting Effects of Child Sexual Abuse. Newbury Park: Sage.

INNOVATIONS IN PRACTICE:

Dziech, B. W. and Schudson, C. B. (1989), On Trial: America's Courts and Their Treatment of Sexually Abused Children. Boston: Beacon Press.

Whitcomb, D. (1985), Prosecution of Child Sexual Abuse: Innovations in Practice. Washington: U.S. Department of Justice. (Available without charge from the National Institute of Justice/NCJRS, Department AAK, Box 6000, Rockville, MD 20850.)

White, K. M., Snyder, J., Bourne, R., and Newberger, E. (1989), Treating Child Abuse and Family Violence in Hospitals: A Program for Training and Services. Lexington: Lexington Books.

11

Termination of Parental Rights and Adoption

DIANE H. SCHETKY, M.D.

I. CASE EXAMPLES

A. Case Example 1

Protective Services referred Mrs. N., age 26, for assessment of her ability to care for and protect her sons, ages 5 and 7 years. Mrs. N. was born with hereditary, congenital deafness and spent her early years in an abusive, hearing family. She was then placed in an institution for the deaf that stressed lip reading, and her signing skills remained rudimentary. She lacked intelligible speech. At age 18 she moved to a halfway house, became pregnant, and married a drug addict. Upon learning that he was sexually abusing their eldest son, she left him. She promptly moved in with another man who had charges pending regarding sexual abuse of his daughters. He soon became physically abusive with her youngest son. A neglect petition was filed and her children were placed in foster care. A psychiatric evaluation of her was requested regarding her ability to parent.

B. Case Example 2

Jim and Grace, both chronic schizophrenics, met on the day treatment unit. Jim's assignment for the day was to practice socialization skills. He proposed marriage to Grace, whom he'd only known for three days, and she accepted. In the next five years they produced two children, neither of whom they could care for. The state built a strong case for termination of parental rights, but wondered about the adoptability of the children who showed serious developmental lags. Their 4-year-old had a mental age of 2 and the child psychiatry fellow who evaluated her thought she might be borderline psychotic.

C. Case Example 3

Ten-year-old Peggy and her 8-year-old brother, Lucas, had been in foster care for four years following sexual abuse by their grandmother. The head of the state's adoption unit thought it was time to free the children for adoption and was convinced she could find a home for them in spite of their attention deficit disorders, possible fetal alcohol syndrome, and serious behavior problems. Both children resisted adoption and regarded their foster parents as their own. Their baseline hyperactivity would escalate whenever a foster child left their home. Their foster mother described them as "wired." A child psychiatry consultation was requested regarding their long-term needs.

II. LEGAL ISSUES

A. Balancing the rights of parents, children, and the state

1. THE RIGHTS OF PARENTS

The right of parents to control their children's upbringing without intrusion by the State is rooted in the 14th Amendment of the U.S. Constitution. This has subsequently been confirmed in case law (*Meyer v. Nebraska* 262 U.S. 390, 1923; *Stanley v. Illinois* 405 U.S. 645, 1972, and *Smith v. OFFER* (Organization of Foster Families for Equity and Reform) 53L Ed. 2d 14, 1977. In *Smith v. OFFER* the Supreme Court held that the right of natural parents to custody of their children is a "constitutionally recognized liberty interest that derives from blood relationship, state law sanction, and basic human right." These rights were strengthened further in 1982 by the decision of the U.S. Supreme Court (*Santosky v. Kramer* 102 S. Ct, 1388, United States) which raised the standard of evidence needed to terminate parental rights to clear and convincing evidence.

2. THE RIGHTS OF THE STATE

The concept of *parens patriae* originally referred to the king's guardianship over people legally unable to act for themselves. In the early 20th century the juvenile court took on this role in regard to abused and neglected children. As noted by Judge Cardozo, "When parents fail to protect their children the state must take over in the role of the parent and do what is in the best interests of the child (*Finlay v. Finlay*, 148 NE 624, N.Y. 1925)." The state may intervene in matters of custody and visitation only when the parents have subjected themselves to the jurisdiction of the court. The usual circumstances in which this occurs include paternity cases, death of a parent, divorce, or when a parent fails to provide adequate parenting.

3. THE RIGHTS OF CHILDREN

Children per se are not afforded any rights under the U.S. Constitution. However, under case law, in face of abuse, neglect, or abandonment the "right of family integrity" must yield to the state's interest in protecting children. The standard of "the child's best interests" has been accepted as a guiding principle in custody decisions and one that takes precedence over parental interests. A court order is required to remove a child from the parents' home except under emergency situations or when a parent consents.

4. REACHING A BALANCE

The rights of a child to his or her psychological home, to some home, or to a home free of abuse are in potential conflict with the rights of the biological parent to possess the child. Two underlying social considerations govern the outcome of this conflict. On the one hand is a well-justified apprehension concerning the coercive arm of the government entering into the private domain of the family. It is the family, more than any other factor, that deprives the state of a monopoly of unfettered power. Any diminution of the prerogative of parents is a corresponding and ominous increase in the power of the state. On the other hand, the interest of society is not served when children are mistreated, grossly neglected, or allowed to languish in the limbo of foster care. Unless the chain of mistreatment is broken, abuse breeds abuse from one scarred generation to the next. As noted by Goldstein, Freud, and Solnit, "Each time the cycle of grossly inadequate parent-child relationship is broken, society stands to gain a person capable of becoming an adequate parent for children of the future" (1973, p. 7).

B. Protective services intervention

Children come under the care of Protective Services following a complaint of neglect or abuse or when parents voluntarily seek services. Recognizing that states have different acronyms for this agency we will refer to it as the state. If a complaint is substantiated the case is continued and the child may or may not be placed in foster care. If the child goes into an involuntary placement the state may assume temporary custody of the child through a court order.

Persons reporting child abuse or neglect in good faith and those participating in the investigation of the charges are immune from any related criminal or civil liability.

When a child has been ordered into the state's custody the responsibility for reunification and rehabilitation of the family is shared between the parents and the state.

1. DEPARTMENT'S RESPONSIBILITIES

The state is expected to develop a plan for rehabilitation and reunification that spells out the reasons for the child's removal, changes that must occur in order for the child to return home, services that the parents are expected to avail themselves of, a schedule of visitation, and delineation of financial responsibilities during the reunification process. In addition, in most cases the parents are apprised of where the child is living and of any medical problems the child develops. Periodic departmental and judicial reviews are scheduled to monitor progress of the plan.

2. PARENTS' RESPONSIBILITIES

Parents are expected to maintain contact with their child through scheduled visits, seek and use appropriate services, maintain contact with the department, make good faith effort to cooperate, and pay designated sums toward their child's support. They are usually requested to sign a contract to this effect.

3. EXCEPTIONS TO PURSUING PARENTAL REUNIFICATION

The state is entitled to file a petition to terminate parental rights if it is determined that family reunification efforts are not succeeding and that termination of parental rights is in the child's best interests. This also occurs if parents decide to relinquish parental rights, or when the parent cannot be located or abandons the child.

In addition, in some states certain heinous crimes against children such as murder, rape, and sexual abuse constitute automatic grounds for pursuing termination of parental rights.

If the state discontinues efforts to reunify, it must give written notice of this decision to the parents including reasons for the decision.

C. Criteria for termination of parental rights

The wording of termination of parental rights statutes varies from state to state but generally includes the following components:

1. VOLUNTARY RELINQUISHMENT

This may occur on the part of one or both parents. For instance, a noncustodial father may relinquish in order to allow for adoption by a stepfather. The termination of one parent's rights does not affect the rights of the other parent. In order for a child to be freed for adoption both parents need to relinquish parental rights.

2. INVOLUNTARY TERMINATION

As noted, the standard of evidence requires clear and convincing evidence that:

a. Termination is in the child's best interests

b. One of the following:

1) The parent is unwilling or unable to protect the child from jeopardy.
2) The parent is unable or unwilling to take responsibility for the child.
3) The parent has abandoned, i.e., failed to maintain contact with the child.

4) The parent has failed to make a good faith effort to rehabilitate and reunify with the child.

Aside from abandonment, the courts will usually require demonstration that the parent's conduct or condition is such as to render him or her incapable of caring for the child and that such conduct or condition is not likely to change within the foreseeable future.

3. Problems with existing statutes

Many statutes are exceedingly vague and do not specify what they mean by "the child's best interests" or "reunification within a reasonable time." What is "reasonable" to a 10-year-old is not necessarily so for a 2-year-old. California includes a "return detrimental" clause which states that failure to return a child home after 2 years might be grounds for terminating parental rights, if the parent has not progressed within that time frame. In contrast, in Massachusetts, a similar clause specifies 12 months (Langelier and Nurcombe, 1985).

Some termination statutes have been criticized because they are unduly focused on parental fault rather than upon the child's needs. Critics such as Wald (1976) argue that it should be made more difficult to place a child in foster care and easier to terminate parental rights once the child has been placed in foster care. He further advocates that termination be automatic, in some cases, at the initial neglect proceeding if there has been prior abuse or removal from the home or if the child has been abandoned. However, this seems unduly harsh if, for instance, the parent is suffering from a recurrent but treatable mental illness that may have contributed to his or her negligence.

D. Due process rights

1. The parents

The parents are entitled to legal counsel in child protection proceedings and may request the court to appoint counsel for them. If they are indigent, the court may pay their costs. Parents are entitled to an evidentiary hearing or trial in which they may contest the allegations made against them.

2. The child

Recognizing that the child's interest is not always synonymous with the parent's or the state's, children in most states are entitled to representation by a guardian *ad litem* or an attorney during adjudication hearings and proceedings to terminate parental rights. The guardian *ad litem* is entitled to access to relevant medical and mental health records, school records, and may interview child, parents, and foster parents. The guardian may subpoena, examine, and cross-examine witnesses and is expected to act on behalf of the child's best interests. The guardian must make the child's wishes known, but also must make an independent recommendation.

3. Foster parents

Foster parents are not a party in proceedings to terminate parental rights. They may petition the court for standing and intervenor status that is limited to that proceeding. The court will consider whether to recognize them, taking into consideration the strength and duration of their relationship with the child and the child's best interest.

The case of *Smith v. OFFER* asked whether foster parents had a right to be heard prior to the removal of a foster child from their home. The Supreme Court held that no additional safeguards were needed beyond the existing foster care termination procedures which were adjudged to be sufficient to protect their limited interests. This decision, although viewed by some as a setback for children's rights, was significant in that it recognized the psychological ties that develop between foster parent and child. The court noted that "The importance of the familial relationship to the individuals and to society stems from the emotional attachments that derive from the intimacy of daily association. No one would seriously dispute that a deeply loving and interdependent relationship between an adult and child in his or her care may exist in the absence of a blood relationship."

In a related case, *James v. McLinden* (341 F. Supp 1233 D. Conn, 1969) a district court overruled a juvenile court's refusal to allow a foster mother access to a hearing to remove her foster child, stating that her due process and equal protection rights had been violated. The court reasoned, "The policy of our law has always been to encourage family relationships even those foster in character."

E. Special situations

1. THE RIGHTS OF UNWED FATHERS

In 1972, *Stanley v. Illinois* (405, U.S. 645) extended due process rights to the father of an illegitimate child in custody proceedings. Many states now require parental notification and the birth father's consent, if he can be identified and located, prior to terminating his parental rights. Courts are questioning the constitutionality of laws that deny parental rights to unwed fathers. Recent case laws have taken into consideration the extent of the father's prebirth involvement and support and should be weighed in determining his standing in adoption. In N.Y. State an unwed father successfully blocked the adoption of his 7-month-old daughter and ultimately gained custody of her. In Wisconsin unwed fathers may assume parental rights if they sign affidavits of paternity (Dullea, 1988). Courts have also determined that failure on the part of the unwed father to provide support can constitute abandonment (*Roe v. Doe*; FLA 5th Dist. Ct. App, 87-1277, 3/24/88; Fla. Sup. Ct. 4/89).

2. THE RIGHTS OF GRANDPARENTS

Historically courts have tended to recognize the rights of grandparents as derivatives of parent's rights rather than inherent rights. Thus, adoption of a child would usually result in termination of visitation privileges by the grandparents. Grandparents may petition the courts as third parties requesting the right for visitation in all 50 states. Some states deny visitation following adoption feeling it would undermine the adoption. Other courts have made exceptions when it is in the child's best interests and where there is consent from the adopting parents. This is more likely to occur when older children are adopted and have significant positive ties to a grandparent.

3. INDIAN CHILD WELFARE ACT

The Indian Child Welfare Act of 1978 (P.L. 95-608) gives authority to tribes to determine the best interests of Indian children. This act resulted in part from the U.S. recognition of tribal sovereignty and the importance of Indian children preserving their roots by remaining within their Indian culture. Title I of the act recognizes that tribal courts have exclusive jurisdiction over custody proceedings, other than divorce, involving children residing on reservations. If children are living off the reservation it requires the state courts to transfer custody proceedings to the tribal courts. In addition, in cases of involuntary termination of parental rights, it requires evidence beyond a reasonable doubt. This is a higher standard than is used elsewhere in the country for termination of parental rights.

Title II of the act provides for the establishment of various programs to meet the needs of Indian children and families living both on and off the reservation. Indian children have been overrepresented in foster and adoptive care and institutions, and the majority of Indian children in foster care have been in non-Indian homes. The act has been very controversial, has triggered numerous administrative problems, and has raised concerns regarding the ability of Indians to provide the needed welfare services.

F. Alternatives to absolute termination of parental rights

1. LONG-TERM FOSTER CARE

In some cases children may not be adoptable or may resist adoption because of loyalty binds or the wish to maintain some contact with the parent. Foster care with tenure allows them to experience stability and permanency without fears of having their ties disrupted. Such an arrangement often works well for foster parents who may be reluctant to adopt because of the extent of a child's medical or emotional problems or because they cannot afford the cost of raising another child.

2. GUARDIANSHIP

The legal establishment of a guardianship affords the rights and responsibilities of a parent without the duty to support. It allows the child to maintain contact with the original parent while relieving that parent of the above obligations. Such an arrangement might be preferred by a relative caring for a child who does not wish to alienate the child's parents by pursuing termination of parental rights.

3. EMANCIPATION

Teenagers who can fend for themselves may request emancipation. Emancipation requires the consent of the teenager's parent or legal guardian. Emancipation is usually not considered unless there is evidence that the teen is competent, self-supporting, and able to live on his own or is married. Parents also may initiate emancipation proceedings. Once legally emancipated, a minor no longer needs parental consent for medical care and may sign contracts. The parents are, in turn, freed of any liability for the child's actions.

G. Adoption

1. HISTORICAL FRAMEWORK

Historically, under Roman law, adoption existed primarily for the benefit of the adopter, i.e., it was a means of preserving family lines and property. It was not recognized under English common law until 1926. As noted by Derdeyn (1977) apprenticeship was a precursor of adoption in the U.S.A. and work was the primary function of this arrangement. Child labor laws interrupted this practice, and children whose parents were unable to care for them were placed in orphanages. The first adoption law was enacted in Massachusetts in 1851 and those that soon followed in other states tended to be informal. The rights of the biological parent to custody were generally held superior to the interests of the child.

The 20th century has seen growing emphasis on children's rights and the emotional needs of children. The concept of the child's best interest has gained favor in the courtroom, and adoption proceedings have become more rigorous. Adoptions in the U.S.A. are subject to state laws that vary considerably from state to state. Families who wish to adopt a child out of the country are subject to U.S. immigration law.

2. PURPOSE

"Adoption is the legal proceeding in which a person takes another person into the relation of child and thereby acquires the rights and incurs the responsibilities of parent in respect of such other person" (New York State Domestic Relations Law Sec. 110). The purpose of adoption has shifted from meeting the needs of parents to those of children. Children are no longer viewed as mere property and increasingly their rights and need for permanency are being recognized. Adoption has also become a means of meeting the needs of persons who are unable to bear children.

3. CHANGING TRENDS

The market of children available for adoption has shifted dramatically in face of the availability of abortion, altered attitudes toward out-of-wedlock pregnancy, the educational mainstreaming of pregnant teenagers, and the trend for unwed teenage mothers to keep their babies. Infant adoptions now comprise only 48% of unrelated domestic adoptions or 0.7% of live births, and 97% of babies born to unmarried mothers remain with their mothers (National Committee for Adoption, 1989). Increasingly, couples seeking to adopt healthy newborns are forced to look abroad, primarily to Korea, China, and Latin America, or pursue private adoptions. These options are also being sought out by couples who are discouraged by the long waiting periods they must face with most private and state adoption agencies. Korea, owing to an improved economy and lower birthrate, has drastically cut back the number of babies available for overseas adoption.

Adoption agencies are increasingly focusing on special needs children, i.e., older children, sibships, children of mixed race, and those with emotional, intellectual, or physical handicaps. Approximately 36,000 special needs children are in foster care awaiting placement, and special needs children constitute about 60% of the children in foster care (National Committee for Adoption, 1989). In an effort to place these children, agencies are becoming more flexible in their criteria for adoptive parents, making exceptions to traditional notions about what constitutes a family. Case workers have become more aggressive and recognize that adoptability is often a function of who will have the child. Hard-to-place children are now being adopted by single, older, and gay and lesbian parents who in the past would have been rejected or overlooked. Several states prohibit adoption by homosexuals, though many are coming to recognize that there is no discernable difference between the parenting done by homosexuals and heterosexuals. Recently, there have been several adoptions by parents of the same gender (*Ms*, Oct. 1989).

In an effort to find permanent homes for difficult-to-place children many states are offering subsidized adoptions. The state in these cases continues to pay the family a stipend after the adoption has been finalized.

In the past, foster parents were discouraged from becoming too attached to their foster children, and adoption of them was discouraged or forbidden. Presumably this thinking was intended to prevent them from getting into an adversarial relationship with the child's parents. Agencies and courts have come to recognize the inevitable attachments that form over time and that it is often in the child's best interests to preserve them. Adoption by foster parents of children who have been in their long-term care is becoming increasingly common. Another new trend has been toward the use of open adoptions.

4. THE SEALED RECORD VERSUS OPEN ADOPTIONS

The country's first sealed records law was enacted in 1917 in Minnesota, and most states soon followed suit. The traditional secrecy that has surrounded adoption was intended to protect the birth mother from the stigma of out-of-wedlock pregnancy, the child from the knowledge of his or her illegitimacy, adoptive parents from the shame of infertility, and to promote the solidarity of the adoptive family. Traditionally, the sealed record could only be broken by court order and then by a showing of "just cause" such as a medical necessity to get information about the birth parents. More recently, adult adoptees have successfully argued in some courts the psychological need to know their past as grounds for opening the sealed record. Three states now have open records that permit adoptees to see their original birth certificates. The Adoptees Liberty Movement Association (ALMA) has chapters around the country that help adoptees find their birth records and parents, and is working to repeal sealed records laws. In addition, many states have mutual consent adoption registries for adoptees and birth parents who wish to seek out each other. As attitudes toward sexuality and secrecy are altering, many are coming to question the need for the sealed record. The Child Welfare League, a long time proponent of secrecy in adoptions, has altered its position stating, "Openness, while protecting the rights of the individuals involved, should be an integral part of all adoption services" (Reuben, 1989).

Open adoptions permit mothers to have a more active role in selecting and even meeting prospective parents. In many cases they may stay in touch with their child following placement. Birth parents who have been through open adoptions feel that it eases the surrendering process for them and gives them more peace of mind. Those opposed to open adoption feel that free access to the child may create confusion and disruption in the child's life and add to the insecurities of the adopting parents. At this time there is insufficient information available on which to formulate any opinions about the impact of open adoptions on the child and adopting parents.

5. PRIVATE ADOPTIONS

Private or independent adoptions now constitute about half of adoptions in the U.S.A. (Mansnerus, 1989). In private adoptions couples bypass home studies and go through physicians, ministers, friends, and want ads (illegal in 19 states) to find a child. Because there is no agency screening of adoptive parents or counseling of pregnant mothers, these adoptions tend to be client centered. Consequently, they may put the needs of the adopting parents ahead of the child's. Private adoptions are illegal in many states and in some states (Connecticut and Massachusetts) they are illegal unless an agency finalizes the adoption.

Of concern has been the extent to which couples will go in aggressively marketing themselves to prospective birth mothers. They may even consent to continued contact by the mother and then renege on the agreement. There is risk that the birth mother who has not received adoption counseling may decide not to surrender. This occurs in about 5% of open adoptions. Several studies confirm a higher failure rate for independent adoptions compared to agency adoptions.

Adoptive parents are expected to pay for the mother's expenses even if she changes her mind, which occurs in about 5–20% of cases (Mansnerus, 1989). States prohibit payment to persons, other than agencies, acting as intermediaries in these transactions though gray and black markets in adoption persist.

The tragic death of Lisa Steinberg brought to a focus the problems of illegal adoptions. A study of adopted parents by Katz found that one in seven suspected that their private adoptions had involved some illegal activity (Mansnerus, 1989). For instance, the legal process may be incomplete, as when the father's parental rights have not been terminated. Many states are now tightening up their adoption laws, e.g., New York prohibits an attorney from representing both birth mother and adoptive parents and now mandates home studies on all prospective adoptive homes.

6. WRONGFUL ADOPTION SUITS

Wrongful adoption suits are beginning to appear in which adoptive parents have charged agencies with deliberately withholding information about their adopted child. In *Burr v. Stark County Board of Commissioners* (491 NE2d 1101, 12 FLA 1343, Ohio, 1986) an agency assured the adopting parents that the child in question was a healthy baby boy. Following adoption, the parents discovered that he was retarded and, further, that the agency had known of tests documenting this all along. The court ruled in favor of the Burrs and concluded, "In no way do we imply that adoption agencies are guarantors of their placements. . . . However, just as couples must weigh the risks of becoming natural parents, taking into consideration a host of factors, so too should adoptive parents be allowed to make their decision in an intelligent manner."

Similar problems may arise if agencies fail to disclose information to adopting parents about children who are HIV positive or children who have been sexually abused and may require years of treatment later on.

III. CLINICAL ISSUES

A. Role of foster care and rationale for termination of parental rights

Foster care is defined as a service "which provides substitute family care for a planned period for a child when his own family cannot care for him for a temporary or extended period and when adoption is neither desirable or possible" (Child Welfare League, 1959). In spite of this, Wald (1976) found that a child in foster care has a 50% chance of remaining there three years or longer. Several studies have demonstrated extensive physical, emotional, and developmental pathology in this population which more often than not goes untreated (Frank, 1980; Swire and Kavaler, 1978). Swire and Kavaler (1978) found moderate to severe impairment in 70% of the foster children surveyed in New York City. Only 4% of these children were judged to be free of mental problems. They concluded that the level of pathology in this sample of children in foster care was roughly comparable to that of other disadvantaged populations. The child in foster care must contend with separation from biological parents, fear of the unknown, feelings of being different, shifting agency personnel, loyalty conflicts over having to relate to two sets of parents, hesitant or ambivalent attachments, and the fear of rejection, separation, and yet another move. Given these stresses, it is difficult for most children in foster care to maximize their potential for normal emotional growth.

Permanent placement is an alternative to indefinite foster care for children unable or unlikely to be returned home. The rationale for termination of parental rights is based upon the beliefs that children are entitled 1) to have some adult function on a permanent basis in the role of nurturing parent, 2) that the child is entitled to maintain such a relationship once it has been ratified by time, and 3) that the child is entitled to a minimal level of freedom from abuse and exploitation within that relationship. When those rights are not being served by the relationship between child and parents and when they would be better served by severing that relationship and freeing the child for adoption, it is the child's right for that separation and reattachment to occur.

B. Assessment of parenting

There is very little in the literature about assessing parenting, yet the child psychiatrist or psychologist may often be called upon to do such an evaluation in the context of an agency deciding whether or not to pursue termination of parental rights.

1. FRAMING THE QUESTIONS

The following questions may be helpful in focusing such an evaluation:
a. Is the parent currently able to meet the child's needs?
b. What is the parent's current level of functioning, and does this represent an arrest in development or a regression?
c. Is the parent's condition treatable, and, if so, is the parent motivated to change and willing to accept therapy?
d. What is the parent's record with respect to following through with recommendations for treatment?
e. If the parent is treatable, will help improve the parent sufficiently in time to meet the child's needs within the child's time perspective?
f. What is the impact of the parent's pathology or conduct on the child, and what ameliorating factors might be present such as the protection of a spouse or grandparent?
g. Does the child have special needs or problems that require exceptional parenting skills?
h. Why does the parent want to regain custody?

2. OBTAINING A HISTORY

Histories obtained from parents will often be self-serving. A parent who has not had good experiences with the state is likely to be mistrustful of the evaluator. Some parents may reveal much incriminating information about themselves which may raise questions about their judgment and motivation.

a. Past history

Abusive histories are common in this population. It is important to determine how much parents may have worked through their own abuse and to what extent they are continuing to enter into abusive relationships. Mothers who are unable to protect themselves from abuse are likely to have trouble protecting their children from abuse and exploitation. One must consider what sort of role models the parents had, and in turn what they offer to the child in this regard. One also needs to look to history to determine the parent's strengths, e.g., the mother who was able to stop drinking and leave an abusive marriage. If there has been a history of mental illness, one needs to determine the parent's perception of it, what they found helpful in treatment, and whether they suffer from residual symptoms, and what effect the illness has had upon their children.

b. Parent-child relationship

A history of the child's development should be obtained with an eye toward what the parents know about parenting and child development, how the parents have handled the stresses of child rearing, and what the child means to them. Parents in this population may view the child as there to meet their needs and may have very unrealistic expectations of them. One father, harking back to earlier times in history, said the main reason he wanted his four sons back was to preserve the family name. Can the parent allow the child to separate and be his own person or is the parent overcontrolling and fused in her identity with the child? What is the parent's capacity for empathy and can she differentiate her needs from those of her child? Has the parent been able to offer reasonable consistency and continuity of care? Has the parent been able to set limits, encourage the child to develop internal controls, and buffer him from excessive stimulation in the environment?

c. Current functioning

Assessment should be made of the parent's current functioning and ability to work and manage everyday affairs. An estimate of intelligence is relevant as is mental status exam and substance abuse history. Who does the parent turn to for support and has she been able to benefit from help? Asking about future orientation and goals is helpful. Many parents live from day to day, have no idea how to go about bettering their lives, and feel as if they have little control over their lives.

Psychological testing is very helpful to corroborate the clinician's impressions and to delineate those areas of functioning that are likely and unlikely to change. If a parent resists testing it may be necessary to get a court order, although whether a court can order such tests to be used in a termination proceeding remains controversial.

C. Assessment of the child's needs

1. SPECIAL NEEDS OF CHILD

Does the child have special needs? A hyperactive child might require parents with exceptional patience, whereas the child with developmental delay might do best with parents who do not hold out high expectations for him. The child who is acting out sexually will probably do best with parents who can set limits but at the same time are not too prudish about sexual matters.

2. CAPACITY FOR OBJECT RELATIONS

Some children have great difficulty attaching, either because they have experienced repeated disruptions in their attachments or because they have not yet obtained the capacity for object relations. Children who have experienced repeated placements often become stand-offish as a way of protecting themselves from future losses. History of past and present attachments will often help differentiate what is a defensive posture from the inability to attach. If a child cannot attach and is placed in an adoptive home, the adoptive parents are likely to become discouraged and feel as if they have failed.

3. EXTENT OF EMOTIONAL OR INTELLECTUAL IMPAIRMENT

Assessment of intellectual and emotional functioning is critical to determining what type of care, treatment, and remediation the child needs. Routine testing of IQ is not necessary unless one suspects developmental problems or learning disabilities. Developmental testing may be used to document where the child is and subsequent gains that she might make in placement. It is imperative that the adoption agency level with prospective adoptive parents about the extent of the child's impairment and let them know what the prognosis might be. Some severely disturbed children may need a period of emotional grooming in therapeutic foster care before they are adoptable. This also allows the psychiatrist to form a clearer picture of the child's diagnosis, e.g., differentiating mental retardation from environmental deprivation.

4. ADOPTABILITY

As noted, increasingly, adoptability has become a function of who will have the child. Previous barriers to adoption such as Down syndrome are disappearing as are prejudices against physically handicapped children. Capacity for object relations remains a major criteria for placement in an adoptive home. The most difficult children to place are those with severe behavior problems including children who are acting out sexually. One must always consider the risk of failed adoption with these children and the devastating effect of yet another rejection.

D. Assessment of the parent-child relationship

1. QUALITY OF ATTACHMENT

This can be obtained by history and by direct observation. One needs to assess the impact of parental separations on the child and how the child reacts to visitations. That a child is upset following visits does not necessarily mean that the visits went poorly and may even be a sign of attachment. Also, one must consider that the child might be reacting to inappropriate behavior by the parent, e.g., the mother who keeps telling her young child that she'll soon be returning home when the parent is not making any effort toward reunification.

Direct observation of parent and young child is invaluable. Home visits can be fruitful, as one can see how the parent handles distractions and to what extent he or she protects the child. For example, during a 30-minute home visit a psychiatrist observed an 18-month-old get into her mother's cigarettes, try to take a drink from a can of gasoline left in the living room, and toddle up a darkened staircase all in full view of her mother who sat smoking and did nothing. The mother insisted she was a good parent because her kids hadn't "torched the house" (yet) and she always took them to the doctor when they were sick. The child was also indiscriminately affectionate with the psychiatrist whom she'd never met before.

How the parent and child play together may provide clues to their relationship How attentive is the parent? Can she talk at the child's level? Does she offer encouragement or berate? Does the child seek out the mother or is she used to solitary play?

2. ROLE REVERSAL

Often one may see the young child waiting hand and foot on the parent, and being exquisitely attuned to the parent's emotional needs. The parent may inappropriately confide in the child and treat her as a much older child. If the child fails to please the parent she may be harshly reprimanded. The parent may demand displays of affection when the child resists.

3. EMPATHY

Capacity for empathy, or lack of it, can be assessed through direct observation of parent and child. One might expect parents to put their best foot forward when they are being observed, yet all sorts of unwitting behaviors may emerge. For example, parents may be overly aggressive with puppets or tickling and may show intimidating behaviors and oblivion to the child's ensuing distress.

E. Possible contraindications to termination of parental rights and adoption

1. CHILD LIVING WITH RELATIVES WHO DO NOT WISH TO ADOPT

If a child is in a satisfactory long-term relationship with relatives who do not wish to adopt, the need to preserve that relationship must be weighed against the child's need for permanency. Relatives may not wish to adopt for fear of alienating a parent. One also needs to assess how intrusive the parent might be in the child's life and whether the contact is a positive or negative one.

2. CHILD STRONGLY BONDED TO THE PARENT

Some children may remain strongly bonded to their parents even after years of foster care. This may occur when past relationships were loving and/or abusive and often when the child continues to fantasize, counter to reality, about the parent improving and coming to get them. One very oppositional 10-year-old strongly identified with all of his mother's passive-aggressive traits and anti-social behavior to the point where he wore out all of the available foster homes. He made no attempt to adjust to foster placements, remained attached to his mother albeit in an unhealthy way, and ultimately was returned home for lack of a better placement. He has since sexually abused his little sister. A strong bond to the parent and loyalty conflicts may prevent a child from attaching to new parents. In one study of termination of parental rights only 5% of 61 children maintained positive ties with their parents at the time of termination and for most of them the ties were tenuous, ambivalent, or nonexistent (Schetky et al., 1979).

3. THE CHILD WHO IS ACTING OUT

The child who is acting out sexually or aggressively is not likely to be a good candidate for adoption and probably needs continued therapy and foster care before he is ready for adoption. This is particularly true for the child going into a home where there are other children whom he or she might victimize. Even if adoptive parents are willing to work with the child around these behaviors, there is risk that they may not appreciate what they are in for and have second thoughts once the child is placed with them.

4. THE CHILD WHO DOES NOT WISH TO BE ADOPTED

Older children may be quite vocal about their preferences. Some may resist adoption because of their fear of the unknown or yet another rejection, whereas some truly do not wish to leave their foster parents whom they have come to regard as their parents. Loyalty to their parents or foster parents also may be a factor, and some may not wish to sever those ties. One also needs to explore the meaning of sibships. It is not always possible to keep sibs together though often it can be arranged for them to maintain contact following adoption. How much weight to give to the child's wishes will depend upon her maturity and stated and likely unstated reasons for her preference. With most teens one would give strong consideration to their wishes and with school-age children some consideration. Preschoolers do not have sufficient maturity to make an informed decision about such matters. Nonetheless, it is always worthwhile exploring their feelings about adoption in order to help them deal with them.

F. Weighing the child's best interests

Having assessed parent, child, and the parent-child relationship, the clinician needs to arrive at recommendations. Factors to be considered include the child's need for permanency, continuity of relationships, and relationships with sibs and extended family. One must look to the quality of the parent-child relationship and what impact severing that relationship would have on the child. Readiness for adoption is another factor, as some courts may be reluctant to terminate if a child is not adoptable. In terms of the parent, the bottom line is whether the parent can be rehabilitated, and, if so, in time to meet the needs of the child.

IV. PITFALLS

A. Countertransference issues

1. Rescue fantasies

It is easy to have rescue fantasies in which we overidentify with a child and want to save him from his miserable environment. Some clinicians may even fantasize about adopting the child and a few have actually acted upon these fantasies. While adoption of a patient is not prohibited in the APA code of ethics, it clearly represents a boundary violation and acting out of countertransference on the part of the therapist. More commonly rescue fantasies take the form of wanting to see the child in a nurturing, intellectually stimulating foster or adoptive home. It is important not to let value judgments polarize thinking and see competing families in black and white terms. We are often privy to much information about the child's family of origin and know very little about the foster family, which may also tend to skew our thinking.

2. Fear of doing harm to parent

Because we are trained to be helpful and empathic it is exceedingly difficult to arrive at a decision that nothing more can be done to reunify a family. Termination of parental rights counters our notions of being helpful and raises concern about how such a drastic action will affect a parent. This is particularly difficult if the parent suffers from a mental disorder that could be exacerbated by termination of parental rights. There is a terrible finality in termination and unlike making psychiatric diagnoses, we do not have time in which to rectify erroneous opinions. The danger is that our apprehensions may lead us to water down our findings or stall in order to spare the parent's feelings or to buy time. The risk to the child is that of prolonging the search for permanency and leaving her in limbo.

A tactful way to deal with this situation is to address the parents' limitations within the context of their own deprived childhoods. For example, it is possible to say that a mother truly loves her child and has tried to the best of her ability, but that her parenting capacities have been adversely affected by her abusive childhood. Further, one might add that she needs to apply her limited emotional resources to her own healing and not be saddled with responsibilities for a child for whom she is unable to care.

B. Role conflict

Double agentry may occur when we confuse treatment with evaluation or when case workers are assigned to work with a client and then must testify against her. This can be clarified at the onset by informing the patient who we are working for and whether communications are confidential. We need to keep the child's interest primary and avoid holding out the child as a therapeutic incentive for the parent.

V. CASE EXAMPLE EPILOGUE

A. Case Example 1

The psychiatrist could not help but feel sympathy for this woman, to whom life had dealt a bad hand. She also had to decide whether she held deaf parents up to the same standard of parenting as hearing parents. Mrs. N.'s dependency issues were very real and it was not clear to what extent they might be altered by psychotherapy. The eldest child was evaluated, and it was apparent that he had assumed a very parental role with his mother. He was literally her mouthpiece as she relied heavily upon him to negotiate with the outside world. He revealed that, several years earlier, he had witnessed his mother inflict multiple bites upon his infant sister. Records were obtained from the state where they formerly resided, and his story was corroborated. The mother's parental rights to this child had been terminated.

Mrs. N. was evaluated with the help of a translator. Her manner was angry and defensive and she expressed her belief in the innocence of her present boyfriend. Her credibility was judged to be poor. Psychological testing showed borderline intelligence, low frustration tolerance, and emotional lability. The prognosis for change was felt to be guarded, but it was recommended that she pursue psychotherapy with a goal of gaining independence. She was also urged to explore job training and work on developing more proficiency in signing. A year later, she continued in therapy, but little had changed in her life, and she remained with her abusive boyfriend. She and her ex-husband, who was awaiting sentencing, then agreed to relinquish parental rights. Her eldest son was adopted by his foster parents and her youngest son remains in foster care.

B. Case Example 2

The foster parents of these little girls were eager to adopt them. The child psychiatry fellow shared his concerns regarding genetic loading and the effects of early deprivation. The foster parents remained steadfast. Parental rights were terminated and the foster parents adopted the children. When reevaluated one year later the 4-year-old's IQ had risen 20 points, and her behavior appeared to be within normal limits as did her sister's.

C. Case Example 3

The child psychiatrist and the children's therapists recommended against placing the children in adoptive homes but were not heard. An adoption worker was assigned to the children and pursued their life history books with them. The children's behavior regressed severely and they became almost unmanageable around the adoption worker's visits. Peggy began setting fires and stealing and Lucas was not able to focus in school. A team review was held six months later. The consulting child psychiatrist and both therapists reiterated the need for long-term permanent placement of the children in their present foster home. Plans for adoption were dropped; the children were told they would remain with their foster parents, and their behavior improved. The foster parents were willing to keep the children, but were understandably reluctant to adopt, given the extent of the children's behavior problems.

VI. ACTION GUIDE

A. Understand the law

Laws regarding termination of parental rights and adoption vary from state to state, and anyone who does this type of work needs to be acquainted with them. The state's assistant attorney general or the state's protective services office can usually direct one to the appropriate statutes.

B. Careful documentation

Successful terminations are built upon careful documentation of efforts to help parents. This includes recording missed and cancelled appointments and documenting recommendations that have been made to parents and whether they were acted upon. Further, the psychiatrist needs to be able to give examples illustrating why the parent continues to be unable to care for the child in question and why that parent's conduct or condition is harmful to the child. The judge who sees that no stone has been left unturned is more likely to terminate than in a case where parents have not had the opportunity to avail themselves of services or visitations.

C. Humility

Mental health professionals need to recognize the limits of their expertise and that they do not have all the answers. Humility goes a long way. It is the judge who is the ultimate decision maker, and we are but one cog in the wheel.

D. Ethical issues

We need to work toward the availability of support systems for families so that foster care and termination of parental rights do not become alternatives to intervention with multiproblem families.

E. Professionalizing foster care

As case worker loads increase, foster parents are assuming more and more responsibilities for their charges. In turn, as more women enter the job market, the pool of competent foster parents is bound to shrink unless something radical is done soon to remediate the situation. Recognizing that not all children are adoptable, and that many need extensive foster care before they are adoptable, we need to recruit more foster parents and dignify the vital work they do. Several measures in this direction would include special training, ongoing support and guidance to foster parents, and paying them salaries with fringe benefits and paid vacations. In closing, I am reminded of a wonderful monument to foster parents that dominates the central square in Tashkent, U.S.S.R. Unfortunately, few foster parents in this country receive that sort of recognition nor do they have the time or money to travel to Tashkent.

VII. SUGGESTED READINGS

OVERVIEW:

Goldstein, J., Freud, A., and Solnit, A. (1973), Beyond the Best Interests of the Child. New York: Free Press.

Hersov, L. (1985), Adoption and Fostering. In: Rutter, M. and Hersov, L., ed: Child and Adolescent Psychiatry. London: Blackwell.

Kessel, J. A., and Robbins, S. P. (1984), The Indian Child Welfare Act: Dilemmas and Needs. Child Welfare Vol LX III (3):225–232.

FOSTER CARE AND TERMINATION OF PARENTAL RIGHTS:

Derdeyn, A. P. (1977), A Case for Permanent Foster Placement of Dependent, Neglected and Abused Children. Am J Orthopsych 47:604–613.

Derdeyn, A. P., Rogoff, A., and Williams, S. (1978), Alternatives to Absolute Termination of Parental Rights after Long-Term Foster Care. Vanderbilt Law Review 31(54):1165–1192.

Dullea, G. (1982), Unwed Father Given Custody Despite Adoption. New York Times, Dec. 9, B13.

Fanshel, D. and Shinn, E. (1978), Children in Foster Care. New York: Columbia U. Press.

Frank, G. (1980), Treatment Needs of Children in Foster Care. Am J Orthopsych 50:263–265.

Hardin, M., ed. (1983), The Legal Framework for Ending Foster Care Drift: A Guide to Evaluating and Improving State Laws, Regulations, and Court Rules. Chicago: ABA.

Horowitz, R., Hardin, M., and Bulkley, J. (1989), The Rights of Foster Parents. Chicago: ABA.

Langelier, P. and Nurcombe, B. (1985), Residual Parental Rights: Legal Trends and Controversies. JAACP 24(6):793–796.

Mnookin, R. (1973), Foster Care in Whose Best Interest? 43 Harvard Ed Rev 599:606–638.

Schetky, D. H., Angell, R., Morrison, C. V., and Sack, W. H. (1977), Parents Who Fail: A Study of 51 Cases of Termination of Parental Rights. J Am Acad Child Psychiatry 18:226–653.

Swire, M., and Kavaler, F. (1977), The Health Status of Children in Foster Care. Child Welfare 56:635–653.

Wald, M. (1976), State Intervention on Behalf of Neglected Children: Standards for Removal of Children from Their Homes, Monitoring the Children in Foster Care, and Termination of Parental Rights. Stanford Law Rev 28(4):623–705.

ADOPTION:

Adoption Fact Book (1989), Washington, DC: National Committee for Adoption.

Adoption Magazine. Ulick Publishing Co, P.O. Box 8551, Bartlett, Il. 60103.

Angell, R. (1985), The Rights of Grandparents. In Schetky, D. H. and Benedek, E. P., (eds.) Emerging Issues in Child Psychiatry and the Law. New York: Brunner/Mazel, Inc.

Brodzinsky, D. M. and Schecter, M. D. (1990), The Psychology of Adoption. New York: Oxford University Press.

Derdeyn, A. P., Wadlington, W. J. (1977), Adoption: The Rights of Parents versus the Best Interests of Their Children. JAACP 16:238–255.

Feigelman, W. and Silverman, A. (1977), Single Parent Adoptions. Social Case Work, July 416–425.

Kadushin, A. (1970), Adopting Older Children. New York: Columbia U. Press.

Mansnerus, L. (1989), Private Adoptions Aided by Expending Network. New York Times, 10/5/89, p. 1.

Reuben, D. (1989), Adoption, The Open Option. Parenting, Nov. pp. 88–96.

Segal, E. C., ed. (1985), Adoption of Children with Special Needs: Issues in Law and Policy. Chicago: ABA.

12

Post-Traumatic Stress Disorder

ELISSA P. BENEDEK, M.D.

I. CASE EXAMPLES

A. Case Example 1

Marissa, an 8-year-old girl, was playing tag with friends in her neighborhood. The game had elements both of tag and hide and go seek. The leader, by agreement, would cover his eyes and all children in the game would hide. The leader would then try to find and catch them. Marissa ran by a basement window where a 13-year-old neighbor was experimenting with what he believed was an unloaded B-B gun. Tragically, the gun was loaded, and Marissa received multiple skin lacerations and abrasions which needed in-hospital care. Marissa was hospitalized precipitously and separated from her parents. Subsequent to surgical repair of her wounds, she suffered a wound infection and spent seven more days separated from her parents. After her return from the hospital, her parents described a young girl who both walked and talked in her sleep, wet the bed, and described nightmares in which she was being chased by a clown with a hideous face. The nightmares diminished over time as did the sleep-walking and talking. Her parents described no school problems, no peer relationship problems, no problems with depression or phobias. Marissa talked freely about the accident and hospitalization for a brief time. Marissa's parents were angry because the neighbor's insurance company would not pay for her hospitalized treatment, and they instituted a suit. Their attorney requested an evaluation for post-traumatic stress disorder (PTSD).

B. Case Example 2

Cecilia, a 17-year-old, sued her stepfather alleging that she suffered serious emotional damages because her stepfather repeatedly sexually abused her from ages 7 to 14 years of age. She alleged that her stepfather would enter her room every other night and abuse her. The abuse progressed from voyeurism to exhibitionism to petting and frank intercourse when she was 14. Cecilia did not tell any other family members about the intercourse. The family recollected that she became progressively more depressed, withdrawn, and isolated. They also noted repeated and frank sexual play with dolls. She lost interest in boys and in her peer group. Her grades in school dropped. She had trouble sleeping. She attempted suicide by overdose. At age 16, she ran away from the home of her natural mother and stepfather, and she went to the home of her natural father and stepmother. She did not tell her natural father why she had run away, but he noted that she seemed changed. She had lost weight and seemed listless, apathetic and depressed. She told the examining psychiatrist for the first time about the sexual abuse in a clinical examination. The psychiatrist revealed the abuse to her natural father, who consulted an attorney. Cecilia was anxious to sue her stepfather, believing that "he destroyed my life." A forensic psychiatrist was consulted after the treating clinician refused to testify. The attorney claimed post-traumatic stress disorder following sexual abuse.

II. LEGAL AND ETHICAL ISSUES

A. History

The role of PTSD syndromes in clinical practice and forensic evaluation is an issue of increasing theoretical and practical importance. Some forensic child experts insist that PTSD in children is a well-researched and clinically proven entity. Citing child emotional and sexual abuse, they point to the current diagnostic nomenclature, DSM-III-R, which sets specific inclusion criteria for the diagnosis of PTSD and makes brief reference to children. Others argue that PTSD still lacks clinical specificity for children and is a syndrome relying too heavily on self-report of a child who is easily suggestible or a parent who has motivation for secondary gain. They suggest that PTSD as a legal concept is one which is ripe for abuse, particularly when there is the possibility of accruing a large reward for civil damages.

Prior to 1980, when DSM-III was published, the symptoms that are now grouped under PTSD were not included in a single diagnostic heading. The result was that prior to 1980 mental health professionals and attorneys lacked an identifiable and accepted description of the symptoms now known as PTSD which could be used in litigation. However, prior to 1980, the concept of traumatic neuroses allowed some information with regard to the role of trauma and the development of psychiatric syndromes to be introduced into the courtroom.

B. Uses of post-traumatic stress disorder in the law

Post-traumatic stress disorder has been introduced primarily by defense attorneys in criminal cases to support claims of self-defense, diminished capacity, or insanity in Viet Nam veterans charged with crimes. Several Viet Nam veterans have gained acquittal by reason of insanity with a PTSD defense. The defense has been less successful in traumatized women who claim that repeated brutal beatings have led to an anticipation of danger and chronic PTSD in order to explain their violent actions. PTSD has also been used with mixed success in a defense in children who, subsequent to repeated emotional, physical, and sexual abuse on the part of their parents, ultimately either attempt to murder or in fact do murder their parents.

PTSD can also be used to attempt to establish liability and to help to define damages in personal injury cases and to establish need for psychiatric care and vocational rehabilitation. PTSD has also been used to establish those personal injury claims based on the psychological sequelae of automobile accidents and emotional damages to witnesses of trauma who have not been actually physically injured.

Although the DSM-III-R states quite explicitly that the use of the manual for nonclinical purposes such as "determination of legal responsibility, competency or insanity, or justification for third party payment must be clinically examined in each instance," the manual has been a boon to the civil defense bar.

C. Legal causation and PTSD

Legal causation is defined by two component parts: (a) direct causation and (b) proximate causation. Direct causation refers to phenomena that can be empirically proven, such as laws of physics, chemistry, astronomy, or in medicine and genetics. Because direct causation is rarely encountered in personal injury tort law (the sponge in the abdomen) or criminal law, the legal concept of proximate cause has been developed.

In essence, proximate causation reflects a social policy decision having to do with determining the limits of liability. It is based on the legal doctrine of foreseeability which creates a method for assessing causation, taking into account a complex nature of human behavior and variables. The doctrine of foreseeability, according to attorneys, holds liable for damages those whose behavior produces injuries which are reasonably expected to flow from either negligent or illegal acts. With regard to PTSD, one must show that the stressor was responsible for the psychological damages. However, attorneys must consider the issues of individual susceptibility, the nature of the traumatic stressor, and assessment of the symptoms and factors that intervene between the stressor and the development of the symptoms. These issues are discussed further in Chapter 21.

D. Susceptibility to PTSD

Not all victims exposed to overwhelming trauma develop PTSD, and not all victims of trauma have pretraumatic healthy personalities. Attorneys who seek to minimize the importance of the stressor in the development of PTSD postulate that the premorbid personality is responsible for impact of the stressor. That is, that the child came from a chaotic, disruptive home environment and that the symptoms the child exhibits are not related to the stressor (flood, sexual abuse, burn) but are more likely than not related to a previous home environment. However, most courts support what is known as "the eggshell theory." That is, that the plaintiff may have been fragile beforehand for whatever reason, but the stressor was the ultimate cause of the collapse of the youngster. Thus, the defendant generally cannot successfully assert that the young victim had a predisposition to injury or "a neurotic constitution."

With regard to the nature of the traumatic stressor, the diagnostic criteria suggests that the person must experience an event that is "outside the range of usual human experience" and that would be markedly distressing to almost anyone, e.g., serious threat to one's life, physical integrity; threat or harm to one's children, spouse, or close relatives; sudden destruction of one's home or community; or seeing another person who has recently been or is being seriously injured or killed as the result of an accident or physical violence. Thus, certain kinds of common experiences are excluded by definition from PTSD. Such experiences as nontraumatic death of a parent or loved one; divorce; and separation from family, such as being lost in a crowd, do not seem to be included as traumatic stressors.

E. Specific problems with PTSD in court

Problems specific to the admissibility of PTSD testimony center around expertise of clinicians in such testimony and, more specifically, whether there is adequate scientific grounding for such testimony. Domestic violence, battered wife system, child sexual abuse syndrome, and trauma syndrome have all been subjected to critical analyses by courts who cannot find sufficient valid scientific research to establish a relationship between a traumatic stressor and the subsequent symptoms of a child. In addition, in some situations where the stressor is obvious, such as the Kansas City Hyatt Regency disaster, the courts do not need expert testimony to establish the existence and nature of the stressor. In other cases regarding pollution, while an expert may testify that exposure to pollution is outside the range of one's usual experience, courts do not generally believe that in today's society such exposure is an extraordinary stressor. Although mental health experts may be qualified to determine whether symptoms exist and whether such symptoms in children can reasonably be interpreted as PTSD, a judge or jury alone is responsible for assessing the nature and extent of the trauma and the credibility of the complainant. The requirement of a connection between a traumatic stressor and the PTSD-specific symptoms states a greater probability that the testimony may implicate the role of a judge or jury than for most other DSM-III-R diagnosis.

III. CLINICAL ISSUES

A. Symptoms and definition

1. Existence of a recognizable stressor that would evoke significant symptoms of distress in almost anyone. It does not take a trained mental health clinician to recognize that war, natural disasters, malignancy, incest, kidnapping, and observation of suicide, homicide, or rape are recognizable stressors evoking distress in almost anyone. These are the stressors described in this volume. In fact, if a child

patient denies distress after one of these experiences, one must wonder about the possibility of pathological denial.

2. Reexperiencing of the trauma as evident by at least one of the following: (a) recurrent and intrusive recollections of the event; (b) recurrent dreams of the event; (c) suddenly acting or feeling as if the traumatic event were reoccurring because of an association with an environmental or ideational stimulus. Although children do have recurrent nightmares in which there may be exact repetitions of the traumatic event or symbolic and actual attempts at mastery, children's recurrent and intrusive recollections are more like daydreams and fantasies. In addition, as primary-process thinking is so close to the surface in young children, environmental or ideational stimuli reminiscent or symbolic of the trauma may be directly responsible for behavioral changes. Children often are unable to link their changed affects, moods, thinking, and behavior to loud noises, darkness, or sudden visual or auditory stimuli which may "remind" them of the traumatic event, but an astute clinician can note the linking.

3. Numbing of responsiveness to or reduced involvement with the external world, beginning some time after the trauma, as shown by at least one of the following: markedly diminished interest in one or more significant activities, feelings of detachment or estrangement from others, constricted affect. Information about this symptom can be obtained from children or from their friends, relatives, or caretakers. These symptoms have been described repeatedly (Freud and Burlingham, 1974; Terr, 1979). Emotional numbing may make children appear as if they are uninvolved or disinterested subsequent to trauma, but, in fact, the numbing is defensive.

4. At least two of the following symptoms which were not present before the trauma: hyperalertness or exaggerated startle response, sleep disturbance, guilt about surviving when others have not or about behavior required for survival, memory impairment or trouble concentrating, avoidance of activities that arouse the recollection of the traumatic event, intensification of symptoms by exposure to events that symbolize or resemble the traumatic event. Particularly prominent in children are sleep disturbances, with inability to fall asleep, night terrors, and nightmares. Traumatized children are described as regressing in the following ways: climbing into bed with their parents, sleeping in strange places, sucking their thumbs, and becoming enuretic.

Terr (1979, 1981) reports some special criteria, while describing symptomatology following psychic trauma in children: (a) fear of death, separation, and further trauma; (b) misidentification of perpetrators and/or hallucinations of perpetrators; (c) no disavowal or traumatic amnesia; (d) absent vegetative or nervous effects; (e) no visual flashbacks; (children are more likely to daydream and fantasize at will; conscious daydreaming, she believes, may partially block the chances for gruesome visions to intrude;) (f) work performance (school) rarely suffers for more than a few months after psychic trauma as opposed to long-term decline experienced by adults; (g) time skew; (h) shortened sense of the future.

Terr has also suggested new forms of PTSD in children. One form, Type I disorder, follows exposure to a single traumatic event (dog bite, accident), while Type II disorders result from multiple or long-standing experience with extreme stress such as prolonged sexual or physical abuse. Terr differentiates between Type I and Type II disorders suggesting that all PTSD children experience visualization, reenactment, fear, and futurelessness, but children exposed to Type II trauma attempt to cope with ongoing stressors. In that attempt, they develop additional problems such as denial, rage, and unremitting sadness which may become characteristic personality styles for children with Type II disorder.

B. Assessment of symptoms and factors which may affect symptom development

Assessment of symptoms poses two difficulties. One is the veracity of the complainant. Most PTSD symptoms are subjective and not objective. Thus, even in children, attorneys, to up the ante with regard to damages, suggest that symptoms are magnified, embroidered, or exaggerated. Even more importantly, the symptoms of PTSD are not necessarily specific to the diagnosis, although clinical studies of post-traumatic stress disorder in children consistently list the following symptoms: development of trauma-related or mundane fears, sleep disturbances including difficulties in going to bed and falling asleep, nightmares, regressive bedwetting, eating disturbances, acting out or withdrawal behavior, depressive symptoms—sadness, madness, badness, mistrust, personality problems. Terr has described certain phenomena which seem to be exclusive to childhood PTSD including posttraumatic play, reenactment behavior, emotional numbing, time distortion, and belief in omens. Terr has also categorized these behaviors into four general areas—visualization, reenactment, fear, and futurelessness. Many of these symptoms are PTSD-specific in children but are not related as yet to any specific form of trauma.

C. Intervening factors

It is not sufficient legally to show that "but for the stressor" PTSD would not have occurred. The attorney must also demonstrate that no foreseeable intervening act could break the chain of causation between the stressor and the PTSD symptoms. However, in children, factors such as change in appearance, school failure, or loss of a peer group may develop along with the traumatic event (flood, airplane crash) and exacerbate the symptoms of PTSD which are due to the original trauma. Specifically in children, parents often do little to empathize with the feelings of responsibility and condemnation that the child experiences, and family dynamics and intrapsychic functioning of parents may be significant in the formation of PTSD in children.

Burgess and Holstrom suggest that the family is probably the strongest potential source of support available to the sexually abused child. Benedek too (1985) finds a strong correlation between the child's psychiatric symptoms and home environment. Friends and relatives of a traumatized child may turn their frustration into blaming the victim, accusing the child of being irresponsible, of provoking an attack, of failing to do all she could to prevent it, or of actually enjoying the attention. Parents might be overprotective or patronizing to a victim. Thus, it is often not clear whether it is the traumatic event itself or its indirect consequences that caused the symptoms of PTSD in a child. Additionally, in children a clinician may confuse problems in living (poor peer relationships, school difficulties) with PTSD symptoms. These clinical errors may have grave legal consequences.

D. Developmental factors

It is also generally assumed that the impact of a trauma will be a function of the child's developmental stage and be related to (a) whether the trauma is manmade or of natural causes (compare flood to sexual abuse); (b) the degree of ambiguity surrounding the source of the trauma; (c) the outcome of the traumatic event; (d) the proximity to the trauma; (e) co-morbidity; (f) previous life events; and (g) personal impact on the child. Pynoos and Eth (1985) have described special interview techniques they use which permit children to spontaneously and fully describe their subjective experiences. Those techniques encourage children to re-call the central event of the trauma, their own perceptual experience, the worst moment of the trauma, the details including sight and smell of the trauma, and to report ongoing traumatic reminders. Their strategies for interview and closure have been described in great detail (1985).

E. Treatment

Treatment techniques for psychic trauma in children are very preliminary. There is no one certain established standard technique. Possibilities for treatment of childhood post-traumatic stress disorders cluster into individual, family, and group treatment using standard treatment modalities such as play therapy, psy-chodynamic psychotherapy, cognitive and behavioral therapy, and medication. Treatment considerations suggest that all those involved in the child's immediate environment, including parents, teachers, religious counselors, girl and boy scout leaders, and significant others, may be important in treatment. It is also important not to allow treatment to be delayed by pending litigation.

IV. EPILOGUE

A. Case Example 1

Marissa's attorney was specific with regard to the evaluation he requested and presented a possible diagnosis—post-traumatic stress disorder. Although a clinician might empathize with Marissa and her family because Marissa indeed did suffer a traumatic injury, the diagnosis of PTSD would not be appropriate. The stressor was outside the range of normal experience for a child (a wound from a B-B gun); however, Marissa suffered none of the cardinal features of PTSD. She had a brief period of bad dreams and enuresis. Her academic performance and peer relationships were not disturbed. Marissa talked freely about the accident, the hospitalization, and her feelings. She developed no symbolic post-traumatic play.

B. Case Example 2

Cecilia was sexually abused for 7 years by her stepfather. Clinical evaluation revealed suicidal ideation, depression, nightmares, and posttraumatic play at an early age. The treating clinician diagnosed post-traumatic stress disorder appro-priately and appropriately declined involvement in Cecilia's suit. It is difficult, if not impossible, for a treating clinician to remain objective and to wear both the hat of an expert in a forensic case and that of a treating clinician.

V. PITFALLS

A. Inadequate review of preexisting documents

This pitfall has been described in other chapters. All existing documents, including hospital and treatment records, must be reviewed. In certain cases in toxic tort, specialized documents such as air and water assessments, flood patterns, and toxicology literature must also be reviewed.

B. Inadequate interview

The interview in forensic cases has been discussed in other chapters. Once again, time and care must be taken in the clinical interview or interviews to elicit factual and nonsymbolic data from parents and child.

C. Nonobjective interview

If a child has been physically injured (i.e., badly burned, suffered an amputation, etc.) countertransference feelings may be strong, and the clinician may wish to "help" the child and proffer a diagnosis which does not fit with diagnostic criteria. This is of particular relevance in child psychiatrists who may wish to help the family recoup financial losses suffered in a natural disaster. The results of the interview may be prejudged or predetermined because of clinician bias and lack of objectivity.

D. Financial fee splitting

Attorneys may suggest to clinicians that their fees may be paid at the conclusion of a case depending on the result of the case. While this may be ethical behavior for attorneys who accept cases on contingent fees, such behavior is not ethical for psychiatrists.

VI. ACTION GUIDE

1. A discussion of the neurobiology of PTSD is beyond the scope of this chapter. Anyone working in the area should become familiar with the emerging literature on the pathophysiology of PTSD.

2. Do not be afraid to consult with colleagues. A second opinion in this area is often useful. In addition, medical colleagues in other disciplines may provide helpful information.

VII. SUGGESTED READINGS

Eth, S. and Pynoos, R. (1985), Developmental perspective on psychic trauma in childhood. In: Figley (ed.): Trauma and Its Wake. New York: Brunner-Mazel.

Eth, S. and Pynoos, R. (1985) Psychiatric interventions with children traumatized by violence. In: Schetky, D. H. and Benedek, E. P. (eds.): Emerging Issues in Child Psychiatry and the Law. New York: Brunner-Mazel.

Goodman, R. and Rosenberg, M. (1987), The child witness to family violence. In: Sonkin, D. J. (ed.): Domestic Violence on Trial: The Legal and Psychological Dimensions of Family Violence. New York: Springer.

Malmquist, C. P. (1985), Children who witness violence: tortious aspects. Bull Am Acad Psychiatry Law 13(3):221–230.

Malmquist, C. P. (1986), Children who witness parental murder: post traumatic aspects. J Am Acad Child Psychiatry 25(3):320–325.

Pynoos, R. and Eth, S. (1984), The child as witness to homicide. J Soc Issues 40(2): 87–108.

Pynoos, R. and Eth, S. (1986), Witness to violence: the child interview. J Am Acad Child Psychiatry 25(3):306–309.

Schetky, D.H . (1978), Preschoolers' responses to murder of their mothers by their fathers: a study of four cases. Bull Am Acad Psychiatry Law 6:45–57.

Terr, L. (1983), Chowchilla revisited: the effects of psychic trauma four years after a school bus kidnapping. Am J Psychiatry 140:1542–1550.

Terr, L. (1984), Time and Trauma. Psychoanal Study Child 39:633–665.

Terr, L. (1984), Time sense following psychic trauma: a clinical study of ten adults and twenty children. Am J Orthopsychiatry 53(2).

Terr, L. (1988), What happens to early memories of trauma? A study of twenty children under age five at the time of documented traumatic events. J Am Acad Child Adolesc Psychiatry 27(10):96–104.

13

Juvenile Delinquency

MICHAEL G. KALOGERAKIS, M.D.

I. CASE EXAMPLES

A. Case Example 1

Thomas is already in trouble by the age of 13. Always a poor student, he begins to be truant in the seventh grade, "hanging out" with older adolescents. One of seven children born to a widowed seamstress, he is not missed when he begins to stay out late at night. Neither is his mother aware of the extent of his truancy until the school guidance counselor initiates action to declare Thomas a person in need of supervision or a status offender.

His first appearance in court results in returning home despite the fact that the probation officer at intake notes a history of severe learning disability, a borderline IQ, troubled sleep marked by nightmares, and poor judgment in managing peer relationships. He is admonished to attend school and is referred to his school district's Committee on Special Education.

A year and a half later Thomas is returned to court by the police, charged with delinquency. He is apprehended with some older youths dealing drugs. He is assigned a lawyer and is remanded to a detention center pending adjudication.

B. Case Example 2

Roger and his siblings are removed from the care of an alcoholic mother, are separated, and are placed in various foster homes. This leaves Roger lonely and bitter. He becomes increasingly defiant of authority in a succession of foster homes and is frequently disruptive in class. Despite this, numerous teachers see him as a bright youngster whose academic underachievement seems more related to personality problems than to intellectual deficiency. In his last foster home, he is frequently in difficulty with his foster mother's boyfriend who seems to take special pleasure in baiting him.

On one occasion, after Roger has a few beers at a friend's house, he returns home to find his foster mother being beaten by her lover. Roger goes "crazy," attacks the man, and beats him into unconsciousness. In court, the seriousness of the assault and Roger's age (16 years) raises the question of waiver to adult court, in spite of this being his first offense.

C. Case Example 3

By the time of his sixth appearance, Vincent is well-known to the court. As a child of 7, he and his immigrant parents were referred by the state's child protective services unit on charges of child abuse. Referral of the family to a community mental health center was the disposition at the time. On subsequent returns to the court, it is noted that even though gross abuse by the parents has been controlled, Vincent continues to show signs of disturbance: he is frequently disruptive in class, has started a fire in the basement of his buiding, shows cruelty to animals, and is a loner. This changes when, at the age of 14, he becomes a member of a local gang and gradually establishes a reputation of being fearless during turf wars with other gangs.

After adjudication as a delinquent, Vincent spends 4 months in a residential treatment center. He runs away. Reports from this facility indicate that he has never fit into the program and seems unable to take advantage of the educational and vocational opportunities available. Apprehended by the police while committing a robbery at gunpoint, he is returned to court just before his sixteenth birthday.

II. INTRODUCTION

A. Definition

Juvenile delinquency is a crime committed by a minor which would constitute a felony if committed by an adult. A minor is defined in most states as anyone under the age of 18 years. In a few states, "adulthood" in the eyes of the court is reached at 16 or 17 years of age.

Delinquency is punishable under the law, with individual states determining the range of punishment that may be applied. Jurisdiction over juveniles falls to the juvenile or family court. Most courts permit the transfer of jurisdiction, also known as waiver, to the adult court when older minors commit specific, serious crimes (Case Example 2).

B. Dimensions of the problem

1. NATIONAL STATISTICS

In 1984, the juvenile courts in the United States handled 1,304,000 delinquency and status offense cases. Of these, some 5 percent were for violent crimes, 34 percent for property crimes, 40 percent for other delinquent offenses, and about 21 percent for status offenses (noncriminal behavior such as truancy and running away). According to Gardner (1987), violent juvenile crime rose by 250 percent between 1960 and 1981.

2. IMPACT

One cannot overestimate the toll taken on the individual child, on families, on neighborhoods, and on society as a whole by youthful delinquency. The disruption, the pain, and the economic hardship are incalculable; the cost to the nation is in the billions of dollars. Though found everywhere, it is overwhelmingly the scourge of our cities, where it is endemic. It has resisted all efforts to reduce it, and, if anything, it has taken on more virulent forms in the last decades. Delinquency affects our youth directly and shapes the future of our society. Juvenile delinquency is the apprenticeship for adult crime, and few adult criminals did not begin their careers during adolescence.

3. ASSOCIATION WITH POVERTY AND URBAN SLUMS

Although white-collar crime has its juvenile counterpart, delinquency remains quintessentially a phenomenon of the impoverished, unskilled, and semi-literate masses, most particularly in our urban slums. This is not surprising since delinquency is fundamentally an expression of resentment by the youthful offender: resentment at society for the way in which it discriminates in its distribution of wealth, resentment of authority for its abuse and exploitation, resentment of fellow citizens for their rejection and hostility, and resentment, too, of their own families for failing to meet their responsibilities after bringing a child into the world. Most delinquent acts are either attempts to redress what are perceived as economic injustices or expressions of anger at those seen as responsible for their misfortune.

Yet there is no simple equation between poverty or living in a slum on the one hand and delinquency on the other. Research remains to be done that will provide definitive explanations for how some families in urban ghettos manage to avoid significant antisocial patterns or how a child in a delinquent family emerges unscathed by the lifestyle of the others.

4. VIOLENCE

The most disturbing development in the history of delinquency in this country has been the sharp increase in violence committed by youth. More recently this has been closely associated with the epidemic of drug abuse, notably the use of crack cocaine. But the trend has manifested itself earlier, and other factors are also responsible. For some, the gradual erosion of respect for authority (witness the surge of previously rare attacks on the elderly) has had an important impact. For others, the failure of the civil rights movement to achieve its goals has led to despair and rage which often gets expressed indiscriminately. It is uncertain whether trends in the nature of emotional disturbances are playing a role, but it is clear that the ranks of the violent draw heavily from the more disturbed population.

5. THE RISK FACTORS

Overall the risk factors for delinquency include social, familial, biological, and psychological contributions which have been studied and identified by numerous researchers (Glueck and Glueck, 1950; Lewis, 1983; Offer et al., 1979; Benedek and Cornell, 1989; and others). Considerably more research needs to be done to identify new issues as well as to test out the validity of existing hypotheses. As of this writing, the National Institute of Justice and the MacArthur Foundation have launched a major 5–8-year longitudinal study of criminal behavior covering 6000 individuals from birth to age 18, integrating biological, behavioral, and sociological perspectives (*NIJ Reports,* May/June 1990).

C. Juvenile court

1. ESTABLISHMENT AND STRUCTURE

As noted in Chapter 1, the juvenile court was established with an air of optimism if not naiveté. From the outset, the juvenile court functioned as part court, part social agency concerned as much with assuring the best interests of the delinquent child as with protecting the community from his/her actions. As originally conceived, the new court assumed a *parens patriae* role (the state acting in the role of parent) and embodied a number of major departures form criminal court philosophy (Whitebread and Heilman, 1988). Rehabilitation replaced punishment as a goal. All records and proceedings were kept confidential. Sentencing, renamed disposition in the new court, was exclusively to facilities for juveniles, thus assuring separation from adult criminals. Finally, proceedings were carried out informally, not in the adversarial climate of adult courts. Thus lawyers were not generally involved, and even the judges of the juvenile court commonly lacked legal training.

2. PROCEDURES

Children brought to court by a police officer or sent by school officials would be seen by an intake worker who would decide whether to dismiss the case, divert it to another agency, or move it forward to the adjudicatory (trial) phase. At adjudication, a finding of juvenile delinquency would lead to the disposition phase which replaced the sentencing of the adult court. At each step in the process there was considerable discretion, both judicial and nonjudicial, leading to unavoidable abuses.

3. LATER HISTORY

a. *Parens patriae* and the rehabilitation ideal

As the court developed, the original concept of a social service agency was expanded. Probation officers and social workers were brought in, and child guidance clinics took shape around court-related youth. The notion predominated that delinquents were troubled children who needed a healthy atmosphere in which to grow, as well as some form of psychiatric treatment. However, combination of exaggerated expectations of the juvenile court and increasing abuses inherent in its loose structure led by mid-century to mounting criticism of the juvenile justice system. The rates of delinquency were rising, not decreasing. Among those adjudicated, recidivism was common, regardless of the treatment. More virulent forms of criminal behavior were emerging. Disenchantment with the promises of the mental health professions was widespread. In addition, lawyers and children's rights advocates were expressing alarm at the absence of minimal due process procedures in the juvenile courts (Feld, 1980).

b. Due process and procedural reform

By the late 1960s, constitutional issues which had surfaced in lower courts reached the United States Supreme Court. Three major decisions led the way to a far more vigorous juvenile court.

Kent v. United States (1966). This case concerned the issue of waiver of juveniles to adult courts. The Court ruled that the procedure was so serious as to require, as a guarantee of adequate constitutional protection, a hearing and a statement of reasons prior to transfer.

In re Gault (1967). Widely regarded as a landmark decision, *Gault* involved a 15-year-old Arizona youth who was adjudicated for making obscene phone calls and remanded to the state industrial school until adulthood. He was facing incarceration for a 6-year period for an offense which would have earned an adult 2 months in jail. The Court recognized the injustice in the handling of juveniles and mandated a number of due process requirements at all adjudicatory hearings on delinquency petitions. It called for an adequate and timely notice of charges, the right to subpoena witnesses, and the right to confront and cross-examine them. The court also established the privilege against self-incrimination for juveniles. Last and most important of the rights guaranteed by *Gault* was the right to counsel.

In re Winship (1970). Only the right to trial by jury remained as a point of distinction with adult criminal court. The Court, in a subsequent decision, *McKeiver v. Pennsylvania* (1971), failed to extend this right to juveniles. However, in *In re Winship* (1970), it held that the standard of proof for delinquency adjudication must be the most rigorous, "beyond a reasonable doubt," the standard applicable in adult criminal cases.

c. Juvenile Justice and Delinquency Prevention Act

Other developments were beginning to have an impact on the original juvenile court, effecting significant changes. Judges began to be drawn from the ranks of the legally trained (Smith, 1974). In many states, those who had interest or experience in juvenile matters began to specialize as juvenile court judges. The federal government, responding to public concern, set up a number of presidential commissions which ultimately resulted in the passage of the first legislation specifically related to juvenile delinquency, the Juvenile Justice and Delinquency Prevention Act (1974). This act established the Office of Juvenile Justice and Delinquency Prevention which was given the responsibility of funding and overseeing programs emphasizing community-based treatment and prevention. A major aim of this legislation was to deinstitutionalize status offenders and to remove them from the jurisdiction of the court (decriminalization).

d. ABA/IJA Standards

The American Bar Association, working with the Institute of Judicial Administration, also addressed the procedural concerns with the juvenile court. Beginning in 1977, its "Standards" were published which advocated a number of radical revisions in the operation of the court. Though not all of these were ultimately approved by the ABA, the thrust with regard to delinquency was unmistakable: individualized treatment and rehabilitation were rejected and in their place a philosophy of least possible intervention emphasizing "just deserts" and proportionate and determinate sentencing emulating the adult criminal court was urged (Morse and Whitebread, 1982). They also supported the decriminalization of status offenses and jury trial for delinquents. Criticism of these radical proposals came from many quarters, including the American Psychiatric Association (1978), which deplored the abandonment of the rehabilitative ideal and the virtual elimination of distinctions between adult and juvenile offenders.

e. Emergence of a punitive model

In the wake of the ABA/IJA Standards, a number of legal scholars have continued to advocate a more punitive approach to delinquents (Gardner, 1987). The rationale for this approach is that the rehabilitation model has been tried and has proved a failure and that punishment meted out in proportion to the crime committed would at least be fair to the juvenile and at the same time protect the community. Some even subscribe to a belief in the deterrent value of punishment.

f. Increase in violent crime; waiver; the move to eliminate the court

The sharp increase in violent crime committed by juveniles—250% between 1960 and 1981 (Gardner, 1987)—has generated considerable fear in the public and has led to a demand for stiffer penalties for offenders. As more and more youngsters are being waived to adult court—where paradoxically they often end up with lighter sentences than they would have received in juvenile court—some have wondered whether there is any purpose in keeping the juvenile court at all

(Wizner and Keller, 1977). It is not clear, however, what some of those who advocate eliminating the juvenile court would propose to do with abuse and neglect cases. Nor is it clear what importance they give to developmental factors as issues relevant to the commission of crimes or to the dispositions that are meted out (Melton, 1984; Morse and Whitebread, 1982; and Gardner, 1982).

III. LEGAL ISSUES

A. General issues and concerns of the court

1. PROCEDURES REQUIRING CLINICAL EVALUATION

a. Waiver

From the earliest days of the juvenile court, it was apparent that the paternalistic approach was not suitable for all delinquents. Some were already functioning as adults and retained little of the developing child in them. Their crimes were serious, even atrocious, and they showed little amenability to rehabilitation. A mechanism for dealing with such youth in the criminal court was needed. Waiver, or transfer, became that approach and was incorporated as a regular procedure in the juvenile courts of most states.

Generally, the factor leading to the consideration of waiver, in addition to the aforementioned age of the youth, heinousness of the crime, and amenability to treatment, were the mental and physical condition of the youth, his or her previous record, and the danger posed to the public (Whitebread and Heilman, 1988). Assessment of the unknowns among these factors fell to the mental health professional or forensic clinician.

b. Competency

The issue of competency to stand trial, applied to juveniles as well as adults prior to 1899, fell into disuse as the *parens patriae* purposes of the juvenile court made it unnecessary. With the increasing criminalization of the court, however, competency again became an issue. Today it is arising with greater frequency. At present, more than one third of the states provide for the defense to be used in juvenile court (Grisso et al., 1987). Most of these states use the adult standard (*Dusky v. U.S.*, 1960) of ability to consult with one's lawyer and rational and factual understanding of the charges and proceedings as the criteria for determining competency.

Noting that adequate research does not exist to guide courts in assessing what is relevant to a determination of competency, Grisso and his associates nonetheless offer guidelines for selecting *classes* of juveniles who are at greater risk of being incompetent. A youth 12 years of age or younger, or one with a history of mental illness or mental retardation, a borderline IQ (71–80), or a learning disability may qualify. In addition, problems in interpreting reality that are observed by the court can lead to a finding of incompetence. Youths found to be incompetent after clinical evaluation are remanded to an inpatient psychiatric service for treatment and further disposition. A number of states bar mental health evaluations prior to adjudication, in which case a competency determination as such cannot be made. Disposition may, nonetheless, be to a psychiatric facility. If this could be assured in all cases where it is clinically indicated, pre-adjudication competency determinations would serve no practical purpose (Fitch, 1989). There remains, however, the important legal consideration that juveniles are entitled to every opportunity to defend themselves against charges of delinquency.

c. Diminished responsibility

Responsibility for criminal behavior has, from the earliest times, received special treatment when the offenders were children. Their punishment was often harsher than that imposed on adults. Under Roman law, immunity from criminal prosecution existed until speech was attained. This translated in Anglo-Saxon law to the age of 7; and later became the basis for total absence of responsibility in American jurisprudence. Puberty was often the time when full criminal responsibility began. The years 7 to 14 constituted a period of relative or partial responsibility (Drukteinis, 1986). In the Case Examples, Vincent (Case Example 3) might reasonably be defended on grounds of diminished responsibility, particularly at an earlier appearance in court.

Besides age, the youth's level of maturity, ability to distinguish right from wrong, evidence of criminal intent (*mens rea*), and the nature of the crime were taken into consideration in determining what responsibility to allocate.

Infancy defense. Prior to the establishment of the juvenile court, the infancy defense by which a youth can be deemed accountable only if able to know what he or she is doing and that it is wrong, was the standard method of protecting offenders who, because of their immaturity, were thought to be incapable of knowingly doing wrong. After 1899, and especially since *Gault*, most authorities, and indeed most states, view the infancy defense as redundant. Some scholars continue to see a place for the doctrine in juvenile court proceedings (Walkover, 1984). Others point out that, in contrast to the insanity defense which permits treatment of the juvenile, the infancy defense precludes such treatment (they are not ill) and would consequently be unacceptable to a "safety-conscious society" (Fitch, 1989).

Insanity defense. The most widely accepted standard for use of the insanity defense in adult criminal cases is that of the American Law Institute (1962). This standard states that a criminal defendant may be found not guilty by reason of insanity if at the time of committing the crime (s)he "lacked substantial capacity either to appreciate the wrongfulness of his conduct or to conform his conduct to the requirements of the law" because of "mental disease or defect." Those exculpated by this defense are generally hospitalized in a psychiatric hospital as the alternative to serving a prison term.

Since treatment still remains a major consequence of adjudication as a juvenile, there is little interest in engaging in a defense that guarantees such an outcome except in jurisdictions or cases where punishment is the likely disposition. As with the infancy defense, the clinical assessment of the forensic expert is crucial for establishing insanity.

Though the legal arguments for permitting use of the insanity defense in juvenile court are compelling (e.g., fundamental fairness), from a practical standpoint the defense seldom arises. This experience notwithstanding, Weissman (1983) believes that "proof of any incapacity diminishing the juvenile's ability to morally appreciate delinquency prohibitions or to volitionally conform with the dictates of law merits formal attention." He recommends the responsibility determinations be transferred to the dispositional phase as a way of extending more effective protection to the juvenile (p. 516). Conceivably, Roger (Case 2) could benefit from such a defense, possibly on the grounds of temporary insanity.

2. MATTERS FOR THE FORENSIC EXAMINER

a. Double agentry

This addresses the question, "Who is my client?" In the court, a mental health professional may serve numerous masters: the accused juvenile, the court, the public, or the youth's parents. It is clear that to serve two clients in such a situation is to serve neither well. As the Hastings Report on double agentry (1978) points out, a forensic psychiatrist is often involved in multiple agentry: evaluating a patient in need who may pose a serious threat to the community, wishing to produce a report helpful to a lawyer, etc.

Simon (1987) elucidates the problem in the context of the fiduciary relationship existing between psychiatrist and patient. This is defined as "every case where confidence is placed by one person and accepted by another with resulting dependence of one party on the influence of another." The author warns against converting a psychiatric examination into a criminal investigation, obtaining information from a defendant that might subsequently be used against him or her.

Of paramount importance is the juvenile's understanding of the purposes of the examination which is being conducted.

b. Validity and reliability of the mental health examination

Critics of the juvenile court have often focused their attention on the utility of the forensic evaluation, pointing to the literature on the difficulties of diagnosis, especially with adolescents, the problems with predicting future behavior, frequent disagreements between experts, etc. The high variability in the level of competence of forensic clinicians has fueled such criticism and is an argument for improving training for such specialized work.

c. Prediction of dangerousness

Here, too, an extensive literature has cast serious doubts on mental health professionals' ability to predict violence. Although the American Psychiatric Association has issued a clear disclaimer regarding such a capability (1974), the courts continue to request a statement from the evaluating clinician about a juvenile's potential for violence. The relevance of such an opinion to disposition is obvious, as is the public's interest in reliable prediction.

d. Admissibility of expert opinion

Aber and Repucci (1987) have called attention to an increase in reliance on mental health issues to decide legal issues at the same time that skepticism about the value of such expertise has grown. Given that "wholly objective or value-free empirical data does not and cannot exist in the social sciences" (p. 169) and that judges will continue to use expert opinion with broad discretion, these authors issued an appeal to mental health professionals to be aware of their limitations and to make them clear when they offer opinions in the courtroom.

Although severe critics of the admissibility of mental health opinion have stated, "there is no reason to consider such testimony as other than highly speculative" (Ziskin, 1981), others, such as Bonnie and Slobogin (1980), have found utility in "informed speculation." These authors note that it is customary in legal matters to deal with different standards of proof and that it is, therefore, appropriate to allow different standards of evidence for different cases with regard to mental health testimony.

e. Dispositional recommendations

Disposition is the end-point of all the activity that has gone before in juvenile court proceedings. Whether the juvenile gets help or not, whether liberty is sacrificed or not, how punitive the court will be, and how long the youth will remain in the custody of the court are all questions that are likely to be answered at disposition.

The contribution of the forensic specialist has the greatest practical value at this stage. Despite this, in some jurisdictions the mental health expert is barred from making recommendations stemming from the evaluation. Diagnosis and a report on the findings of the direct examination may be all that is permitted. More commonly, dispositional recommendations are welcomed and have a great influence on the court. In homicide cases, for example, identification of mitigating factors can play an important role in deciding ultimate disposition. This has become vital in waiver cases now that the Supreme Court has decided in favor of allowing the death penalty for juveniles 16 or 17 years of age, even if handicapped (*Stanford v. Kentucky*, 1989; *Wilkins v. Missouri*, 1989).

The ABA/IJA Standards (1977) recommend equal access to public "services" for delinquents and nondelinquents but want such services to be voluntarily accepted by the juvenile (informed consent). The Standards also draw the distinction between custodial and noncustodial dispositions and secure and nonsecure placement. Secure placement should be reserved for those cases when no other disposition will protect the public sufficiently.

f. Confidentiality

Since a report will be written to the court, the usual doctor-patient privilege that is present in a therapeutic relationship does not exist between the clinician evaluating a juvenile and the client. On the other hand, in contrast to adult criminal court, juvenile court records and proceedings are private and not open to the public.

B. Issues of primary concern to the prosecution

1. WAIVER

The transfer of jurisdiction over a juvenile to the adult criminal court is a very serious proceeding. A youth who is waived loses a number of protections: confidentiality of the proceedings, the special status of adjudication rather than conviction (it usually cannot be used against the youngster in future court appearances), the more benign dispositions of the juvenile court (including no death penalty) and the limitations on length of detention (to majority in juvenile court, for life in adult court).

Except in states which mandate waiver statutorily, the prosecutor usually initiates the procedure. After a "probable cause" hearing, probation and mental health reports are requested, and, using a preponderance of the evidence standard, the attempt is made to demonstrate that the youth is not suitable for juvenile court dispositions because he or she is already operating like an adult criminal. In Case Example 2, Roger was being considered for waiver to the adult criminal court because of the seriousness of his assault and his age (16), but the mitigating factors (his mother being beaten) and this being his first offense reduced the likelihood of transfer. In all such cases, the protections laid down by *Kent v. U.S.* (1966) apply.

2. PUNITIVE MODEL AND PRETRIAL DETENTION

Sensitive to public clamor and mindful of the evidence that the rehabilitation model has failed, prosecutors often are inclined to think of restrictive placement such as training schools rather than the traditional "least restrictive alternative" for any youth posing a continuing danger to the community. In addition, they are likely not to release such a youth pending adjudication. Such "pretrial detention" has been found to be constitutionally permissible by the Supreme Court (*Schall v. Martin,* 1984).

Consistent with the concept of diminshed responsibility, most punishment theorists concede that being an adolescent is per se reason enough to reduce punishment levels that operate in the adult system (Gardner, 1987; Zimring, 1982). Still, with the Juvenile Justice Standards leading the way (American Bar Association, 1977), proportionate sentencing and other adult techniques such as restitution have been applied increasingly in juvenile courts.

3. PROPORTIONALITY AND DETERMINANCY

These concepts are aimed at increased fairness in an arbitrary and frequently discriminatory court. Punishments are, as in adult courts, set according to the seriousness of the offense, and individual considerations (mitigating factors) are minimized. It is apparent that if such an approach is rigorously applied, disposition is arrived at without the need for input from probation officer or mental health professionals.

4. ACCESS TO PAST RECORDS

Although readily accessible to court personnel involved in the case, court records are not made available to the public or the press. The questions of stigma and labeling have figured prominently in the literature on children's rights and have also been addressed by the Supreme Court. The prosecution has an interest in highlighting prior delinquent activity and also may wish to make hospital and other medical records available to the clinician evaluating the youth.

C. Issues of primary concern to the defense

1. LIBERTY INTERESTS

The defense attorney usually has an *a priori* commitment to advocate for the client's retention of maximum freedom. For juveniles, this generally involves being allowed to remain at home, attending a normal school in the community, with little or no imposition of "special services." The latter includes psychiatric treatment which, if not voluntarily sought by the youth, is viewed as coercive and an example of overzealous intervention by the state.

Secure facilities are opposed regularly as the settings which limit the juvenile offender's freedom most severely. Hospitalization also is likely to be opposed unless it is viewed as a less punitive alternative to an industrial or training school.

2. WISHES VERSUS BEST INTERESTS

Adolescents' wishes with regard to what is done with them are not always consistent with what is in their best interest as an adult would construe it. For the delinquent, the stakes are higher than usual. Defense lawyers are divided as to whether they should promote "best interests" dispositions with their clients or simply do their best to obtain the disposition desired by the youth. The more formal or legalistic practitioner opts for the latter course leaving best interest advocacy to a guardian *ad litem*, if there is one, or to the judge. This choice often puts the defense attorney at odds with the child's parents, the probation officer, or the mental health expert who may recommend some form of placement.

A doctrinaire approach on this issue occasionally leaves the defense attorney in a difficult quandary or untenable position, e.g., when the juvenile insists on returning to a home that has been found to be severely abusive.

3. LEGAL REPRESENTATION DURING THE MENTAL HEALTH EXAMINATION

Concern that unwitting admissions by the juvenile client being examined clinically might jeopardize the case or that the expert might seek to intimidate the youth led many defense attorneys to demand to be present during the examination. A recent court ruling (*Matter of Jose D.* (1985), Vol. 66, N.Y. 2nd, p. 638) has ended such efforts and established an important precedent which preserves the integrity and privacy of the psychiatric examination.

4. PRIVACY

Civil libertarians have broached the issue of privacy from another standpoint. Some view the mental health evaluation as an intrusive violation of a youth's right to remain silent which contributes little, if anything, to the court's deliberations. They would prefer to eliminate such examinations altogether. Failing that, they are likely to advise the juvenile not to respond to the psychiatric inquiry. This is a puzzling tactic since the mental health expert is more likely to produce information that will help the juvenile obtain the needed services than otherwise. Once again, however, this seems to hinge on the question of wishes versus interests and how the defense attorney defines his or her role.

5. DOUBLE JEOPARDY

In *Breed v. Jones* (1975), the Supreme Court ruled that once an adjudicatory hearing has begun, the juvenile may not be tried subsequently on the same charges. This has, for example, been applied to status offender adjudications which later resulted in delinquency charges.

IV. CLINICAL ISSUES

A. Performing a competent examination

1. THE REFERRAL

The mental health professional who performs examinations for the juvenile court may be contacted by different parties: the court itself (judge's request), the prosecuting attorney, the defense attorney, or occasionally the family. Depending on who is requesting the examination, the task of the clinician will differ. It is essential, therefore, to be clear about who the client is and what is being asked of the expert. Although the basic requirement of a thorough, careful, competent examination is standard, specific emphases will vary. The prosecution will have a special interest in the issues of concern to the community, chiefly the nature of the danger posed by the youth or the likelihood of recidivism. The defense, on the other hand, would be eager to identify mitigating factors in the commission of the crime of which the juvenile is charged or strengths which might justify a less restrictive disposition.

2. Obtaining previous records

The value of obtaining all previous psychiatric, medical, social, and educational records (full disclosure) cannot be overemphasized. In a given case, a particular item of history may be more important than any findings emerging in the direct examination. This is all the more true if, as is often the case, the adolescent is withholding information or lying. A longitudinal picture is also invaluable for all speculations about prognosis.

3. Getting a reliable history

a. From family

It is as essential to meet with significant family members as it is to procure past records. Not all jurisdictions facilitate such contacts, and some may actually oppose them. The mental health professional may have to spell out the rationale for the request to see the parents. What they have to contribute will not be just historical data. Their own beliefs, attitudes, personality structure, and psychopathology are relevant information. Their awareness or lack of awareness of their child's delinquency is significant, as is their response to the court involvement. Since most parents of a youth charged with delinquency are likely to feel very guilty about their role in causation, skillful and sensitive handling of the interview is of the greatest importance. In all three Case Examples, interviews with the family are critical, most importantly with Vincent where early child abuse was an etiological factor.

b. From the juvenile

The youth being seen will seldom feel comfortable about the examination. Apprehensiveness is built into the situation, and many do not believe the examiner can be objective and dispassionate. One should assume a certain amount of withholding, some distortion of facts, particularly around the alleged crime, and both conscious and unconscious denial. Developing skills to get around such impediments is essential for working with this population.

4. Tailoring examination to the needs of the court

A proper referral will spell out the court's or lawyer's particular interest and should be specific to the youth being examined. The more refined the questions, the easier the task of the clinician. Many varieties of questions may arise. Among the most common are:

a. Diagnostic issues

These are especially important when disposition hinges on the diagnosis. "Dual" diagnoses such as mental illness with either mental retardation or a substance abuse problem are particularly difficult for the court unless the clinician delineates the relative importance of each and the implications for dispositional planning. Borderline retardation was a factor with Thomas (Case Example 1) and required special attention during evaluation.

b. Dangerousness

Despite the hazards of predicting future violence, the court may look to the examiner for any indication that permits placing the juvenile in either a high risk or a low risk category. Taken together with other data, these impressions may permit the judge to arrive at a decision that serves the interests of the youth and the community. A history of increasing violence, evidence of poor impulse control, pervasive hostility, and open admission of intent to commit violence constitute a serious syndrome and should be highlighted in any report. How much of a continuing threat, for example, was posed by Roger who pommeled his foster mother's lover into unconsciousness?

c. Recidivism

Here again the clinician is being asked to opine on prognosis. The best indicator of future delinquent activity is probably past history, especially if nothing has occurred (e.g., treatment) that might justify a revised outlook. Returning to the same criminogenic environment, a personality structure that is associated with delinquent activity, and the absence of realistic alternatives for the youth all make for a poor prognosis. It is the responsibility of the examiner to point up such reasoning. The court will ultimately decide what importance to ascribe to various aspects of the report.

B. Special evaluations

1. WAIVER

The examination for waiver of jurisdiction to the adult court, it will be remembered, occurs prior to adjudication or at the intake phase. Because of its serious implications, the clinician's report can have a major effect on the life of the juvenile. A careful, thorough assessment of the relevant factors is essential (Barnum, 1987). Developmental level, mental status including DSM-III-R diagnosis, prior record of mental illness and delinquent activity, history of previous interventions, special characteristics of the crime (bizarreness, mental state at the time), dangerousness, and treatability with itemizing appropriate modalities should all be taken into serious consideration. The examiner should not comment on the proposed transfer per se but, data permitting, develop the rationale for or against treatability within the juvenile justice system.

2. COMPETENCY

To review, competency is defined as the ability to understand the charges against oneself, the court proceedings and possible consequences, and capacity to cooperate with one's lawyer. It is these capabilities that must be assessed in the examination. Stein (1983), cited in Grisso et al. (1987), offers an interview schedule for use with juveniles based on adult schedules in general use. Space does not permit reproduction here, but the reader is referred to Grisso et al. (1987), Table 1, page 11, for details. See also Grisso (1981) and Grisso (1986) for further elaboration of that author's belief that existing techniques of clinical evaluation, which should include psychological and educational testing, do not actually address the competency issues. McGarry et al. (1977) have provided excellent semi-structured interviews for use with adults.

3. DIMINISHED RESPONSIBILITY

a. Infancy defense

The factors to be evaluated in the unlikely event that the infancy defense will arise are intelligence, cognitive development, prior contact with the law, moral development, and presence of mental illness (Leong, 1989). The expert is expected to relate these findings to the juvenile's degree of awareness of the wrongfulness of the delinquent act. Immaturity that precludes real understanding of the irreversibility of death would be a relevant development issue in a homicide, for example. Partial understanding of the lethality of a particular weapon could be a mitigating factor.

b. Insanity defense

An examination that establishes the presence of psychosis, particularly if one can document chronicity that suggests strongly it was present at the time of the alleged crime, can justify acceptance of the insanity defense. It is also likely that when lesser states of disturbance, e.g., dissociative state, a post-ictal state, can be shown to impede significantly the youth's ability to evaluate reality, this can support the defense (Case Example 2). Care must be taken by the clinician to preserve the treatment option for a disturbed youth. Dismissal of charges based on the insanity defense, against a youth who is not committable under local statutes, may mean that the youth will get no treatment at all.

C. Psychological testing

Psychometric examination is employed frequently in the court. It requires the availability of a competent clinical psychologist. It is *not* a substitute for the clinical interview but is used in conjunction with a standard (or modified) psychiatric evaluation and can contribute important data. The mental health professional responsible for the complete evaluation must decide when to request testing and the purposes to which the data will be put. As an example, testing is essential whenever intellectual development, attention deficit disorder, specific learning disabilities or deficiencies, and, generally, level of psychological maturity are at issue. Testing may also be required as part of the referral material for certain placements.

Judges are often confused if separate reports of the clinical examination and psychometric testing are submitted, particularly if they seem to contradict one another. This can be avoided if the court requires a single report which pools all of the data and interprets them as a whole.

D. Physical and/or neurological examination

1. INDICATIONS

There are many instances in which children before the court should receive physical examinations: those with a chronic illness such as diabetes or congenital heart disease; those with seizure disorders; drug abusers; and psychotic adolescents. All these and selected others require careful examination. Lewis (1983) has shown that a high proportion of delinquents display neurological dysfunction or psychotic symptomatology, especially those who are violent. Other researchers (Benedek and Cornell, 1989) have not been able to confirm these findings. Though it is not feasible to routinely give every delinquent a psychiatric or neurological examination, criteria should be developed for deciding who should have more extensive investigations.

2. USEFULNESS

The most important consequence of conducting adequate physical and neurological examinations where indicated is that appropriate treatment can be provided and inappropriate placements avoided. A hospital or drug rehabilitation program may be chosen over a state training school, anticonvulsant medication may be prescribed in addition to behavior modification therapy, etc.

E. Assessing developmental level

1. THE ISSUE OF MINORS' AUTONOMY

There are compelling reasons for fostering adolescents' growth towards autonomy and independence. "To shape their inchoate identities, perceive themselves as being in control of their lives, and nuture their sense of self-worth, adolescents need to act independently" (Tremper and Kelly, 1987). At the same time, such efforts must be consistent with developmental *capacity,* physical, intellectual, social, and emotional (Group for the Advancement of Psychiatry, Reports No. 68, 1968, and No. 126, 1989). Prematurely granted independence regularly leads to psychosocial maladjustment, especially with regard to decision making and organizing one's life, identity issues, the sense of competence, and locus of control. This can result in anxiety and depression. Failure to permit appropriate development of autonomy at each stage, on the other hand, may result in rebellion, academic failure, and delinquency.

2. ITS IMPORTANCE TO CRIMINAL RESPONSIBILITY

There is no disagreement that developmental factors are both psychologically and legally relevant to the question of responsibility. Controversy arises with regard to where to draw the line concerning different kinds of responsibility. The clinical evaluator is called upon to assess cognitive, moral, and biopsychosocial development of all juveniles examined, but especially those for whom an infancy defense is being mounted. Despite the recent Supreme Court decisions (*Stanford v. Kentucky,* 1989; *Wilkins v. Missouri,* 1989) permitting capital punishment for older minors, assessment of developmental stage is of the greatest urgency in homicide cases (Fitch, 1989).

3. THE STANDARD MEASURES

Invariably, the most important measures of criminal responsibility from the developmental perspective involve cognition. The Piagetian stages of intellectual growth leading, ultimately, to the capacity for formal or abstract reasoning are the most often cited. The clinician must relate cognitive level to the capacity to understand the nature and consequences of the delinquent acts and must consider the juvenile's judgment as well as the ability to form intent (*mens rea*). Other questions may arise, for example, the younger child's capacity to conceptualize death as an irreversible state.

Kohlberg's scales for moral development have less weight in the courtroom but may be especially relevant in particular cases.

4. LINKING STAGE OF DEVELOPMENT AND DELINQUENT ACTS

One of the most important aspects of the mental health report is the reasoning that relates the findings to the acts committed. This applies to all findings, of course, but the degree and nature of the psychopathology and the level of development are paramount considerations. The cogent argument, thoughtfully presented, will be more likely to influence the court to pursue an appropriate disposition.

F. Disposition

In summing up his discussion of criminal responsibility and the "niceties of legal doctrine," Fitch (1989) firmly underscores the importance of the disposition phase and the role of the mental health professional in the juvenile court: "Without a doubt, the most significant contribution that the mental health community can make to the juvenile justice process is to identify the needs of troubled youths and to provide services responsive to those needs" (p. 160).

Although the individual clinical consultant to the court is rarely in a position to fulfill the latter part of that mandate, identifying the needs, formulating recommendations (triage), and developing the rationale for them are major responsibilities.

1. RANGE OF OPTIONS: COMMUNITY OR INSTITUTIONAL PLACEMENT

(Many of these dispositions are effected by the probation officer or the court without participation of the mental health expert.)

Dismissal—Usually decided at intake by the probation officer (P.O.) for lack of evidence. Occasionally this happens at adjudication.

Diversion—Again, a P.O. function, with or without mental health input, usually for lesser crimes, younger children, or first offenders. These youths are generally referred to the social services or the mental health systems. In some states, admitting to the allegations is a prerequisite.

Probation—By far the commonest disposition, this is usually decided by the court (in the disposition phase) and applied if there is little question of safety and the youth is capable and willing to abide by the laws and conditions of probation. These include attendance at school, reporting to the P.O., respecting curfews, and living at home. Restitution may be made a condition of probation or made a separate disposition. Community service, a common sentence in the adult court, has been increasingly used in some states, notably California, and has distinct benefits for the juvenile and for society. The clinical report may be instrumental in fostering this choice.

Residential treatment—For youths who cannot remain in the community if they have the wherewithal to profit from a loosely structured, non-secure, therapeutic setting. Assessing the youth's resources and danger potential as well as the degree of support available in his or her home, neighborhood, and school is essential to this recommendation.

Training school—For the more dangerous, the recidivists, and those not amenable to a "therapeutic" approach, a more controlled, often more punitive, and sometimes highly secure setting is called for. Careful documentation of the reasons for making this recommendation is absolutely essential for the clinician, inasmuch as it is the disposition that most interferes with the youth's liberty and is anathema to most defense attorneys.

Psychiatric hospital or developmental center—These are reserved, respectively, for the mentally ill and for the mentally retarded juveniles. Evaluation by a psychiatrist or psychologist is essential and may involve carefully drawn diagnostic differentiations.

Drug rehabilitation center—For the youth whose delinquency has drug use as its basic problem and possible cause, this disposition is used. It is necessary to rule out a more general personality disturbance.

2. TREATMENT METHODS

The full range of psychiatric modalities may have application to the juvenile population inasmuch as delinquent behavior can be a part of almost any psychiatric syndrome. Thus, behavior therapy; individual, group, and family psychotherapy; pharmacotherapy; and cognitive or relationship therapy all have their value. Selectively used, they can ameliorate both the delinquent propensity and the coexisting psychopathology.

3. TREATABILITY

The court expects and needs a statement of the capacity of the youth to respond to the proposed therapeutic interventions. This is as important when specific treatment is being urged as when the clinician thinks that the youth is not amenable to treatment. A realistic appreciation of the difficulty of altering the well-established personality structure that often underlies delinquent patterns of behavior is of vital importance. The mental health field's failure to recognize this reality was largely responsible for the increasing hostility to and ultimate discarding of the treatment model in many quarters. This problem was evident in the case of Thomas (Case Example 1) on his first appearance in court which led to inadequate treatment.

G. Prognosis

Clinical evaluations are incomplete without some indication of the outlook for the patient, generally assuming implementation of the treatment plan. Where it concerns the juvenile offender, two separate prognostic statements are required. One is for the psychiatric condition, if any, the other for the delinquency. It is quite possible to improve in one regard while not changing at all in the other.

1. Psychiatric condition

An anxious, depressed, or agitated youngster may respond very quickly to a pharmacologic approach. An angry or hostile youth may be able to abate some of these feelings in individual or group psychotherapy. One who is being abused at home can benefit by intervention with the family (Case Example 3). Improvement of such symptoms may, in turn, diminish the impulse to behave in an antisocial manner. This is likely to be seen whenever a direct relationship can be drawn between the delinquency and specific psychopathology, i.e., when the behavior is but one symptomatic manifestation of an identifiable psychiatric disorder.

2. Delinquent behavior

Recidivism is the bane of the criminal justice system. It is only slightly less so in juvenile justice. Like psychiatric disturbance, delinquency is greatly dependent on the pathogenic qualities of the environment to which the adjudicated youth sooner or later returns. This is the major reason why intervention with the individual delinquent is so frustrating. The therapeutic task that confronts those working with such youths is often how to shore up their defenses to be able to resist the temptations they face when they return to their criminogenic environments. When the temptations are measurable in huge sums of money—as is currently the case with those involved in the drug trade—the outlook is gloomy indeed. The clinician must be keenly aware of these realities in venturing predictions. It is also important to be as specific as possible about such predictions. A youth who has committed a violent act under great duress may not pose a threat for further violence, yet may remain fundamentally antisocial, continuing to steal or to deal drugs.

V. PITFALLS

A. The referral

Clinicians who work in the juvenile justice field may in some ways be said to be entering a minefield. Armed with a good map that points out the danger spots, they may be able to thread their way without serious mishap. Being unprepared, on the other hand, is hazardous (Kalogerakis, 1991).

The problems can start at the very outset. If employed as staff of the court, it is important for the clinician to have a clear contract that permits maximum flexibility to carry out one's work in a competent professional manner. If recruited from private practice for a particular case, a clinician should establish who the client is, who pays the fee, what is being requested of the expert, whether old records have been obtained and informed consent forms signed, who is to get the report, and whether court testimony is likely to be needed.

It is best to review all court records and decide who it will be necessary to see in addition to the youth. Any uncertainty should be cleared up with the probation officer or the lawyer making the contact.

B. The examination

The juvenile (or other interviewee) should be told the purposes of the examination and should be informed that what the examiner is told is not confidential in that it will form part of the report to the court. At the same time, every effort must be made to reassure the youth that it is in his or her interest to be as open as possible with the clinician.

Comprehensiveness is essential in both history taking and clinical examination. Major omissions of any relevant items weaken the report and leave one open to attack as a witness. Good lawyers will attempt to discredit any witness whose testimony hurts their case, experts included.

Finally, specific questions raised by the court must be given particular attention. If one is unable to shed light on a given issue, this should be clearly stated and the reasons given.

C. The report and testimony

Herein lie the most dangerous parts of the minefield. There should be full disclosure of the sources of facts presented, whether hearsay or direct observation. Factual information should be carefully distinguished from opinion. Opinion offered should consider various possible interpretations and provide a detailed rationale for choosing a particular hypothesis. References to authoritative studies, not anecdotal literature, should be cited to back up these opinions.

Grisso (1984, cited in *Aber and Repucci*, 1987:180) offers some guidelines for the expert formulating recommendations. The factors that should be considered are the potential harm that may result from the recommendation, its finality, the reliability of the information on which the recommendation is based, and the degree to which autonomy is compromised. Recommendations also cannot be made in a vacuum or a fictitious universe. They must be consonant with relevant local statutes and be at least partially realizable within the court's jurisdictional area.

Lastly, the clinician must remember that, in contrast to the psychiatric clinic, the courtroom is a place where the ultimate decisions are made by judges and juries. The expert's testimony, however important, is but one of the sources of information that must be weighed before a final disposition is reached. Psychiatrists and other mental health professionals are no more immune to omnipotent strivings than other participants in the courtroom drama.

VI. CASE EXAMPLE EPILOGUES

A. Case Example 1

Status offenders are no longer adjudicated by the court and, as noncriminal offenders, are usually handled by the local social services agency. Yet their truancy or running away are often precursors of more serious antisocial behavior. Careful evaluation, including a mental health examination, is essential when these youths are first identified. In Thomas' case, although some attention was paid to his educational needs, the implications of his sleeping disturbance and poor social judgment were not fully appreciated and therefore not addressed. A thoughtful treatment plan early on might have averted subsequent maladjustment.

B. Case Example 2

Clinical evaluation prior to adjudication would be of great value to the youngster and to the court in this case. Waiver to the adult criminal court might not only alter radically the sentence imposed, but could preclude a rehabilitative effort with a youth known to have significant personal resources. Roger was obviously the victim of intolerable provocation. Though guilty of a major delinquent act, not taking into account the overweaning psychological turmoil can lead to a meaningless, punitive disposition. Such punishment could reinforce the development of a criminal lifestyle rather than redirect the youth to more constructive pursuits.

C. Case Example 3

The history of maladjustment and the apparent failure of earlier treatment initiatives stand out in Vincent's case. An abused child from the start, he suffered early and persistent personality damage. A rather chronic, schizoid course marked by increasing antisocial activity was the unfortunate outcome. A major question for the clinician here is whether Vincent is still amenable to change. Is Vincent treatable? If so, by what means and in what setting? His ability to cooperate with a treatment plan, his motivation for change, and his personal resources all require careful examination. A pessimistic assessment emphasizing the recidivism would discourage further efforts to rehabilitate the boy. Adjudication as a delinquent and long-term commitment to a training school or waiver to an adult court would be the options. On the other hand, a clinician taking a more optimistic view would outline constructive forces in Vincent's personality and would explain the failure of prior therapeutic efforts. This could form the basis for a carefully drawn treatment plan that might be acceptable to the court.

VII. ACTION GUIDE

A. Preexamination

1. Be thoroughly clear about the stipulations of the contract with the court, if an employee, or with the lawyer or court if called in as a consultant.
2. Develop a consultation request form to be used by the court or others on each case.
3. Check time frame for submitting report during initial contact and be certain your schedule permits you to take on the case.
4. Arrange with probation officer or lawyer to obtain prior records.
5. Obtain assurances that all parties to the case will be available for examination.
6. Know the local statutes that may apply, especially the juvenile court law and civil commitment laws.
7. Be familiar with the placement options locally available and their current situation with regard to beds, etc.
8. Be aware of any biases that may operate in the particular court with regard to utilization of the mental health expert and make the necessary adjustments.

B. Examination

1. Decide what questions are pertinent in the specific case, who should be seen, and how much time is likely to be needed.
2. Arrange for the most favorable conditions for the examination, assuring privacy, no interruptions, etc.

3. Over time, hone skills for interviewing uncooperative adolescents.
4. Inform the patient that confidentiality does not apply and explain.
5. Obtain an impression of the reliability of the particular informant, whether the juvenile or a parent.
6. Be certain that, in addition to general thoroughness, the items that are particularly relevant or of specific interest to the court are carefully addressed.
7. Every examination must include an assessment of developmental level, a mental status, relevant individual and family psychodynamics, and a DSM-III-R diagnosis, where appropriate.
8. A protocol should be developed for the assessment of dangerousness and used in all cases where the question exists.

C. Report

1. Consider all likely hypotheses for collating data, and spell out the reasons for choosing a particular formulation. A thoughtful discussion, free of obvious bias, will encourage a favorable reception of the report.
2. Distinguish clearly between the "facts" and the "opinions" in the report.
3. Do *not* attempt to address the question of guilt or innocence of the charges. That is a legal matter for the court to decide.
4. Develop recommendations after giving some attention to the specific needs of the youth and ruling out unsuitable dispositions.
5. Although the recommendations made may reflect what is *ideally* indicated, they should end by providing the court with a *realistic* treatment plan.
6. If possible, the clinician should be available to facilitate placement once the court has reached its decision.

VIII. SUGGESTED READINGS

Aber, M. S. and Repucci, N. D. (1987), The limits of mental health expertise in juvenile and family law. In J Law Psychiatry 10:167–185.

American Bar Association (1977), Juvenile Justice Standards: Summary and Analysis. Cambridge, MA: Ballinger Press.

American Law Institute (1962), Model Penal Code, Sec. 401. Philadelphia: The American Law Institute.

American Psychiatric Association (1974), Task Force Report 8, Clinical Aspects of the Violent Individual. Washington, D.C.: American Psychiatric Association.

American Psychiatric Association (1978), Response to Juvenile Justice Standards Project of the ABA/IJA. Washington, D.C.: American Psychiatric Association.

Barnum, R. (1987), Clinical evaluation of juvenile delinquents facing transfer to adult court. J Am Acad Child Adolesc Psychiatry 26:922–925.

Benedek, E. P. and Cornell, D. G. (eds.): (1989), Juvenile Homicide. Washington, D.C.: American Psychiatric Press.

Bonnie, R. J. and Slobogin, C. (1980), The role of mental health professionals in the criminal process: the case for informed speculation. Virginia Law Rev 66:427–522.

Breed v. Jones 421 U.S. 519, 1975.

Cressy, D. R. and Ward, D. A. (1969), Delinquency, Crimes and Social Process. New York: Harper and Row.

Drukteinis, A. M. (1986), Criminal responsibility of juvenile offenders. Am J Forensic Psychol 4(2):33–48.

Dusky v. U.S. 362 U.S. 402, 1960.

Feld, B. (1980), Juvenile court legislative reform and the serious young offender: dismantling the rehabilitative ideal. Minnesota Law Review 65:165.

Fitch, W. L. (1989), Competency to stand trial and criminal responsibility in the juvenile court. In E. P. Benedek and D.G. Cornell (eds.): Juv Homicide. Washington, D.C.: American Psychiatric Press.

Gardner, M. R. (1987), Punitive juvenile justice: some observations on a recent trend. In J Law Psychiatry 10:129–151.

Glueck, S. and Glueck E. (1950), Unraveling Juvenile Delinquency. New York: Commonwealth Fund.

Grisso, T. (1981), Juveniles' Waiver of Rights: Legal and Psychological Competence. New York: Plenum Press.

Grisso, T. (1984), The interpretation of clinical data in legal assessment: ethical issues. Paper presented at the American Psychological Association Meeting, Toronto: Ontario, Canada.

Grisso, T. (1986), Evaluating Competencies: Forensic Assessments and Instruments. New York: Plenum Press.

Grisso, T., Miller, M. O. and Sales, B. (1987), Competency to stand trial in juvenile court. Int J Law Psychiatry 10:1–20.

Group for the Advancement of Psychiatry (1968), Report No. 68, Normal Adolescence. New York: Group for the Advancement of Psychiatry.

Group for the Advancement of Psychiatry (1989), Report No. 126, How Old is Old Enough? New York: Brunner/Mazel.

Hastings Center (1978), In the Service of the State: Psychiatrist as Double Agent, Special Supplement to Hastings Center Report. Hastings-on-Hudson, N.Y.: Hastings Center.

In re Gault 387 U.S. 1, 1967.

In re Winship 397 U.S. 358, 1970.

Juvenile Justice and Delinquency Prevention Act of 1974: 88 Stat 1109.

Kalogerakis, M. G. (ed.) (1991) Handbook of Psychiatric Practice in the Juvenile Court. Washington, D.C.: American Psychiatric Press.

Kent v. United States 383 U.S. 541, 1966.

Leong, G. B. (1989), Clinicolegal issues for the forensic examiner. In Benedek, E.P. and Cornell, D. G. (eds.): Juvenile Homicide. Washington, D.C.: American Psychiatric Press.

Lewis, D. O. (1983), Neuropsychiatric vulnerabilities and violent juvenile delinquency. Psychiatr Clin North Am 6:707–714.

McGarry, A., Lipsitt, P. and Lelos D. (1977), Competency to Stand Trial and Mental Illness (DHEW Publication No. ADM 77-103) Rockville, MD: Dept. of Health, Education, and Welfare.

Melton, G. B. (1984), Developmental psychology and the law: the state of the art. Fam Law 22:445–482.

Morse, S. J. and Whitebread, C. H. (1982), Mental health implications of the juvenile justice standards. Child Youth Serv 5(1-2):5–27.

Offer, D., Marohn R. C., Ostrov, E. (1979), Psychiatry of the World of Juvenile Delinquency. New York: Basic Books.

Schall v. Martin 467 U.S. 253, 1984.

Simon, R. I. (1987), Clinical Psychiatry and the Law. Washington, D.C.: American Psychiatric Press.

Smith, K. (1974), A profile of juvenile court judges in the United States. Juv Jus 25:27–42.

Stanford v. Kentucky 109 S Ct 2969, 106 L Ed 2d 306, 1989.

Thompson v. Oklahoma 101 L. Ed. 2nd 702, 1988.

Tremper, C. R. and Kelly, M. P. (1987) The mental health rationale for policies fostering minors' autonomy. In J Law Psychiatry 10:111–127.

Walkover, A. (1984), The infancy defense in the new juvenile court. UCLA Law Rev 31:503–562.

Weissman, J. (1983), Toward an integrated theory of delinquency responsibility. Denver Law J 60:485–518.

Whitebread, C. H. and Heilman, J. (1988), An overview of the law of juvenile delinquency. Behav Sci Law 6(3):285–305.

Wilkins v. Missouri 109 S Ct 2669, 106 L Ed 2d 306, 1989.

Wizner, S. and Keller, M. F. (1977), The penal model of juvenile justice: is juvenile court delinquency jurisdiction obsolete? New York University Law Rev 52:1120–1135.

Zimring, F. (1982), The Changing Legal World of Adolescence. New York: Free Press.

Ziskin, J. (1981), Coping with Psychiatric and Psychological Testimony (Vol. 1, 3rd ed.). Venice, CA: Law and Psychology Press.

14

Adolescent Homicide/Victims and Victimizers

ELISSA P. BENEDEK, M.D.

I. INTRODUCTION

Reports of adolescent homicide find their way to the front pages of newspapers, television programs such as "60 Minutes," and radio news reports. The public and profession are alternately fascinated and horrified by the details of a particular adolescent homicide, particularly when the homicide is intrafamilial and the victim is a relative. Public debate ranges from extreme responses, such as a recommendation for psychiatric treatment, medical hospitalization for treatment, or incarceration and capital punishment. Homicide is one of the five leading causes of death for all persons in the United States who are between 1 and 17 years of age. Juveniles who kill present a major challenge to courts and clinicians. We know very little about such youngsters. We know less about whether an individual adolescent who commits a homicide will behave violently in the future.

II. CASE EXAMPLES

A. Case Example 1

Alex, a 16-year-old youth, was charged with first degree murder in the death of his 14-year-old brother. Alex's brother was found by his father at home, lying on the bedroom floor. He had been stabbed and struck repeatedly on the head with a metal pipe. Alex was also found on the floor with minor lacerations.

Alex told police that he and his brother had been attacked by two intruders, two schoolmates who had teased them and picked fights in the past. On further questioning by the police, there were multiple inconsistencies in his account and officers began to suspect that he might have been his brother's assailant.

During the forensic evaluation, Alex reported visual and auditory hallucinations which had begun shortly prior to the homicide. He describes "evil guy," a little green man who stood on his finger and told him to do "bad things," such as smoke dope, drink, and kill his brother. Alex claimed that all of the voices which were outside of his head bothered him continuously and that he always obeyed them. He also claimed that he was powerless to disobey them and had no strategies to diminish them. Alex claimed a minimal understanding of his legal situation and talked to examiners in a childlike manner. For example, when asked what might happen if he was convicted of a homicide, Alex said, "They will probably send me to a summer camp; then, my mother would come and get me."

Alex was admitted to a psychiatric hospital for observation and continued to claim that "evil guy" disturbed him on the unit. However, unit staff and patients observed that Alex showed no unusual behavior or signs of distraction by internal stimuli. He interacted well with the other patients and took part in all the ward activities. No medication was prescribed, and he seemed to improve during the course of his treatment.

Alex received psychological testing prior to the offense by his outpatient clinician. On a Wechsler Intelligence Scale for Children-Revised (WISC-R) he obtained a full scale IQ of 118, placing him in the high average range of intellectual functioning. On the Minnesota Multiphasic Personality Inventory (MMPI), his clinical scores were all within the average range. However, during hospitalization, he was retested three times. He refused to answer many of the WISC-R questions that he had answered as an outpatient and he took the MMPI on three occasions, each time producing an invalid profile with extreme elevations on all clinical scales.

B. Case Example 2

Fifteen-year-old Bob was charged with the murder of his mother. When Bob's father returned home from work he discovered his wife stabbed to death. Bob was found by his father hiding in the basement, reading the Bible and chanting "kill the Devil.'' On evaluation, Bob professed a strong and enduring belief in witchcraft. He told the examining clinician that he listened to rock music in his head every day and that music and voices had suggested to him that he kill his mother. He had not listened to the voices for a period of time, but on the day of the offense there were a variety of signs which he believed were clear indications that he must kill his mother. He stated that he knew his mother was an agent of Satan and that she would ultimately seduce him if he did not kill her.

Bob's father had described him as becoming progressively more withdrawn, violent, and apathetic. His father described him as remaining secluded in his room for several months prior to the alleged crime, listening to music and pacing. He had stopped seeing any of his friends, and his school attendance was sporadic. He had refused to eat, claiming that his mother had poisoned his food.

C. Case Example 3

Carol was a 16-year-old girl charged with killing her mother and father. On the day of the homicide, Carol had had a violent argument with her mother. They quarreled about her boyfriend, 21-year-old Dan, who was a known drug dealer. Carol's mother had grounded Carol for 2 months. Carol took the family shotgun and waited for her father to return home from work and shot first her mother and then her father. In an attempt to escape, she then drove the family car into a ditch, returned and took her mother's purse, money, and keys to the second family car. She drove to her boyfriend's house and demanded that he help her, stating that she believed she had just killed both of her parents. Her boyfriend drove her to a gas station, called the police, and Carol was arrested. Carol explained that she saw no way of avoiding ongoing conflict with her parents except to kill them and that she had thought about murder for several months and had even questioned a schoolmate about how to use a rifle properly.

III. PSYCHIATRIC LEGAL ISSUES

Psychiatric legal issues that are raised for juveniles currently include both those that are common with adult defendants and those unique to juveniles. Competency issues include competency to stand trial and competency to waive Miranda Rights. Criminal responsibility issues include the insanity defense and diminished capacity. One issue unique to juveniles is the question of waiver to adult courts. A second issue unique because of the issues of developmental immaturity to juveniles is the question of capital punishment.

A. Competency to stand trial

The concept of competency to stand trial is deeply rooted in the traditions of English common law and has been described as having both ritual and fairness functions. Court procedure required a plea from an accused person. Early on, courts recognized that certain lunatics or deaf mutes could not plead because of their affliction or disability, and provisions other than trial were developed for such persons. Additionally, it has long been held that it is necessary for a criminal defendant to present his case in court, in that it is unfair to try an individual whose mental disturbance or youth prevents such participation in his or her own defense.

In contemporary criminal law, the function or role of competency to stand trial has been described as continuing the tradition of preserving both ritual and fairness in trial proceedings, including (1) the safeguarding of the accuracy of the criminal adjudication; (2) guaranteeing a fair trial; (3) preserving the integrity and dignity of the legal process; and (4) ensuring that defendants found guilty understand why they are being punished.

The modern standard for competency to stand trial was contained in the 1960 U.S. Supreme Court decision of *Dusky v. the United States* wherein the court defined the test for competency as ". . . whether a defendant has sufficient present ability to consult with his lawyer within a reasonable degree of rational understanding and whether he has a rational as well as factual understanding of the proceedings against him." The language in *Dusky* with its emphasis on a defendant's cognitive capacities (". . . rational as well as factual understanding . . .") and communicative abilities (". . . ability to consult with his lawyer . . .") has become the minimal constitutional requirement for competency to stand trial.

The laboratory of community psychiatry at Harvard Medical School developed a competency to stand trial assessment instrument (C.A.I.), a survey of 13 areas of functioning relevant to the role of a criminal defendant. This C.A.I. includes the following areas of functioning: (1) appraisal of available legal defenses; (2) unmanageable behavior; (3) quality of relating to attorney; (4) planning of legal strategy including guilty plea to lesser charges where pertinent; (5) appraisal of role of: defense counsel, prosecuting attorney, judge, jury, defendant, witness; (6) understanding of court procedures; (7) appreciation of charges; (8) appreciation of range and nature of possible penalties; (9) appraisal of likely outcome; (10) capacity to disclose to attorney available pertinent facts surrounding the offense including the defendant's movements, timing, mental status, actions at the time of the offense; (11) capacity to realistically challenge prosecution witnesses; (12) capacity to testify relevantly; and (13) self-defeating versus self-serving motivation (legal issue). The Harvard group emphasized that the weight of a given item could certainly vary from defendant to defendant depending on the complexity of the case. Although the C.A.I. can be used as an interview format, it is not determinative of incompetency. Clinical evaluation and an assessment of whether a defendant can be educated is critical.

No strict protocol exists for an actual competency evaluation of a juvenile, but adherence to certain standards will facilitate a thorough evaluation. As in all forensic evaluations, it is critical to review as much background material as possible including court orders for the examination, police reports, treatment records, and other relevant documents. At the onset of the interview, the patient should be informed of the limits of privilege and confidentiality, and the clinician must make sure the patient understands it. A standard mental status evaluation serves as a pool of data regarding a patient's cognitive and affective functioning from which descriptive and diagnostic statements may be generated. Information obtained in the course of competency evaluations is not admissible to establish guilt or as a basis for subsequent determination of criminal responsibility.

Special clinical concerns include malingering, amnesia, and suicidal potential.

B. Competency to waive *Miranda* rights

While competency to stand trial is by far the most common competency referral in the evaluation of the juvenile, another competency is competency to waive Miranda rights. The *Gault* case (*In re Gault*, 1967) extended constitutional rights of the juvenile to include rights afforded to adults such as *Miranda* rights. The landmark *Miranda* case (*Miranda v. Arizona,* 1966) provided that a defendant could waive his rights (right to have an attorney present, right against self-incrimination) as long as the waiver was made voluntarily, knowingly, and intelligently. The *Miranda* ruling has been extended for juveniles. The determination of whether or not a minor has knowingly and intelligently waived his rights depends on the minor's age, degree of intelligence, his familiarity with the law or legal proceedings, the method and duration of the interrogation, and similar factors. Some clinicians suggest that no minor can confidently waive *Miranda* rights (Grisso, 1983). A few minors are competent to waive their rights because of age, intelligence, and level of experience.

C. Criminal responsibility: the infancy defense

The infancy defense refers to the concept that underaged youth are not criminally responsible for their acts. It too has roots in the English common law. Under the age of 7 years, a youth was *legally* incapable of committing a crime. Between ages 7 and 12, and later between the ages 7 and 14, English common law allowed for a guilty finding and even capital punishment. In the United States, between 1806 and 1882, there were 14 recorded cases where the infancy defense was raised for juveniles between the ages of 7 and 14 with eight of these 14 cases involving a charge of homicide (Platt and Diamond, 1966). However, no forensic evaluations were involved in these cases, as forensic clinicians did not exist. The current legal standard of the infancy defense remains similar to that of the English common law. State law is important in determining a local standard for the infancy defense. For example, in California, minors under the age of 14 are incapable of committing a crime. In New York, a child under 7 is presumed incapable of committing a crime, and a child between 7 and 14 is rebuttably presumed to have criminal capacity. The infancy defense is distinguished from the defense of criminal responsibility in that in the infancy defense a showing of developmental immaturity is commonly asserted rather than mental illness.

D. Insanity defense

Insanity is a legal term that denotes mental state (acute psychosis or behavioral condition, severe retardation) that is sufficiently disordered or incapacitated so as to relieve a defendant of blameworthiness or criminal responsibility for an offense. The courts reason that a defendant who was so psychologically disturbed or intellectually deficient at the time of an alleged offense as to be considered insane lacks the moral guilt or evil intent (*mens rea*) that is a necessary element of criminal liability. Traditionally in common law, the finding of guilt requires evidence that a defendant has committed an act (*actus reus*) and has possessed a certain guilty state of mind or intention (*mens rea*). The standards of legal insanity have developed from the M'Naghten test, an 1843 test evolving from the trial of Daniel M'Naghten who was accused of killing the secretary to the prime minister in Great Britain and was ultimately acquitted as insane. This standard has been called the "right/wrong test," and it requires complete noncomprehension of behavior. Presently, approximately 19 states retain some variation of M'Naghten.

The M'Naghten standard was supplemented in many jurisdictions by language intended to broaden the scope of insanity to include conditions characterized by impairment or affective or volitional controls. These so-called irresistible impulse rules applied in a situation where a defendant apparently knew right from wrong (was not cognitively disturbed) but lacked sufficient inhibitory capacity as a result of mental disease or defect to refrain from committing an act. The irresistible impulse standard has been difficult to distinguish from an irresisted impulse and to operationalize in terms that are useful and convincing to a judge or a jury. There have been several efforts over the last three decades to eliminate that portion of the insanity standard, including the 1954 Durham rule which swept away the cognitive and volitional standards of M'Naghten and irresistible impulse and offered instead a "product test" in order to allow greater latitude and scope to psychiatric testimony. However, the latitude and scope were too great, and the Durham test was never widely accepted outside of the District of Columbia and was ultimately rejected there in 1972.

The most current standard for an insanity defense is the language in the ALI or American Law Institute test. "A person is not responsible for criminal conduct if at the time of such conduct as the result of mental disease or defect he lacked substantial capacity either to *appreciate* the criminality (wrongfulness) of his conduct or to conform his conduct to the requirements of law." This standard is the one that is most applicable in juvenile cases. However, the insanity defense is rarely raised in juvenile court and is generally raised for psychotic patients. Psychosis generally begins in late adolescence or early adulthood; thus the likelihood of juveniles who qualify for an insanity defense after examination by a trained forensic clinician is rare. Subsequent to a finding of legal insanity, dispositional problems exist. Unless a minor meets civil commitment criteria, a treatment disposition is not possible. Thus, the juvenile may be discharged after the completion of the legal proceedings, and the juvenile justice system is reluctant to release a youngster who has been found guilty of committing a homicide but not guilty by reason of insanity. Even if a placement in a treatment facility is recommended, it is difficult to obtain.

Guidelines for evaluating an adolescent for the insanity defense do not differ from those for evaluating an adult. For example, it is critical to obtain the police reports with regard to the alleged crime, the youngster's version of the alleged crime, important information from parents and/or significant others, past medical history, past legal history, and drug and alcohol abuse history. The events of the alleged crime must be linked to the applicable insanity standard.

E. Diminished capacity

Diminished capacity differs between jurisdictions but generally implies that due to psychological disturbances or impairment the defendant's capacity to form the requisite intent, *mens rea*, required for certain events is somehow affected or diminished. However, the mental incapacity of the youngster is not so severe as to lead to an insanity defense. It may be a mental or emotional disturbance or drug or alcohol intoxication that interferes with the defendant's capacity to form intent. The doctrine of diminished capacity remains controversial. It is most generally used when an adolescent is either inebriated or high on drugs. Defendant's attorneys postulate a defense to show that despite the fact that the defendant committed the crime, he or she did not intend to do so.

F. Guilty but mentally ill

The Guilty But Mentally Ill (GBMI) statutes have been enacted in states as an alternative to the insanity defense. Michigan originated the defense in an attempt to allow alternatives to a finding of insanity. The GBMI verdict implies that the defendant has been proven to be guilty of an offense but has also met statutory criteria to be considered mentally ill but not legally insane. His mental illness is generally not connected to the postulated crime. The GBMI verdict has been criticized as definitely stigmatizing an offender (bad and mad) while providing nothing in the way of treatment.

G. Waiver

In the juvenile court, one of the first hearings generally conducted is on the issue of juvenile fitness or waiver of a juvenile into adult court. The guidelines for waiving a juvenile to adult court include: (1) the prior record and character of the child, his physical and mental maturity, and his patterns of living; (2) the seriousness of the offense; (3) whether the child may be on rehabilitation under the regular statutory juvenile procedures; (4) the suitability of programs and facilities available to the juvenile courts for the child; and (5) whether the best interests of public welfare and protection of public security generally require that a juvenile stand trial as an adult offender.

Waiver of a juvenile into the adult court places the juvenile at risk for more severe legal consequences including life imprisonment in an adult penal institution and, in some states, the death penalty. Defense attorneys for juveniles charged with homicide strategically attempt to keep cases within the juvenile court system. This court has a limited jurisdiction over a juvenile. The jurisdiction terminates in various states from ages 18 to 21. Consultation with a forensic clinician is often necessary to persuade the judge that waiver is not appropriate.

H. Competency to be executed

In *Thomas v. Oklahoma*, the United States Supreme Court examined the constitutionality of the capital punishment statutes which allow death sentences to be pronounced on convicted capital defendants who commit their capital felony under the age of 16. Billy Thompson, age 16, brutally murdered his former brother-in-law. After his first degree murder conviction and death sentence, Thompson challenged the constitutionality of his sentence as a violation of the Eighth Amendment protection against cruel and unusual punishment. The major issue before the court was whether the Eighth Amendment prohibition against cruel and unusual punishment as made applicable to the states by the Fourteenth Amendment, prohibited the execution of a capital felony offender who was *under* the age of 16 at the time of the crime. The court held that such executions did violate the Eighth Amendment and remanded the case to the Oklahoma courts to vacate Thompson's death sentence. The court's decision seemed to be predicated on determining what was a national consensus in regard to what limits should be placed on the use of capital punishment on adolescents. A plurality of the courts in the states saw an increasing reluctance of juries to apply the death penalty to all capital defendants and also a sharp distinction between 15-year-old minors and adults and the total body of law which state legislators were compiling. It also noted that specific state statutes existed which restricted minors in such activities as voting, driving, and marrying without parental consent. Using such trends in the law for guidance,the court held that a 15-year-old was not able to act with the same degree of culpability as an adult even during the commission of a capital crime and that less education and less intelligence and developmental immaturity reduced a teenager's culpability. The court also noted that a teenager still had ability to mature with respect to these clinical issues.

IV. CLINICAL ISSUES

A. Statistics

The homicide rate among young men in the United States is four to 73 times the rate in other industrial nations. Researchers at the National Center for Health Statistics indicate that 4,223 American men from ages 15 to 24 years old were murdered in 1987, a rate of *21.9 per 100,000*. The rate for black men in that group was 85.6 per 100,000, an increase of 40 percent since a low in 1984. In contrast, the homicide rates in 21 other countries for males in the same age group ranged from a high of 5 per 100,000 in Scotland to a low of 0.3 per 100,000 in Austria. Homicide rates vary for whites and blacks. Michigan was considered the most treacherous state, with a homicide rate of 232 per 100,000, largely concentrated in the Detroit metropolitan area. Michigan was followed by California (155 per 100,000), the District of Columbia (139 per 100,000), and New York (137 per 100,000).

California was described as the most risky state for young white males with a homicide rate of 22 per 100,000, which was still less than one-tenth the rate for black males in this age group in Michigan. The next highest homicide rate for white males was described as Texas (21 per 100,000), New York (18 per 100,000) and Arizona (17 per 100,000). The safest states for white males were Minnesota (1.9 per 100,000) and Massachusetts (2.6 per 100,000). For black males, the safest states were North Carolina (34.2 per 100,000) and Kentucky (34.8 per 100,000). Even in these safe states, the homicide rate among young black men was at least seven times that for young men in any foreign country studied (*New York Times*, June 27, 1990).

Not surprisingly, the combination of an available gun and substance abuse is more lethal in adolescents than it is in adults, perhaps because of their developmental immaturity, poor judgment, and lack of training or experience with guns. Handgun violence is a topic about which the psychiatric profession has remained largely apathetic or uncommunicative. In 1981, there were 11,258 murders and a similar number of suicides by handguns. Among these fatalities, 474 were adolescents between the ages of 13 and 18, and 156 were children under the age of 12 (*Handgun Control*, 1981). Handguns are involved in 50% of the homicides in the United States and account for 31 murders per day in the United States (*Handgun Control*, 1981). The United States is the only developed nation that has no restrictions on handgun availability. Industrialized nations such as Japan, Great Britain, Sweden, Australia, Israel, and Switzerland that have strict handgun laws report negligible deaths by handguns.

B. Clinical considerations

Psychosis. Benedek and Cornell, in their study of 72 adolescents referred for evaluation at the Center for Forensic Psychiatry, determined that five patients, or seven percent of their sample, were psychotic at the time of the commission of the crime. The question of psychosis is critical to a forensic evaluation, because the presence of psychotic symptoms can support an insanity defense. In the Benedek-Cornell project, defendants were classified as psychotic at the time of the offense if they met DSM-III criteria for psychosis. The psychosis could be due to drug intoxication, schizophrenia, major affective disorder, or any other psychotic disorder. For the youth in this group who were psychotic, the most common and clear-cut indications of psychosis were hallucinations and delusions. Often, the psychosis was manifested by a grossly bizarre behavior at the time of the crime, for example, tearing off one's clothing, drinking one's urine, or painting a victim's nipples or vagina after a murder. As compared to other youngsters, these youngsters tended to have an earlier history of psychiatric illness and more contact with mental health personnel prior to the commission of the crime.

C. Organic brain damage

A recurrent hypothesis in the clinical literature is that the homicidal behavior in juveniles is a product of brain damage. Lewis, 1981, has championed this position and has clearly articulated the view that homicidally aggressive youths should have received comprehensive neuropsychiatric examinations because of reported high incidence of both hard and soft signs of neurological abnormality. However, the evidence for organic damage remains equivocal and her ideas controversial. As more and more sophisticated evaluations for organic dysfunction become available, the evidence in this area will perhaps become clearer. At the time of Lewis' studies, CAT scans and MRIs were not available, nor were the more sophisticated neuropsychological examinations.

D. Intrafamilial homicides

Sergeant (1962) presented the classic hypothesis that sometimes a child who kills is acting as the unwitting, lethal agent of an adult (usually a parent) who unconsciously prompts the child to kill so that he can vicariously enjoy benefits of the act. In the Michigan group of adolescents, 30 cases, or 42%, were youngsters who had murdered a parent or a familiar person in the course of a conflicted situation. These youngsters were, more likely than not, involved in a prolonged argument or dispute, although the homicide was not necessarily carried out during an argument and could have been planned over a period of time. Frequently, the youngster might have acted in anticipation of a renewal of an ongoing conflict. The paradigmal situation involved an adolescent male who, after years of conflict with an abusive parent, planned and carried out a homicide.

These youngsters almost always had a history of prior conflict with their victims. In rare cases the relationship was brief. In other rare cases, the youngsters attempted to disguise their conflict-motivated murder as a crime-related murder.

E. Homicide committed during another crime

The last group of youngsters were those who committed a homicide in the course of another criminally-motivated act such as a robbery, burglary, or rape. Other investigators noted a similar subgroup (Solway et al., 1981; Xenoff and Zion, 1979). Fifty-two percent of the youngsters in the Forensic Center sample committed their homicides in the course of another crime. The homicide was most often secondary to the other crime and often unplanned. For example, a victim might awaken during a burglary, scream, and as a result of this behavior, be killed.

F. Forensic evaluation

As in all forensic evaluations, it is critical to review as much background material as possible, including court orders for the examination, all police reports, prior treatment records, both inpatient and outpatient, and other relevant documents (such as depositions). At the onset of the interview, the juvenile should be informed in depth of the purpose of the examination and of the limits in privilege and confidentiality. At times, even overtly psychotic or retarded defendants or terrified defendants have concerns about their evaluations that may be productively addressed and understood by the defendants.

A standard mental status evaluation serves as a pool of data regarding the defendant's cognitive and affective functioning from which both descriptive and diagnostic statements may be generated. In addition, it is critical to obtain a defendant's version of the events of the alleged crime. The defendant's version may vary from a total denial of any involvement or claim of amnesia to a detailed statement of great length. The material should first be elicited in a nondirected, open-ended manner and accurately recorded. Subsequently, the clinician must ask detailed questions which cross-check the defendant's version of the events, which may be used to classify ambiguous statements. The use of alcohol or prescription or illicit drugs proximate to the time of the alleged offense should also be carefully ascertained. In addition, it is important for the clinician to specifically inquire regarding the defendant's specific intentions, motivation, cognition of wrongfulness, and capacity to control or conform behavior. Psychological testing may offer a relatively objective, quantifiable data base pertinent to diagnostic, clinical, and treatment issues.

V. GUIDELINES FOR ASSESSMENT

A. Review all medical records

Oftimes, attorneys representing juveniles charged with murder are selective with regard to which medical records they make available to a psychiatrist they wish to enlist as an expert witness. They provide only records which support their client's version of the facts of the alleged crime. It is imperative to have all available information in order to avoid being blindsided and reaching premature or improper conclusions.

b. Speak to important friends, relatives, and significant others

They can provide information about the defendant's state of mind prior to the alleged homicide. Many people, such as police, detention officers, and child care workers, often have critical insights into the patient's state of mind. They also may have had contact with the defendant for a longer period of time than the evaluator. Statements with regard to premeditation and deliberation and evidence of planning can be obtained from significant parties in the patient/client's life.

C. Remember transference/countertransference

The juvenile murderer understandably stirs strong feelings in the most experienced of clinicians. There are three possible biases based on countertransferential feelings. The prosecutorial bias exists in those clinicians who identify with police, investigators, or prosecutors in their attitudes and constant skepticism toward defendants. They consider the defendant's behavior in a condemning rather than a clinical fashion and assume a judgmental role. The helper bias is a countertransference attitude derived from a clinician's basic humanitarian and empathic philosophy that influences the clinician to side consistently with the client offender and to ignore facts which may not be helpful in his or her defense. The uncommitted clinician is a clinician incapable of independent judgment and can form no opinions except to echo those of negative supervisors or no legal standards in particular jurisdictions. The legal standards for all the relevant procedures differ in different jurisdictions. Although a clinician is not expected to be an attorney, he or she can obtain information with regard to the relevant legal standards from an attorney or judge. The clinical examination must be tailored so that relevant questions are asked.

D. Take care in writing reports

The format for a written forensic report is considered in other chapters. However, care must be exercised so that data are presented which lead up to the ultimate conclusion expressed by the expert, with regard to both diagnosis and whether the client/defendant meets the relevant legal standard.

E. Always think about feigning, malingering in adolescents charged with homicide

Although the incidents of feigning and malingering are rare in all criminal defendants (about five percent), there is secondary gain associated with feigning, and the frightened defendant may feign psychiatric symptoms in an attempt to be exculpated and freed.

VI. CASE EXAMPLE EPILOGUES

A. Case Example 1

Clinicians concluded after lengthy psychological testing and clinical evaluation that Alex was malingering and did not meet the criteria for legal insanity. However, an outside clinician not schooled in forensic evaluations recommended that Alex be considered legally insane because of the bizarre nature of the crime. A jury did find Alex not guilty by reason of insanity. Subsequently, a judge found him not committable, as the judge determined he was not mentally ill and Alex was released to the community with no treatment recommended.

B. Case Example 2

Bob was extensively evaluated at a forensic hospital. He continued to profess that he heard the voice of the Devil demanding him to behave in certain fashions. Bob was treated with neuroleptic medications and restored to competency within the period of time allowed through the court. He was subsequently recommended as legally insane and adjudicated legally insane (i.e., mentally ill and unable to appreciate the wrongfulness of his conduct or to conform his conduct to the requirements of law). Bob was then hospitalized and treated in a forensic hospital for a year and a half. Ultimately, he was followed in the community by community psychiatrists and treated with supportive psychotherapy and neuroleptic medication.

C. Case Example 3

An extensive forensic evaluation and a diagnosis of antisocial personality was made with regard to Carol. History revealed that Carol had been involved in a variety of antisocial activities prior to the homicide of her parents which had escalated from truancy to armed robbery to the eventual homicide. Carol was sent to a treatment/rehabilitation/detention facility for adolescents and will remain there until the age of 21.

VII. PITFALLS

A. Conflict of interest

When one is contacted by an attorney, there is always a temptation to be sympathetic to the side of the case the attorney presents. Thus, if the attorney is representing an adolescent who may have emotional problems, it is tempting to suggest that that adolescent fits the pattern conforming to a legal definition of insanity. That may not be the case, and it may be very difficult to "not be helpful."

B. Knowledge of the law

The law, with regard to legal insanity, competency, diminished capacity, guilty but mentally ill, differs in each of the states. Although the clinician is not a lawyer, some general idea of the legally relevant statutes in case law is important. A referring attorney can serve as a mentor with regard to the important issues in a particular case. Conversely, although the psychiatrist may know certain areas of the law better than a novice attorney, ultimate responsibility for the legal issues in any situation lies with the attorney.

C. Seduction

Many situations where an adolescent is either a victim or a victimizer are high profile cases. Occasionally, a psychiatrist gets seduced into participating in such a case because of the notoriety. Before agreeing to participate in such a case, it is critical to examine motivation.

VII. SUGGESTED READINGS

Applebaum, P. S. (1986), Competence to be executed: Another conundrum for mental health professionals. Hosp Community Psychiatry 37:682–684.

Benedek, E. P. (1985), Waiver of juveniles to adult court. In: Schetky, D. H. and Benedek, E. P. (ed.) Emerging Issues in Child Psychiatry and the Law. New York: Brunner-Mazel.

Benedek, E. P. and Cornell, D. G. (1989), Juvenile Homicide. Washington, D.C.: American Psychiatric Association Press.

Cormier, B. I. and Marcus, B. (1980), A longitudinal study of adolescent murderers. Bull Am Acad Psychiatry Law 8:240–260.

Cornell, D. G., Benedek, E. P., and Benedek, D. (1980), Characteistics of adolescents charged with homicide: review of 72 cases. Behav Sci Law 8:240–260.

Cornell, D. G., Benedek, E. P., and Benedek, D. (1987), Juvenile homicide: prior adjustment and a proposed typology. Am J Orthopsychiatry 57:383–393.

Grisso, T. (1981), Juveniles' Waiver of Rights: Legal and Psychological Competency. New York: Plenum Press.

Grisso, T., Miller, M. O., and Sales, B. (1987), Competency to stand trial in juvenile court. Int J Law Psychiatry 10:1–20.

Haizlip, T., Corder, B. F., and Ball, B. C. (1984), The Adolescent Murderer. In: Keith, C. R. (ed.): The Aggressive Adolescent: Clinical Perspectives. New York: The Free Press.

Lewis, D. O. (1981), Vulnerabilities to Delinquency. New York: SP Medical and Scientific Books.

Lewis, D. O., Moy, E., Jackson, L. D., et al. (1985), Biopsychosocial characteristics of children who later murder: a prospective study. Am J Psychiatry 142:1161–1167.

Lewis, D. O., Shanok, S. S., Grant, M., et al. (1984), Homicidally aggressive young children: neuropsychiatric and experiential correlates. Am J Psychiatry 140:148–153.

Lewis, D. O., Shanok S. S., and Pincus, J. H. (1981), The neuropsychiatric status of violent male juvenile delinquents. In: Lewis, D. O. (ed.): Vulnerabilities to Delinquency. New York: SP Medical and Scientific Books.

Palombi, J. J. (1980), Competency and criminal responsibility. In: Schetky, D. H. and Benedek, E. P. (eds.): Emerging Issues in Child Psychiatry and the Law. New York: Brunner-Mazel.

Paluszny, M., and McNabb, M. (1975), Therapy of a six year old who committed fratricide. J Am Acad Child Psychiatry 14:319–336.

Petti, T. A. and Davidman, L. (1981), Homicidal school-age children: cognitive style and demographic features. Child Psychiatry Hum Dev 12:82–89.

Sargent, D. (1962), Children who kill—a family conspiracy? Social Work 7:35–42.

Wolfgang, M. E. (1958), Patterns in Criminal Homicide. Philadelphia: University of Pennsylvania Press.

Wolfgang, M. E., Figlio, R. M., and Sellin, T. (1972), Delinquency in a Birth Cohort. Chicago: University of Chicago Press.

Yates, A., Beutler, L. E., and Crago, M. (1984), Characteristics of young, violent offenders. J Psychiatry Law 137–149.

Zenoff, E. H. and Zients, A. B. (1979), Juvenile murderers: should the punishment fit the crime? Int J Law Psychiatry 2:533–553.

CASE CITATIONS:

Barefoot v. Estelle, 463 U.S. 880, 1983
Commonwealth v. Durham, 225 Pa. Super. 539, 1978
Dusky v. United States, 362 U.S. 402, 1960
In re Gault, 387 U.S. 1, 1967
Jackson v. Indiana, 406 U.S. 715, 1972
Kent v. United States, 383 U.S. 541, 1986
Miranda v. Arizona, 384 U.S. 436, 1966
Thompson v. Oklahoma, 56 USLW 4892 (1988)
In re Winship, 397 U.S. 358, 1970.

15

Countertransference Issues in Forensic Child Psychiatry

DIANE H. SCHETKY, M.D., AND LESLEY DEVOE, M.S.W.

I. CASE EXAMPLES

A. Case Example 1

Dennis Harrison, a Ph.D. who professed to having performed hundreds of sexual abuse evaluations, traveled from his home in Maryland to Massachusetts to evaluate 8-year-old Nicole LaLonde for alleged sexual abuse by her father. He saw her while she was being kept in hiding by her mother, and he videotaped his evaluation of her. Harrison took it upon himself to write the judge concerning the existence of this tape and about a medical examination that had been performed on the child in another state. The court refused to accept his tape or the medical report in evidence. In "a desperation play," Harrison released both the tape and medical report to the media citing the "stonewalling" by the Massachusetts' authorities as a factor that pushed him to this extreme (*Boston Globe*, Nov. 3, 1987). Portions of the video were shown on TV and excerpts of the gynecologic exam were published in the *Boston Globe*.

B. Case Example 2

A child psychiatry trainee has done several child custody evaluations and in each has put inordinate emphasis on the child's stated preference for custody regardless of the child's age. His supervisor calls his attention to this pattern and questions what it might mean.

C. Case Example 3

Jenny, age 3½, peacefully asleep in her mother's bed, was abruptly awakened by her estranged father breaking down the bedroom door. She watched helplessly as her father shot her mother in the head with a handgun. She remained in the room with her dead mother for about 5 minutes until rescued by the police. Play therapy was initiated the following day and continued for 3 years. Her therapist became witness to Jenny's grim drawings and spontaneous statements made with alarming detail. For example, "Yesterday Mom was a baby who threw up. Daddy was yelling and Mom screamed and screamed and screamed. Her head was off. I stayed in bed and watched her." Jenny would engage in delightful age-appropriate play, then suddenly begin to draw her mother's bloody eyeball. Her therapist would wince and conjure up her own disturbing imagery. In addition to listening as the child's therapist, she took careful note of all of this in the event that she might be called as a witness or asked for a victim impact statement by the court.

D. Case Example 4

A social worker is seeing 4-year-old Trina for the first time for evaluation of possible sexual abuse. Trina flies through her office showing no anxiety about this new situation. She seems to be at ease with change and chaos. Trina quickly checks out the room while chatting away and then settles upon play with the doll house. With great enthusiasm she has the dolls perform oral sex on one another and attempts to involve the social worker in this play. The therapist is shocked by this highly eroticized play and struggles to balance her internal reactions with her external presentation. She wonders how she can remain nonjudgmental while contemplating her evaluation of Trina.

II. DEFINITION OF COUNTERTRANSFERENCE

Freud (1910) introduced the concept of countertransference which he used to refer to the "patient's influence on his [physician's] unconscious feelings. . . ." Generally, countertransference reactions include responses to the patient or patient's productions that are based on an object from the therapist's past rather than on the patient, and the therapist in turn projects his own issues and feelings onto the patient. Countertransference also arises in situations wherein the patient is used to gratify the therapist's needs. A broader application of the term countertransference, especially relevant to forensic settings, includes the therapist's reactions to events described by the patient. The uses and abuses of countertransference in psychotherapy have been discussed extensively in the adult psychiatry literature. Relatively little is written about countertransference in child psychiatry and in forensic settings.

III. COUNTERTRANSFERENCE IN FORENSIC PSYCHIATRY

A. Overview

1. COUNTERTRANSFERENCE AND RESISTANCE TO COURT WORK

Most psychiatrists have a need to be appreciated by their patients and may resist adversarial settings where one side is likely to be unhappy with the psychiatrist's findings and possibly angry with him. Psychiatrists are used to being in a position of authority and many do not like having their opinions challenged. Those who are inexperienced or overly invested in a case may view cross-examination as a personal attack. If the expert has conflicts around aggression he may fear doing harm, i.e., depriving a mother of her child or being instrumental in the incarceration of a juvenile. There is also risk of handling anger over abuse or neglect by becoming overly punitive. Potentially violent patients or parents may also stir up fear of being harmed. At times, such fears are realistic, whereas at other times they may be rooted in countertransference.

Kubie (1971) noted that therapy inevitably stirs up pain and that psychiatrists who flee from doing long-term therapy may be running from the inevitable self-confrontation that occurs in therapy. Schetky and Colbach (1982) speculate that some psychiatrists who flee from doing therapy may be attracted to forensic psychiatry, raising concerns as to how introspective they are. They note that countertransference out of control in the courtroom can be much more devastating than in psychotherapy where one has the chance to correct one's course. They urge that forensic psychiatrists continue to stay involved with treatment in spite of scheduling difficulties relating to the need to testify. Firsthand awareness of treatment issues also puts one in a much better position to critique the therapy of others. We will be discussing some of the countertransference issues that arise in psychotherapy with forensic cases as well as in forensic evaluations.

2. THE COURTROOM AS A MINEFIELD FOR COUNTERTRANSFERENCE REACTIONS

The courtroom may recreate family relationships and trigger countertransference reactions that undermine the psychiatrist's intellectual integrity. Judges are seen as authority figures and may resemble parent or grandparent figures. The wish to please such a parent figure and to gain approval may, if not recognized, affect one's statements. Conversely, anti-authoritarian attitudes may also affect the expert's testimony and lead to a lack of humility.

Experts for the other side may be viewed as siblings and generate feelings of competition that could lead to overstatements in an effort to prevail. Performance anxiety and feeling under attack also may trigger aggressive responses on the part of the expert witness. Various courtroom personnel may also become "family," if one frequently testifies in a particular court, and there is the risk of becoming too friendly with them. This could lead to loss of objectivity and to bias in the minds of jurors if they see the expert fraternizing.

An everpresent danger is identifying with the winning or losing side. This represents role blurring and may also indicate self-esteem issues for the psychiatrist.

Highly publicized cases feed exhibitionistic needs. It is a heady feeling to see one's name appear in case law or in the evening news. However, this momentary high should be secondary and not the driving force for testifying. There is always the possibility that the case may be appealed and overturned. It is a humbling experience to see one's testimony implicated as grounds for overruling a decision.

Forensic work is lucrative, and this may fuel greed especially as one discovers that desperate lawyers are willing to pay high sums to help their client. Feelings about money need to be dealt with and fees should remain commensurate with skills and experience. If one sees forensics as a road to paying off debts or making up for earlier deprivations in one's life, there is a risk of becoming a hired gun. Financial interests should never be allowed to interfere with opinions rendered.

3. COUNTERTRANSFERENCE IN CLINICAL SETTINGS

Forensic psychiatry places extreme demands on the psyche of the clinician in that one is forced to come in contact, often in graphic detail, with the intentional and violent acts of one person against another. In the process, evaluators and therapists become witnesses once removed as they share the horrors experienced by victims. Clinicians need to understand how trauma reconstruction affects their own belief systems and their personal lives. They must be prepared to process their own personal traumas that may be stirred up by work with these patients.

The risk of not acknowledging our own responses is that we may play into the patient's need to deny. As noted by McCann and Pearlman (1990), therapists can be vicariously traumatized and their responses should not be seen as pathological, rather they should be acknowledged and used therapeutically. For instance, a therapist working with a woman whose adolescent son had just died from an alcohol overdose dreamed before her next session with the patient that her own adolescent son had died. She awoke with a horrible empty feeling which she was able to connect to her patient's loss. Unaware of the connection, she might have pulled back from the patient. Instead, she shared her dream with this bereaved woman, who had been convinced no one could know her pain, and in doing so conveyed some empathy.

The following section will explore responses to trauma victims in general. We will then deal with specific types of forensic cases. It is recognized that strictly speaking some of the reactions described are not countertransference in that they are solely generated by material from the patient. However, they are included as often they overlap with countertransference reactions. While we believe it is important to make the distinction between evaluator and therapist, these terms may at times be interchangeable in discussing countertransference issues.

B. Working with victims of trauma

1. MIRRORING OF SYMPTOMS

Work with victims can be traumatic especially when the clinician is unprepared to hear or see what the patient presents. The effect upon the therapist may mirror the patient's symptomatology with a range of intrusive and avoidant behaviors that correspond to the denial and reliving phases of post-traumatic stress disorder. At one extreme clinicians may overidentify with the patient, become full of rage, and act like defense attorneys in their overzealous defense of the patient. On the other hand, clinicians may underidentify with patients, become distant, and through passivity and helplessness become professionally and emotionally paralyzed. In their withdrawal, as with their overzealous counterparts, they become ineffectual, and their patients are victimized yet again. Clinicians and patients may experience a parallel order of emergence of feelings and stimulus barriers against similar feelings. If patients are to heal, clinicians must heal as well. One problem faced by the forensic psychiatrist is that evaluations are time limited; hence he may not have the opportunity to heal with the patient through extended contact.

Trauma theory offers a useful framework for analysis in both patient and therapist. It is rare for the therapist to be massively traumatized, rather it is more likely that small attacks occur on the expectations of the therapist that have the effect of cumulative trauma; i.e., the therapist hears and sees more than expected and is left without defenses. As the patient's memory returns he may assault the therapist with intrusive recall. Images of cruelty, violence, and mutilation of one human being by another are terrifying and can result in the clinician feeling a sense of helplessness, danger, and heightened arousal. Intense activation of the nervous system may occur as central organizing schemata are shattered. Therapists, along with patients, are left searching for meaning as a way out of the morass of overwhelming and inescapable feelings and experiences. We have seen some become numb, much like their patients. Others, perhaps as part of mastery, turn to shocking audiences with gory details in didactic presentations on trauma.

2. TRAUMA RECONSTRUCTION

Part of the reconstruction process in therapy involves analyzing the traumatic event frame by frame, over and over, as if it were being photographed by patient and therapist from as many angles as possible. Reconstruction becomes part of the process of mastery and working through and may have to be repeated as the child reaches progressive stages of development. The therapist may initiate the process but can not necessarily control it. Visual images may prove overwhelming for the therapist as well as for the patient, and the therapist may need to pace the process without pushing the patient into denial. Like the victim, the therapist may be left with flashbulb memories (a term introduced by Brown and Kulik) that may unexpectedly intrude. Such was the case when Jenny's therapist visited the small room where Jenny had lain in bed as her mother was shot in the head. The therapist was left with recurring images of the bullet hole in the wall.

The therapist needs to be aware of his own physiological responses to descriptions of trauma. The chill Jenny's therapist experienced at the scene of the crime conveyed empathy for her young patient. Loss of appetite following descriptions of body mutilation may signal disgust and difficulty attending to details. Voyeuristic excitement on the other hand may indicate overinvolvement. An eroticized child may stir sexual feelings in even the most experienced clinician (Berlin, 1986). An expectation that this should not occur could result in premature closure on the subject that would interfere with reconstruction of the trauma.

3. HEIGHTENED VULNERABILITY

Work with trauma victims reminds therapists regularly of their own vulnerability at the hands of others, and of the capriciousness of fate. Added to this is the exposure to dangerous offenders in court which may heighten fears for therapist and patient. The clinician may find herself taking added safety precautions and locking doors where she had not before. Horowitz (1986) suggests that fear of identification or merger with the victim must be addressed with the family members and, we would add, with therapists as well. He relates resistance of trauma patients in treatment to the fear of repeating the trauma, and he stresses that the therapist must push to the core of the trauma. The therapist's fear of repetition and a heightened sense of vulnerability may be additional sources of resistance.

4. SURVIVOR GUILT

Horowitz (1986) suggests that witnesses, victims, and family members of trauma victims must deal with survivor guilt and guilt over aggressivity. We believe that therapists must face similar concerns as well. For instance, Jenny asked her therapist, "Where were you the night my Mommy died?" and later, "Did your Mommy die too?" Without consultation, her therapist would have been at risk of merging guilt with her anger towards Jenny's father and possibly being catapulted into retaliatory behavior in court. Danieli (1988) suggests that survivor guilt may result in therapists being unable to set reasonable limits and in their avoidance of asking important questions for fear of hurting the patient. He notes that guilt may also serve as a defense against total helplessness and passivity (1981).

5. SEARCH FOR MEANING

The patient's search for meaning is likely to trigger a parallel process in the therapist. For the patient, this represents an attempt to master the trauma by seeking reasons for it and hopefully preventing its recurrence. The therapist may experience existential depression from time to time when confronted with man's inhumanity to man. Jenny's therapist struggled with this and had to do all sorts of mental gymnastics to try to explain to Jenny why her father, who loved her mother, had killed her. Therapists who work with children are not given the luxury of time to think in depth about the meaning of an event. Jenny, like other children, needed to know immediately. One of the authors, upon being faced with a murder-suicide involving a child patient, found herself turning to Dostoyevsky and Tolstoy in her attempt to understand the meaning of suffering. Therapists may wonder if they, too, have lost faith in heroes, a characteristic described by L. Terr (1981) in child victims of trauma.

6. VICTIMIZATION BY OTHERS

Psychiatrists may feel used and victimized by others within the legal system, particularly if they allow themselves to be pushed about and are unable to set limits. We see a rather predictable loss of trust and increase in cynicism among some clinicians who do a lot of work within the legal system.

7. POWER IMBALANCE

In forensic work feelings of helplessness may alternate with feeling that one has been given too much power. Confrontation with the question in sex abuse cases as to whether or not a child has been abused may leave therapists feeling ineffectual, particularly when very young children are involved. Helplessness may also arise in response to the impact of cumulative trauma upon children regarding the restorative limits of psychotherapy alone. It behooves the therapist not to convey these doubts to patients nor to hold out expectations for them that are too low.

On the other hand, the forensic psychiatrist may have incredible amounts of influence in the courtroom where his statements may permanently alter the lives of people involved. Impact statements by Jenny's therapist and her brother's therapist resulted in the probation officer extending his recommended sentence for the children's father from 40 to 60 years. Therapists must also worry about how their clinical decisions affect patients. Jenny's therapist worried that she might retraumatize Jenny during a visit to her father in prison if she were not extremely careful. She also worried about traumatizing her with intrusive, "rude" questions concerning the murder she'd witnessed. However, in the course of asking these questions she was able to correct Jenny's mistaken notions about the crime.

8. FAILURE OF EMPATHY

The essence of victimization is the massive failure of empathy from victimizer to victim (Shengold). Jenny's father exhibited this well when, unable to appreciate his daughter's fear of him, he said, "I would never hurt her!" Jenny's therapist's reaction was one of disgust until it occurred to her that he did not understand Jenny's hurt. It was clear that no one had taken the time in the father's childhood to help him understand his feelings, let alone others'. It is vital to understand that we continue that failure of empathy if we distance ourselves, lay blame, experience disgust with patients, or fail to empathize with the parallel pain in their childhoods. Therapists must constantly ask themselves if they become part of the spiral of the failure of empathy or if they indeed offer patients a difference. For many patients, this will be their first experience with empathy.

C. Specific types of cases

1. CHILD CUSTODY

Child custody conflicts stir up unresolved issues with one's own parents such as the need to protect or take sides with one parent as a child, or anger over an absentee or abusive parent. If the psychiatrist is a parent, there is the tendency to identify with parents who share similar views on parenting and to be judgmental concerning other styles of parenting. It is easy for biases about class and education to enter into custody decisions. The childless psychiatrist may have idealistic notions about parenthood. Some child psychiatrists may overidentify with the child and entertain unrealistic rescue fantasies. It becomes easy to blame a parent for the child's problems rather than consider that this may be a very difficult child who would stress the most competent of parents.

The passive psychiatrist who likes to avoid confrontation may become very uncomfortable as divorce situations heat up and sparks begin to fly. Avoidant behaviors may lead to failure to inquire about how family members handle conflict and anger. For some, the risk is that of getting too drawn into the conflicts and the question of whom did what to whom. Balancing objectivity and neutrality with compassion is not an easy task.

2. CRIMINAL OFFENSES AND VIOLENT PATIENTS

Child psychiatrists often have difficulty inquiring about violent tendencies, access to weapons, and homicidal ideation. Perhaps it is because we don't like to think that young people harbor such thoughts, or more likely, it is because our training has not prepared us to deal with the responses we might get. The psychiatrist's discomfort with the topic may lead to denial of the potential for violence and serious omissions in a forensic evaluation that could leave others, as well as the psychiatrist, at risk. Inpatient units and emergency wards are the most common sites for violence, and one study showed that the greatest relative risk of assault (19.4%) was for residents working on a child-adolescent service (Reuben and Yamamoto, 1980). Another study (Dubin et al., 1988) found that the most serious assaults were made by outpatients against psychiatrists in their offices. Both of these studies found that aggressiveness on the part of residents and psychiatrists was likely to provoke these patients into assaultive behavior. Dubin et al. (1988) recommend quietly talking the patient down when confronted with threatening situations.

Judgmental attitudes may lead to punitive responses to the juvenile offender and may preclude consideration of mitigating circumstances in a crime, e.g., mental illness or mental retardation. On the other hand, the psychiatrist who engaged in transient antisocial activity as a teen may tend to minimize the significance of a theft and pass it off as typical adolescent behavior.

Forensic evaluations of juvenile offenders are complicated by the paucity of dispositional options. We may wonder whether we are doing the teen and society any good by sending a youth to a correctional facility and may have rescue fantasies that outpatient psychotherapy may turn him around.

3. RITUALISTIC ABUSE

Ritualistic abuse has emerged as a recognized form of abuse in the 1990s. Just as professionals resisted asking about physical abuse in the '70s, and sexual abuse in the early '80s, we are seeing resistance to becoming involved in cases where there is suspicion of ritualistic abuse. The prevalence of cult activity is not known but is probably more widespread than we care to admit. These cases are difficult to detect and even harder to prosecute, because victims have been so effectively programmed.

Inasmuch as the tenets of satanic cults are antithetical to our beliefs and values, it is understandable why it is easy to deny the existence of practices that shatter our belief in the innocence of children. It is by far easier to turn down a request to evaluate a child involved in ritualistic abuse by pleading lack of experience than to delve into the depths of what amounts to "soul murder" (Shengold, 1989).

Those who dare enter this arena need to suspend disbelief and notions about abuse and abusers. They must not reject information merely because it does not fit their preconceived notions. The seemingly outlandish tales that some children disclose may actually represent a deliberate attempt on the part of abusers to discredit their disclosures; e.g., the abuser may actually have been dressed up like Donald Duck, have simulated taking the children on a trip to the moon, or even simulated surgery. Clinicians need to be prepared to deal with exceedingly painful and disturbing material and have their own supports lined up ahead of time to help deal with their fears and anxieties.

Any patient who has survived ritual abuse deserves our respect and help. Interestingly, those victims who develop Multiple Personality Disorder may be cult failures, as it was through the victims' ability to fragment that they were able to survive and preserve some shreds of their identity.

4. MULTIPLE PERSONALTIY DISORDER

Putnam (1989) notes that patients with Multiple Personality Disorder (MPD) "often evoke unique and complex countertransference reactions from therapists" and that alters "are likely to engender distinct and separate countertransference responses within the therapist." For instance, one may provoke sexual feelings, another anger, another nurturance, and yet another helplessness. The therapist may play favorites and experience a sense of loyalty to the host personality as others start to emerge. He may also feel a sense of loss when one alter leaves or personalities merge, and may feel confusion by the never-ending sea of changes in the patient. The therapist may feel intimidated by the number of personalities and the volume of material that he must process. Putnam (1989) reminds us that the emergence of an alter is a sign of trust on the part of the patient.

These patients, who have almost inevitably been sexualy abused, are adept at pushing boundaries and pulling the therapist out of the therapist's chair. Kluft

(1990) notes that many patients with MPD are likely to go on to become sexually involved with therapists. Some may become aggressively sexual with the therapist. Putnam (1989) stresses that therapists need to be flexible yet very clear about boundaries or else therapy is likely to "degenerate into chaos" (p. 195).

Child alters stir up parental feelings in therapists. The child therapist may be comfortable switching to play therapy and drawing, yet boundary problems may persist. A 4-year-old alter complained that she could not tie her shoe. Her therapist tied it as she viewed this as an act of trust by this alter who had up until then been afraid of her. However, she soon drew the line when the same alter said she did not know how to drive her car home. The therapist suggested that she stay in the waiting room until her host personality returned.

Control issues are ever present with multiples, and the therapist will do well to recognize his limits of control over who comes into his office. The patient's fear of losing control may stir up similar issues in the therapist. These fears and struggles may pose a source of resistance for both patient and therapist in moving on with an evaluation or therapy.

5. PATIENT-THERAPIST SEX

This is an unpopular topic among child psychiatrists who tend not to view it as an issue for child psychiatry. Unfortunately, training in child psychiatry does not offer immunity to sexual involvement with patients, be they adults or children. We are likely at some point in our careers to encounter patients who are highly seductive and some who have been abused by former therapists. We may also encounter these situations as administrators, supervisors, members of peer review committees, and expert witnesses.

Therapists who become sexually involved with their patients tend to be overly controlling and encourage the patient's dependency. Boundary transgressions are common; for instance, they may see the patient at unusual locations, make exceptions to their usual practices, and even begin to confide personal problems to the patient. One therapist would hold hands with his attractive young patient during their 6 A.M. walks in the woods; then they would go out for coffee together afterwards. The patient later commented that these meetings always seemed more like dates than therapy.

The therapist may begin to turn to the patient for comfort at a time when things are not going well in his personal life. Some may truly believe that they are in love with their patients, but as noted by Twemlow and Gabbard (1989), this is often a narcissistic yearning for wholeness in which the therapist sees the patient as a split-off aspect of himself. Smith (1989) notes that more sadistic therapists seduce patients as a means of maintaining control over them. He adds that sexual involvement may also represent a reenactment of childhood seduction. Therapists may attempt to rationalize their sexual involvement under the guise that it is therapeutic. This line of reasoning fails to explain why they only choose to provide this sort of "therapy" to their most attractive patients.

One psychiatrist went so far as to refer to his sexual involvement with his patient, not as sex but as "physical work." Unfortunately, a few naive patients may be initially duped by this, and defer to the therapist as an authority. Other common rationalizations are that the patient initiated the relationship or that it evolved from mutual consent. Given the analogy to incest, there is serious doubt as to whether patients can give truly informed consent to such an exploitive relationship.

The therapist who acts out his own needs by becoming sexually involved with his patient fails to see that in doing so he is abandoning the patient as a therapist and that once he becomes emotionally involved he loses all objectivity. Freud (1915) wisely observed that patient-therapist sex spells death for therapy. As a blatant form of acting out for both therapist and patient it discourages working through of conflicts and prior abuse (often incestuous). The consequences to the patient of this sort of behavior are devastating. Future attempts at therapy are inevitably undermined, as trust has been destroyed.

Countertransference problems abound for the therapist who attempts to treat a patient who has been abused by a former therapist. As Kluft (1989) notes, "The patient may be seen as either overly dangerous (seductive) or overly vulnerable, begetting either a distancing or an extremely protective stance." He points out that either extreme will distort the therapist's empathic stance. These patients may test out the new therapist to see if he can set limits and also because they have learned to relate in a highly sexualized way. Some therapists may shun these patients out of fear that they might falsely accuse them of sexual improprieties.

6. PSYCHIATRIC MALPRACTICE

Being called upon to testify against another mental health professional in a malpractice action is never a pleasant experience. It conjures up feelings of being disloyal to one's brethren and reminds us of our own vulnerabilities. Our protective instincts and wish to deny abuses that go on in the practice of psychotherapy may lead some to believe that the patient is distorting the relationship with the defendant either out of her own psychopathology or wish for secondary gain. On the other hand, bringing a suit is a drastic and painful action for the plaintiff and is likely to stem from a real, rather than imagined, hurt. As physicians we have an obligation to protect patients and our profession from unscrupulous or negligent practitioners. In turn, this requires a willingness to testify as to the standard of practice and to evaluate plaintiffs for psychic harm.

Reviewing another therapist's files is a unique experience that is rather akin to trespassing in someone's house. It may arouse feelings of snooping in what was meant to be private. However, the plaintiff in bringing suit has tendered her medical records. We look to therapy notes as a clue to what was going on and inevitably hark back to our own standards as well as ideal standards for keeping records and conducting therapy. We have the advantage of hindsight and must ask whether we are being too harsh on the defendant or whether he was indeed practicing in a negligent fashion.

Hearing details of a sexual encounter with a therapist from a patient is a disquieting experience and may stir up our own erotic fantasies towards forbidden objects, be they patients, parents, or children. These cases typically, although not always, involve male therapists and female patients. They are likely to be high profile cases in the media. It behooves the forensic evaluator to maintain confidentiality until such a time when there is disclosure within the courts. This often leaves the forensic psychiatrist alone with his outrage over the unethical, exploitive behavior that has been disclosed. Constructive outlets for dealing with anger over these events include joining ethics committees and educating the professional community about the problem of patient-therapist sex. Familiarizing oneself with the emerging literature on the topic of patient-therapist sex helps in processing it on an intellectual level.

IV. PITFALLS

A. Denial

Therapists may wish to deny horrific details that children reveal, because they do not fit in with the therapist's schemata of life and because of their visceral discomfort in dealing with the material. Historically we have seen this in regard to child sexual abuse which was well documented in the 19th century but rarely talked about until the last decade. More recently, as discussed, we are encountering denial in regard to ritualistic abuse of children. Our own denial or nonverbal indicators of discomfort with the material may prevent children from making disclosures and working through material.

B. Overidentification

There is the ever-present risk of overidentifying with the patient. This is easy to do when empathic responses lead to a sharing of traumatic material. The risk increases if the therapist has not yet worked through his own traumas. If the therapist is too emotive the child may feel a need to protect him and begin censoring material. Too much identification may also impede objectivity. Danieli (1988) cautions that "me-too" responses that are intended to be empathic can lead to foreclosure and shut off the patient.

C. Overload

The psychiatrist who fails to keep a lid on his practice or has trouble delegating may feel battered by an avalanche of trauma cases that leave him feeling like a victim. Success with one case may have a snowball effect, and one needs to learn how to put the brakes on. While intellectually stimulating, there is an inevitable emotional toll to pay for accepting too many of these cases.

D. Warning signs

Possible indicators that a therapist is having trouble dealing with a case include symptoms of post-traumatic stress disorder, somatic symptoms, depression, anhedonia, cynicism, abuse of alcohol or drugs, recoiling from intimacy, and sleep disturbance. The therapist may find herself unduly preoccupied with a particular crime or client, or may find a need to compulsively talk about the event. She may experience a sense of loss of control in her own life and be irritable and even explosive. Hopefully, she will be attuned enough to her inner distress to seek support or consultation.

E. Abuse of power

Where there is power, there is always the risk of abusing that power, and the forensic psychiatrist must guard against this. She must keep the legal questions and the patient's needs foremost. The psychiatrist should be guided by ethical codes and be ever vigilant for possible conflict of interest.

F. Boundary problems

The psychiatrist needs to maintain a clear distinction between forensic evaluation and treatment. In our effort to be helpful and supportive, it is easy to stray into treatment while conducting a forensic evaluation. Boundary problems are more likely to ensue when the evaluator is not clear what the purpose of the evaluation is or what his role is.

Some patients who have been victimized may test limits, and those with character pathology may attempt to manipulate. The clinician who is able to see these patterns and appreciate their origins will be better able to maintain boundaries. Unfortunately, as noted by Pope and Bouhoutsos (1986), few training programs adequately address boundary issues.

G. The dysfunctional team

Professionals who work as part of child abuse teams need to deal with the dynamics and cohesiveness of the team. As noted by Fletcher (1982), workers who fail to process anxiety, mistrust, and anger, or those who feel devalued and unappreciated are at risk for becoming "battered professionals." As in dysfunctional families, unrealistic expectations, boundary issues, role misconceptions, scapegoating, backbiting, and collusion all threaten to undermine the efficacy of the team. If internal conflicts within a team are not resolved, the clients/patients will suffer along with the professionals.

V. CASE EXAMPLE EPILOGUES

A. Case Example 1

This case illustrates boundary problems that arise from overzealousness and role confusion. Dr. Harrison strayed in feeling he could act above the law and the code of ethics in order to "protect" the child in question. He colluded in keeping the child in hiding, disregarded rules of evidence, and violated confidentiality and the child's privacy in reporting directly to the media. As often happens, boundary violations lead to more boundary violations, and in a subsequent case Harrison was indicted by the grand jury on three charges of aiding and abetting a kidnapping (*State of Maryland v. Dennis Harrison*, no. 8523, 9/18/89). Charges were dropped when Harrison agreed to reveal the child's whereabouts. Grievances were filed against him with the Maryland Board of Medical Examiners. One can only speculate about what countertransference reactions might have fueled his actions.

B. Case Example 2

The trainee reflects with his supervisor on his own childhood and his parents' protracted divorce. No one ever asked him which parent he wished to live with, and he is still bitter that he was deprived of contact with his father. He agrees to enter into therapy to further resolve this issue.

C. Case Example 3

Jenny's therapist sought out regular consultation to help her be prepared for, and to deal with, the visual assaults that were to become a painful but necessary and regular part of her therapy with Jenny. The therapist was able to deal with the sense of cumulative trauma she felt in working with this child and gave herself permission to ask seemingly rude questions that gave Jenny access to these memories. The more the therapist became aware of her own reactions to these sessions, the less she was governed by her own needs and fears, and the more she was able to respond to those of the patient. She did not have to testify at the trial but was, as noted, asked for a victim impact statement.

D. Case Example 4

The social worker recognized the need to talk to a colleague about the shock she experienced upon seeing such a highly sexualized young child. She shared that she was having a hard time erasing visual images of oral sex with dolls from her mind and discussed how she needed to distance her own sexuality from these sessions. She wondered what the cost might be for her in terms of seemingly leading a double life. Consultation helped her to sort out personal issues and to stay focused on her forensic evaluation. It also allowed her to set limits with the child without inhibiting her play and disclosures.

VI. ACTION GUIDELINES

A. Support/supervision

Developing an ongoing support system with colleagues or ongoing supervision is critical to effectively working in the area of trauma and dealing with the issue of how to act as a trauma membrane around the client while maintaining sufficient space and autonomy. Peer support may occur in the form of a group, e.g., the authors participated in one directed towards helping therapists deal with their feelings about sexual abuse. They have also used one another for help with individual cases. Ongoing supervision of difficult cases can help the therapist process troubling material as well as deal with therapy issues.

B. Consultation

Consultation, in contrast to supervision, is usually time limited and may or may not involve the consultant actually seeing the patient. It is usually more directed towards issues of diagnosis and treatment and management but may also address countertransference issues.

C. Therapy

Working in forensic psychiatry may often trigger unresolved issues in the therapist. These need to be worked through in order that they do not interfere with or contaminate the forensic evaluation and the treatment of the patient.

D. Coping strategies

1. BALANCED CASE LOAD

Too much trauma in one's case load can lead to symptoms of post-traumatic stress disorder as well as to burn out. It is not always easy to predict what traumas may unfold in therapy, but one can do some initial screening before accepting forensic evaluations. It is flattering to be referred high profile or particularly difficult cases, but it is also necessary to accept one's limitations and know when to refer elsewhere.

2. BALANCED LIFESTYLE

The busy clinician may need to book in time out just as he books patients in. We have developed our own coping styles that seem to work. One of us (L.D.) opts for a 4-day work-week that allows her to unwind on weekends and regroup in her canoe on a tranquil lake shared by loons. The other (D.S.) joined an amateur opera company whose rigorous schedule gets her out of the office and forces her to curtail her workaholic tendencies. It transposes her into another world and into the company of persons with whom she cannot talk shop. Although she often sings about death and violence, it is usually in Russian or Italian, and the experience offers catharsis as well as sublimation. She and Dr. Eli Newberger (Chapter 10), who plays tuba professionally with The New Black Eagle Jazz Band, view performing music as a healthy form of dissociation that takes them miles away from the abuse they confront daily in their practices. Exercise, sailing, travel, wilderness experiences, meditation, or creative endeavors that take the mind off work can aid the refueling process and allow one to get back in touch with self.

Clinicians should not depend solely on their work for their self-esteem and need to diversify their emotional investments. Thus, if the "market" begins to fall they still have other resources they can utilize to replenish their sense of self.

3. SOCIAL ACTIVISM

Becoming involved in causes that reduce children's exposure to trauma is one form of dealing with our own helplessness in the face of trauma. Examples of this would be supporting organizations such as ACT (Action for Children's TV) or The National Coalition on TV Violence, giving talks promoting handgun safety, and supporting organizations such as The Center to Prevent Handgun Violence.

4. INTELLECTUALIZATION

If not used excessively to cover up one's feelings, intellectualization can also be a healthy means of coping with trauma. Delving into the literature has stimulated our own interest and ongoing work in this area. Knowing that others have struggled with similar issues can also be a source of comfort. Writing about trauma, as we have discovered, becomes yet another means of mastering it.

VII. SUGGESTED READINGS

Berlin, I. (1986), Some Transference, and Countertransference Issues in the Playroom. JAACAP 26(1):101–107.

Brown, R. and Kulik, J. (1977), Flashbulb Memories. Cognition 5:73–99.

Comas-Diaz, L. and Padilla, A. M. (1990), Countertransference in Working with Victims of Political Repression. Orthopsychiat 60(2):125–134.

Danieli, Y. (1981), Differing Adaptational Styles in Families of Survivors of the Nazi Holocaust: Some Implications for Treatment. Children Today 10(5):6–10, 34–35.

Danieli, Y. (1988), Confronting the Unimaginable: Psychotherapists' Reactions to Victims of the Nazi Holocaust. In: Wilson, J., Hared, Z. and Kahana, B. (eds.): Human Adaptation to Extreme Stress: From the Holocaust to Vietnam. New York: Plenum.

Dubin, R. W., Wilson, S. J. and Mercer, C. (1988), Assaults against psychiatrists in Outpatient Settings. J Clin Psychiat 49:338–344.

Figley, D. R. (1985), Trauma and Its Wake: The Study and Treatment of Post-Traumatic Stress Disorder, New York: Brunner/Mazel, Inc.

Fletcher, L. (1982), The Battered Professional. In: Bates, K. Child Abuse & Community Concern. New York: Brunner/Mazel, Inc.

Freud, S. (1910), The Future Prospects of Psycho-Analytic Therapy. Standard Edition 7:3–122.

Freud, S. (1915), Further Recommendations in the Technique of Psychoanalysis: Observation on Transference-Love In: Rieff, P. (ed.): (1983) Therapy and Technique. New York: Collier.

Horowitz, M. J. (1986), Stress Response Syndromes, 2nd Ed. N.J.: Jason Aronson, Inc.

Kluft, R. (1990), Incest and Subsequent Revictimization. The Sitting Duck Syndrome. In Kluft, R. (ed.): Incest-Related Syndromes of Adult Psychopathology. Washington, D.C.: APPI.

Kluft, R. (1989), Treating the Patient Who Has Been Sexually Exploited by a Previous Therapist. Psychiat Clinics of NA, June 483–500.

Kubie, L. (1971), Retreat from Patients. Arch Gen Psychiat 24:98–106.

McCann, I. L. and Pearlman, L. A. (1990), Vicarious Traumatizations: A Framework for Understanding the Psychological Effects of Working with Victims. J Traumatic Stress 3 (1):131–148.

Pope, K. S. and Bouhoutsos, J. C. (1986), Sexual Intimacy Between Therapists and Patients. New York: Praeger.

Putnam, F. (1989), Diagnosis and Treatment of Multiple Personality Disorder. New York: Guilford Press.

Reuben, I., Wolkon, G. and Yamamoto, J. (1980), Physical Attacks on Psychiatric Residents by Patients. J Nerv and Mental Dis 168:243–245.

Schetky, D. H. and Colbach, E. M. (1982), Countertransference on the Witness Stand: A Flight from Self? Bull Am Acad Psychiat Law 10(2):115–122.

Shengold, L. (1989), Soul Murder: The Effects of Childhood Abuse and Deprivation. New Haven: Yale U. Press.

Smith, S. (1989), The Seduction of the Female Patient. In: Gabbard, G. (ed.): Sexual Exploitation in Professional Relationships. Washington, D.C.: APPI.

Tansey, M. J. and Burke, W. F. (1989), Understanding Countertransference. Hillside: N.J.: The Analytic Press.

Terr, L. (1981), Forbidden Games: Post-Traumatic Child's Play. J AACP 20:741–760.

Twemlow, S. and Gabbard, G. (1989), The Lovesick Therapist. In: Gabbard, G. (ed.): Sexual Exploitation in Professional Relationships. Washington, D.C. APPI.

Wilson, J. P. (1989), Intervention and Treatment. In Wilson, J. P. (ed.): Trauma, Transformation and Healing. New York: Brunner/Mazel, Inc.

SPECIAL ISSUES

16

The Child Witness

KATHLEEN M. QUINN, M.D.

I. CASE EXAMPLES

A. Case Example 1

Aaron, 5, was one of three brothers allegedly molested by an uncle who had lived with them for the past year and a half. He was referred for a competency to be a witness examination pursuant to the state law which required a competency hearing on all children under the age of 10. Aaron was of normal intelligence but presented with severe anxiety, overactivity, and numerous other post-traumatic symptoms. Whenever the possibility of his testifying before the defendant was raised by the examiner, Aaron froze or bolted from the interview room. A written report describing this behavior was delivered sealed to the trial judge.

B. Case Example 2

George, 14, was the only child of a couple undergoing a divorce. State law permitted George to voice a choice of which parent he chose to live with. George's choice would be honored if the court found it to be in his best interest.

George's father was a severe alcoholic who was actively drinking. George stated to the court-ordered examiner that he was choosing to live with his father in order to attempt to get his father to be sober and to care for him. George stated that his mother, an adequately functioning homemaker who had recently returned to school in paralegal studies, could manage on her own without him.

George was a good student with no past history of behavior problems. His social skills and peer relationships were described as good by teachers and by a school counselor he had recently begun to see.

C. Case Example 3

Lisa was a 7-year-old girl allegedly abused by her stepfather for many years. The juvenile court judge ordered a psychiatric examination of the child due to her complex history of hyperactivity and oppositional behaviors. At the time she was seen she was in foster placement. Background developmental history was limited because the child's mother refused to participate in the evaluation, stating through her attorney that Lisa was a liar and could not be believed.

Lisa presented as an overly active child who drew highly sexualized drawings including those of female and male genitalia. She repeatedly and spontaneously stated that "Ed, the boyfriend, did it." The juvenile court clinician seeing the child chose not to redo an investigation of the sexual abuse complaint because an adequate series of interviews had been done by the local protective services.

At times during the interview Lisa made statements such as, "It happened in September," and "It happened in March." Such statements were inconsistent with others she had made in the past.

II. LEGAL ISSUES

A. The child as witness

The mental health professional evaluating or treating a child who may testify is often faced with several forensically important questions: (1) Is this child competent to testify? (2) What data from the child are admissible? (3) How can this child be prepared for the experience of testifying? and (4) Can courtroom procedures be modified for child witnesses? Other roles for mental health professionals in cases involving child witnesses may include the role of expert witness or the investigator of an abuse complaint (see chapter 9). The major clinical events which result in a child becoming a witness include the child who is a victim or witness of a crime and the older child of divorce who is permitted to voice a choice in his/her custodial placement. Different legal principles and clinical issues may govern each of these types of witnessing.

B.   Competency to be a witness

1.   THE PRINCIPLE OF TESTIMONIAL COMPETENCY

Competency is a legal term implying the capacity to perform a particular task. The competency to be a witness or to testify is based upon basic factors including the capacity to observe, adequate intelligence, sufficient memory and ability to communicate, the appreciation of the difference between truth and falsehood, and an understanding of the responsibility to speak the truth. The issue of witness competency is determined by the judge or referee.

A closely related issue to witness competency is the requirement that witnesses testify only to events for which they have direct knowledge. To acquire personal knowledge the witness must have used his/her own senses to perceive the event. In contrast to competency of the witness, the matter of personal knowledge is normally a jury decision.

Competency and credibility are not synonymous. Credibility is the quality in a witness which causes his/her evidence to be worthy of belief. Traditionally, the competency of a witness had to be determined by the judge. Subsequently, the judge or jury weighed the credibility of the witness's testimony during the trial.

2.   HISTORICAL ISSUES

In common law numerous classes of individuals were judged incompetent to testify for a wide variety of reasons, including insane persons, individuals convicted of certain crimes, people unwilling or unable to take the oath, parties to a dispute, being married to the accused, or being a child. Children below a certain age were automatically barred from testifying. In early common law a child below 7 years was believed to lack the capacity to take an oath and was, therefore, unable to testify. As early as 1770, however, the influential English decision *Rex v. Braiser* (11 Leach 199, 168 Eng Rep. 202, 1779) held that there is no arbitrary age below which children are incompetent to testify. In 1895 the United States Supreme Court decision in *Wheeler v. United States* (159 US 523, 1985) upheld a trial court determination that a 5-year-old boy was competent to testify in a murder trial. Therefore, for many years the law has stated that children can testify.

Prior to the adoption of the Rules of Evidence in 1975, the majority of states by statute or case law continued to prescribe an age at or below which a child was presumed to be incompetent to testify. This age varied from 10 years to 14 years. Below the specified age the court held a hearing to determine the child's testimonial capacity

The Federal Rules of Evidence (1975) narrowed the grounds of incompetence by declaring in Rule 601: "Every person is competent to be a witness except as otherwise provided in these rules." Rule 601 was designed to curtail the need for a preliminary inquiry into a child witness's competency and to let the jury evaluate all testimony in terms of the weight it should be given and its credibility. However, Rule 601 did not remove all discretion from the judge to determine that some children lack the ability to give meaningful testimony. Even in states adopting Rule

601, competency hearings remain common for children under 10 years who are to testify.

3. LEGAL STANDARDS

The judicial test for competency of a child is essentially the same in most jurisdictions. The child must possess the ability to perceive, recall, and relate his/her experiences accurately and the ability to understand the obligation to tell the truth and understand the difference between truth and falsehoods. The current law concerning the competency of child witnesses falls into four groups: (1) those states following the Federal Rules of Evidence; (2) states which require an understanding of the oath; (3) states which retain a presumed incapacity below a specified age; and (4) states which permit all alleged victims of sexual abuse to testify (Meyers, 1987).

In jurisdictions following the federal rules approach, a large majority of children are competent. The initial judicial competency examination is usually unnecessary. However, because trial judges retain the authority and responsibility to ensure that incompetent persons do not testify, some children will be evaluated by the judge for competency. Some states have also added exceptions onto Rule 601. The effect of such qualifying language is to preserve the role of the trial judge as the evaluator of a child witness' competence.

A second set of states have laws stating that children are incompetent unless they understand the nature of an oath. In common law the necessity of taking an oath was believed to ensure that fear of divine punishment would prevent false testimony. Today, however, states permit witnesses to substitute a secular affirmation for a religious oath. The purpose of the oath or affirmation is to emphasize to the witness the seriousness of the proceeding and the duty to tell the truth.

A third group of states have laws stating a presumption that children below a certain age are incompetent unless the trial judge determines that they have the capacity to testify. These states adhere to the common law rule which held that children below certain ages were unable to understand the nature of an oath and were therefore incompetent. In states following this approach, the great majority of children over the age of 5 years are found competent to testify after questioning by the court (Myers, 1987).

A new trend in child competency to testify is legislation passed in a growing number of states to permit child victims of sexual abuse to testify regardless of age. It is unclear if such statutes will completely eliminate the traditional judicial role in evaluating the competency of young witnesses.

4. PROCEDURE

Competency examinations should be held at the time of the trial if at all possible, since the issue is whether or not the child can testify at that time. Courts have traditionally held a hearing in chambers to establish a child's testimonial capacity. The defendant does not have a constitutional right to attend a competency hearing. Who questions the child, whether the judge or the attorneys, varies. A prosecutor may request that the judge ask the questions, since this often decreases the amount of questions permitted each of the attorneys. However, some prosecutors request or are permitted to perform the competency assessment due to their relationship with the child and familiarity with the relevant questions to be asked. The questions should be limited to those which assist the determination of whether or not the child meets the minimal requirements of competency. Questions related to the abuse or alleged event should not be permitted. Questions about uncontested facts occurring at about the same time as the abuse can be asked to demonstrate the child's ability to recall accurately and to describe details.

If a mental health examination of the child has been ordered, the report is delivered sealed to the judge since he/she has sole discretion to make the decision based on the examination, observation, and report concerning the child's competency.

A finding of the child's competency is rarely overturned on appeal unless there is a finding of clear abuse of discretion.

C. A child's preference in custody proceedings

At least 30 state statutes and the Uniform Marriage and Divorce Act (1973), a model act endorsed by the American Bar Association, have recognized a child's wishes as a factor to be considered in determining custody (Freed and Foster, 1984). Consensus is lacking, however, on the weight to be given such a preference. Generally the preference is considered depending upon the age and maturity of the child, the strength of the preference, and a consideration of preferences between siblings. Some jurisdictions have an age minimum for consideration of the child's preference, typically 12 or 14 years. Such a choice is called an election. At least 20 states require a judge to interview the older child concerning his or her preference for custody (Franklin and Hibbs, 1980). In a small number of states, a child over 14 years has an absolute right to choose between fit parents. In such states the choice is binding on the court (Siegel and Hurley, 1977).

Most laws governing a child's preference in custody proceedings allow for considerable judicial discretion in weighing the child's choice, along with other factors. A key issue is the reason(s) the child gives for choosing one parent over the other. The method used to elicit the preference is a matter of judicial discretion with little guidance from the law (Lombard, 1984). There is no law establishing standards of competency in these proceedings.

D. Courtroom modifications

In addition to procedural reforms used to shield the child witness from the defendant and to expand the use of out-of-court hearsay statements (See Chapter 9), court scheduling and physical arrangements can be used to aid the child witness. For example, many courts give priority scheduling to cases involving child victims. The timing of the child's testimony can be arranged to maximize his/her performance. This often includes a morning hour, frequent breaks, and little to no waiting. A children's waiting area can be designated which is comfortable for children and separate from the general public or the defendant. Some courtrooms have child-size furniture for the young witness. Judges may choose to not wear robes. At least 10 states permit support persons to be present when a child testifies. At least 11 states permit closure of the courtroom when the child victim testifies.

There are few objections to introducing a degree of informality in the courtroom. Such matters are for the discretion of the judge. However, until recently, certain practices aimed at assisting child witnesses have been found to violate due process rights. For example, in a recent case a 5-year-old witness who had difficulty testifying at the preliminary hearing was permitted to sit with her chair turned away from the defendant. The defendant could hear the child but not see the child. The appellate court overturned the case stating, "A witness's reluctance to face the accused may be the product of falsification rather than fear or embarrassment" (*Herbert v. Superior Court.* 117 Cal. App. 3d 661, 172 Cal. Rptr, 1985:855).

In 1990 in *Maryland v. Craig* (50 USLW 5044 (June 27, 1990) (No. 89–478)) the U.S. Supreme Court held that the Sixth Amendment does not guarantee a criminal defendant the *absolute* right to a face-to-face confrontation with a witness testifying against him. The purpose of the Confrontation clause was interpreted as ensuring reliability of the evidence presented at trial. The elements of preserving reliability included the witness' presence, the taking of the oath, the cross-examination, and the observation of the witness by the judge or jury. Exceptions to the face-to-face confrontation were held as permissible if there had been "an adequate showing of necessity in an individual case."

When the court considers altering the courtroom or its procedures to accommodate a child witness, several factors should be evaluated. The basic issue to balance is any adverse impact of the modification with its need and probable benefit. Will a modification inhibit cross-examination or face-to-face confrontation? Does the child actually need a special accommodation? Will the modification focus unwarranted attention on the child's testimony? Could the child's needs be accommodated through a more traditional means? (Myers, 1987).

The exclusion of the press and the public from the courtroom during the testimony of child witnesses touches on fundamental constitutional rights. The Sixth Amendment gives the defendant a qualified right to a public trial. The public and the press have a limited First Amendment right to open criminal trials. However, a compelling competing right may prevail. The need to protect child witnesses from trauma and embarrassment may be such an overriding interest. The trial judge, however, must decide on a case-by-case basis whether closing the courtroom is necessary to protect the child witness. The 1982 Supreme Court case *Globe Newspaper Co. v. Superior Court* (457 U.S. 596, 607, 1982) stated that the court must consider factors such as the child's age, the nature of the alleged crime, the psychological fragility or strength of the child, the preference of the parents, and the child's wishes. The court must make a specific finding in support of an order to close the courtroom.

III. CLINICAL ISSUES

A. Competency to be a witness

Competency is a legal term encompassing the characteristics which indicate an individual has the mental capacity or ability to perform an act. The capacity to be a witness is the ability to understand the moral obligation to speak the truth and the nature of the questions being asked, and it includes as well the ability to form and communicate an intelligent answer. The psychiatric examination for competency to be a witness should answer two basic questions. (1) Is there a mental disorder or defect? (2) Does this mental disorder or defect directly impair the functions relevant to being a witness?

TABLE 16.1
FORENSIC EXAMINATION FOR COMPETENCY TO BE A WITNESS[a]

Legal Standard	Sources of Data	Psychiatric Assessment of Functioning
Is there a mental disease or defect?	Current mental status examination Clinical interview Caretaker's report Review of documents Relevant past history	Level of anxiety and distractability Presence or absence of unmanageable behavior Presence or absence of significant intellectual deficit Presence or absence of psychosis or other major mental illness Presence or absence of oppositional behavior (refusal to talk) Presence or absence of massive interference by fantasy
Does this mental disease or defect directly impair functions relevant to being a witness?	Same	Basic understanding of court procedure including the role of being a witness Reconstructed mental status examination at time of incident as it relates to memory (both recall and recognition) Intactness of memory of incident Quality of relating to an examiner Capacity to disclose relevant facts Capacity to tolerate cross-examination and confrontation Understanding of difference between truth and falsehood; understanding of responsibility to speak truth Child's willingness to testify

[a] Reprinted with permission from Bull Am Acad Psychiatry Law 14(4):1986.

The competency to be a witness evaluation should be court-ordered. The evaluation is a direct consultation to the judge. Therefore the report should be delivered sealed directly to the judge only.

1. THE EVALUATION

The evaluator assessing the competency of the child witness should review the current legal standard and relevant documents such as the school records, medical records, mental health records, and police reports of the alleged incident. The document review provides an estimate of intellectual endowment, significant health or developmental concerns, or the documentation of past and/or present psychiatric disorders.

Clinical interviews should include a history taken from a parent or guardian in order to review the child's developmental history and the child's current emotional and intellectual functioning. Particular attention should be paid to document incapacitating levels of anxiety, disruptive behavior, significant intellectual deficit, or presence of psychosis or other major mental illness present at the time of the interview or at the time of the alleged event. The evaluator should gather information which can later be used to corroborate the child's answers to questions such as gifts received on holidays or birthdays, family vacations, pets, or major events close to the time of the alleged offense. The adult should be questioned about the child's moral development and any significant history of lying or antisocial acts. A medical history should be reviewed since lapses of consciousness, delirium, organic or functional amnesia, or medication side effects may compromise competency.

The individual interview(s) of the child should produce detailed clinical data to describe the child's current mental status. Is the child hyperactive, disorganized, or unable to separate from a parent? Can the child engage in a focused verbal task (the interview) which is similar to the task of testifying? Can the child relate basic data about neutral events, including events close to the time of the alleged offense? Is the child sufficiently resistant to leading questions on neutral subjects he/she knows well? Can the child relate what will occur if he/she tells the truth? If they lie? Can they identify and give real examples of each? Do they feel an obligation to tell the truth?

No questioning should occur about the alleged offense unless there are stipulated facts.

Both the parent or guardian and the child interviewed must be informed of the purpose of the examination and its lack of confidentiality. Each should also be informed that the determination of competency to be a witness rests with the trial judge based upon the in-chambers examination of the child as well as on any mental health report.

2. THE REPORT

The report should detail the sources of information, a description of the child's current functioning, and relevant past history. Clinical observation should describe the child's mental status, the child's capacity to understand simple questions and communicate coherently, a demonstration of age-appropriate memory, the child's knowledge of truth and duty to be truthful, and ability of the child to use these skills to testify. The child should be given a DSM-III-R diagnosis, if present. However, the behavioral descriptions of the child will most clearly communicate the child's capacity to be a witness. Courtroom modifications which will maximize the child's performance should be described for the court's consideration. The necessity for such recommended modifications for this individual child should be clearly described.

B. Evaluation of the child of election age

A trend in the area of family law is the growing emphasis on the child's preference in contested custody cases. The crucial clinical issue is whether or not the child has the capacity to conceptualize the custodial alternatives and to consider the possible consequences of choosing each alternative. Weithorn (1984) has suggested that based on cognitive-developmental research children of 12 or 14 years are likely to possess such capabilities. However, Wallerstein and Kelly (1980) caution against relying on the expressed preference of youngsters below adolescence in contested custody cases. Their caution is based upon their finding of the long-lasting anger of the children of divorce in the 9- to 12-year-old age group against the parent they held responsible for the divorce. These children often took sides against a parent with whom they had previously had a positive relationship when the family was intact. Wallerstein and Kelly's longitudinal study described a tendency of children of this age to split the parents into the "good parent" and the "bad parent," compromising their capacity to make an informed election.

One study (Greenberg and Rappaport, 1984) has examined the decision making employed by 9- to 14-year-olds in arriving at a custodial preference between divorcing parents. Domestic relation judges evaluated the decisions reached by the children. Demographic variables such as age, IQ, sex, and socioeconomic factors were not found to be useful in predicting competent decision making. The individual child's ability to problem-solve, isolate relevant aspects of the problem, and generate alternative solutions, as well as the child's knowledge about divorce, predicted soundest judgment. This study suggests that clinicians performing such evaluations should attempt to communicate clearly to the court the child's level of cognitive development and a thorough description of how the youngster thought through his/her expressed preference.

Equally important, the clinician should describe the emotional factors which may impact upon the youngster's choice. The child may choose the parent who is most lenient, the parent who is the neediest, the parent whose bribe seems most attractive, or one party to strike out at the other (Moskowitz, 1978; Weiss, 1979).

Eliciting a preference can be a delicate matter. The specific questions about parental preference are best left to the latter part of the custody assessment after rapport is established and other data about the child and his/her experience within the family have been gathered. Gardner (1982) recommends several indirect questions concerning preference in order to protect the child from the feelings of anxiety and disloyalty associated with stating a direct preference and to lead up to a possible direct question about an election. Questions such as, "Which parent is it best for a boy (girl) to live with, the mother or the father?" or "Why does your father (mother) want you to live with him (her)?" or "How do you feel about it?" may lead the child to discuss his or her own preference. Other approaches include asking a series of questions about the preferable custodial parent for children of various ages; often the children shift into discussions of themselves when the interviewer arrives at the age of the child being interviewed. Another useful method is to pose various hypothetical questions to the child. For example, "If the judge asked you where you want to live, what would you say?"

The clinician must choose whether or not to directly ask a child about his or her preference. Some children may not wish to be put in the position of choosing one parent over the other. This wish should be respected. If a direct preference is stated, the interviewer should encourage the child to elaborate upon his/her reasons for the preference so the evaluator can assess the intellectual and emotional reasons for the preference. Gardner (1982) suggests that after the examiner understands the child's own preference a question should also be posed about what the child's preference would be if his/her siblings chose or were ordered to live with the other parent. This question is posed to assess the strength of the child's attachment to each parent as compared to the child's attachment to the sibling group.

C. Preparation for testimony

Testifying is a frightening experience for both adults and children. Some fears can be allayed by appropriate preparation and support of the child witness. Courtroom visits should be a routine aspect of preparation for the child. Either an advocate or the trial prosecutor should assist the child in orienting to the courtroom, its participants, and procedures. Both an empty courtroom and a trial in session should be visited. The empty courtroom will provide an opportunity to explore the room. The child can sit in the witness seat and practice answering selected questions. At times a judge may agree to don robes and sit on the bench, permitting the child the opportunity to experience what testifying is like. A short visit to a trial in session, preferably in the courtroom where the proceedings will take place, will afford the child a chance to see who sits where and who does what. The timing of this visit needs to be considered. It should not be so long before the trial that the child remains too anxious too long. On the other hand, the child should have some opportunity to assimilate the information he/she is given prior to trial.

Mental health professionals involved in cases including child witnesses should advocate for such courtroom visits as well as for adequate opportunity for the child to establish a working relationship with the prosecutor assigned to the case. Commercially prepared books are also available as aids in informing the child about the experience of testifying.

D. The emotional impact of being a child witness

Clinically, it has long been recognized that there can be a widely varying experience of being a child witness (Berliner and Barbieri, 1984). Although stressful, testifying can be experienced as an opportunity to feel less powerless and helpless. If a prosecution results, a child may feel that some adults can listen and believe children. However, for other children, facing the defendant, feeling discredited by cross-examination, or learning of an acquittal can be devastating. Little research has been available to demonstrate this range of reactions. However, the courts have repeatedly asked for more data in order to justify courtroom modifications.

Two recent studies have attempted to answer the question of the impact of legal intervention on sexually abused children. Runyan et al. (1989) did a prospective study of 75 children assessed to be sexually abused. Their data indicated an adverse effect of lengthy delays in the legal resolution of the cases. However, testimony in juvenile court was not found to be harmful. In contrast, Goodman and her colleagues demonstrated a subset of children who testified in criminal court proceedings who showed continuing emotional disturbance after testimony. These included children who testified multiple times; those who lacked maternal support; those whose cases lacked corroborative evidence, thereby placing greater weight on the child's testimony; and those who were most frightened by the defendant (Goodman et al., 1989). This study is the first controlled study to demonstrate the need for greater protection of at least a subgroup of child witnesses. These studies also raise the question of the difference in experience of testifying in juvenile court, which may be more informal than criminal court.

IV. CREDIBILITY OF THE CHILD WITNESS

Two major issues impact upon the credibility of a child witness—the quality of the child's disclosure and the quality of the investigations which document the child's statement. Numerous developmental issues may be raised as compromising the credibility of the child witness. Limitations of memory, vulnerability to suggestion, and the capacity to lie are some of the issues which may need to be addressed in evaluating or testifying about a child witness. Clinicians who become involved in such cases are urged to keep abreast of the rapidly changing research in this area. In addition, the quality of the past investigations may be raised as having compromised the child's disclosures.

A. Memory

Memory consists of free recall and recognition. Free recall is quite age-sensitive (Marin, Holmers, Guth, Kovac, 1979), making it more difficult for a young child to give an organized statement about an event in reply to open-ended questions. Increased retrieval strategies and selective attention develop between the ages of 5 and 10 years (Brown, 1979). Another factor that affects recall is that the young child may not have prior knowledge that would assist him/her in organizing an account relating one set of events to another. This less developed capacity for recall does not, however, represent a defect in the memory system itself. When children are asked to testify about activities with which they are quite familiar, their memories are at least as good as, and occasionally better than, adults' (Johnson and Foley, 1984).

The legal profession has been greatly concerned with the possibility that children will embellish memories or have difficulty distinguishing fact from fantasy. However, children are much more likely to make errors of omission than errors of commission (Goodman and Reed, 1986). Research also demonstrates that children as young as 6 years are as able as older children and young adults to distinguish the origins of memories, whether they be internal to the child or external. The major area of confusion for children is to distinguish memories of ideas which they acted upon from memories of ideas alone (Johnson and Foley, 1984).

Children generally remember more about the central event rather than peripheral information. Memory for actions is better than memory for surroundings (Goodman, Aman, Hirschman, 1987).

Clinically, these findings suggest that children are best approached during both investigatory interviewing and testimony with structured questions aimed at eliciting the who, where, and what of the alleged events. Questions should focus on the main events in order to maximize the child's performance. Questions about what the child thought about another's actions or his/her own actions are not developmentally appropriate for the young child.

B. Suggestibility

Preschoolers are more suggestible than older children or adults (Goodman and Reed, 1986). However, a substantial number of preschoolers are able to avoid the harmful effects of leading questions (Ceci et al., 1987). Leading questions are less detrimental if they deal with an event with which the child is very familiar and if the questions deal with the central aspects of the event (Yuille, 1980).

The vulnerability of the younger child to leading or suggestive questions increases the burden on those who do investigatory interviewing with children. The most counterproductive interviewing takes place when the interviewer has a strong preconceived notion of what occurred. When the interviewer seeks to have the child confirm these notions, leading and coercive interview techniques are more likely to be used.

Clinicians may be asked to critique the quality of past investigations involving child witnesses. Both the quality and quantity of leading or coercive techniques should be assessed as well as the child's response to such techniques. All interviews are likely to include some problematic techniques. Rarely do these contaminatory interview approaches rise to the level that the entire interview appears invalid. Mental health professionals asked to do such critiques should attempt to reconstruct the content of the past investigations through all available tapes, transcripts, and documents. The child's replies may be particularly revealing, demonstrating whether or not the child was able to withstand the problematic techniques.

C. Deception

Current studies indicate that preschoolers are unlikely to be successful telling lies (Morency and Krauss, 1982). By fourth and fifth grades, however, children are more proficient telling lies (Allen and Atkinson, 1978). Avoiding punishment is the main reason why children lie. Other motives to lie include to protect friends from getting into trouble, to protect oneself or someone else from harm, to get something one won't get otherwise, to avoid embarrassment, to maintain privacy, or to demonstrate power over those in authority (Ekman, 1989).

Clinicians conducting medical-legal assessments of children should include lying in their differential diagnosis. The evaluation should address the following questions (Quinn, 1988):

1. Does the child have the developmental capacity to deceive others?
2. Does the child have a persistent history of lying? Is it likely that this statement is also a lie?
3. Does the child have a psychiatric disorder which would alter the child's reality-testing or cause severe distortion or fantasy?

4. Is there a psychosocial stressor such as a domestic relations dispute or other family conflict which would promote the child's lying or minimizing of the family situation?

5. What would be the motive for lying?

Not infrequently it may be an adult who is lying for a child or distorting the child's communications. Such events may occur in custody/visitation battles or in Munchausen syndrome by proxy. Meadow (1977) coined the term to describe a clinical situation in which a child's symptoms were systematically factitiously reported or produced by the child's parents or other caretakers. The older child may ultimately join the parent in falsely reporting symptoms.

Finally, previous mental health assessments may cause an erroneous or premature conclusion about an allegation not attributable to a child's deception.

D. Cognitive development

The child's cognitive stage will affect the quality of the child's communication about the events. Most notably, the preoperational (ages 2–7) child's statements are likely to be fragmented and egocentric. The lack of conservation characteristic of this age prevents the child from understanding that objects and people remain the same despite a change in physical appearance. These children are unable to appreciate that objects may have more than one function. For example, a child may refer to ejaculation as urination because the child perceives urination as the sole function of the penis.

Time and sequence are also difficult concepts for the preoperational child. In addition, the traumatized child may experience distortions of duration and sequence beyond expected developmental limitations (Terr, 1981, 1983).

Interviewers must adjust their questions with these developmental issues in mind. For example, the young child's account may be best anchored by reference to major events related to holidays, birthdays, births, or death. Another strategy which may prove useful is to inquire about the major people in the child's life when the event took place such as the identity of the child's teacher or the presence of pets in the home. Interviewers should avoid questions such as how many times or how long the abuse took place, since for most children this is a developmentally inappropriate inquiry.

Clinicians may also be asked to consult with lawyers who must examine child witnesses. Numerous suggestions can help maximize the child's performance. For example, lawyers often ask questions with multiple clauses, passive voice, and a buried subject. The use of simple words in short sentences is helpful in communicating with the child witness. The examiner should repeat names rather than rely on the child's ability to keep track of pronouns. The tenses should be simple past, present, or future, not past perfect, which is confusing to children. Repeating a question may be experienced by the child as indicating that their initial answer was wrong. If questions are to be asked again, they should be rephrased.

V. CASE EPILOGUES

A. Case Example 1

The judge chose to attempt an in-chambers interview of Aaron who demonstrated similar behaviors. The judge found Aaron not competent to testify due to his inability to communicate his experiences to the court. Aaron's older brother later testified, resulting in a conviction of the defendant.

If this case had occurred today, attempts at courtroom modification, such as the use of one-way television but with full cross-examination, might have been permitted after an individual finding that Aaron would be traumatized by the defendant's presence and that a lesser modification such as two-way television would not be an adequate safeguard.

B. Case Example 2

The evaluator wrote a report describing the reasoning behind George's election to live with his father, as well as George's individual and family history. The evaluator was not able to endorse this choice as being in George's best interest. The evaluator argued that living with his father would impede George's developmental tasks of increased independence and the attainment of individual identity. Because George was a compliant adolescent who recognized and followed adult authority, the examiner stated that George could tolerate the court ordering him to live with his mother and permitting generous visitation with his father. George was also urged to join Alateen.

C. Case Example 3

The evaluator wrote a report to the court diagnosing Lisa as having a presentation consistent with post-traumatic stress disorder and most likely a preexisting attention deficit hyperactivity disorder. Lisa was articulate and in reasonable control during the assessment. She was eager to testify and tolerated questioning about unrelated topics well, giving age-appropriate examples of memory. The evaluator summarized the adequate techniques of the original investigation which had yielded an explicit and detailed description of sexual acts that Lisa had experienced. Her tendency to give inconsistent dates and at times statements about time not age-appropriate were described as the child's attempts to please interviewers and as the way she believed her statements would be more credible. Apart from these inconsistencies, the central aspects of the abuse she described remained the same.

Despite these data the juvenile court and criminal court proceedings were dropped due to the judge's perceptions of Lisa as a not competent or credible witness. She was placed in a residential center due to her ongoing behavior problems.

VI. ACTION GUIDE

A. General principles

1. Establish focus of the evaluation concerning the child witness.
2. Clarify role of mental health professional.
3. Obtain court order for competency or custody assessments.
4. Continue to update knowledge base about child witnesses and their capacities.

B. Competency to be a witness

1. Obtain necessary background data including school, medical, and mental health records.
2. Interview parents or guardians concerning child's development and relevant background.

3. Evaluate child individually:
   a. Assess basic elements of mental status both at time of alleged offense and currently.
   b. Screen capacity to recall neutral events dating from time of offense.
   c. Note child's capacity to communicate.
   d. Examine child's appreciation of the difference between a truth and a falsehood.
   e. Assess child's appreciation of the obligation to speak the truth.
   f. Obtain psychological testing if any evidence of intellectual deficit.
   g. Discuss child's willingness to testify.
   h. Avoid direct discussion of the facts of the case in child interview.
4. Report:
   a. Discuss any mental disorders present and their impact upon child's capacity to testify.
   b. Describe the necessity for any courtroom modifications.
   c. Have sealed report delivered directly to judge.

C. Evaluation of the child of election age:

1. See both parents to obtain individual and family history.
2. See child separately to thoroughly explore the decision-making process which has lead to the election.

D. Preparation of the child witness:

1. Encourage preliminary visits to both an empty and an occupied courtroom.
2. Advocate for an early establishment of a working alliance between the prosecuting attorney and the child witness.
3. Consider use of educational materials for the child.
4. Support family members who are supporting the child.

VII. REFERENCES

Allen, V. L. and Atkinson, M. L. C. (1978), Encoding of nonverbal behavior by high achieving and low-achieving children. J Ed Psychol 70:298–305.

Berliner, L. and Barbieri, M. K. (1984), The testimony of the child victim of sexual assault. In: G. S. Goodman (ed.): The Child Witness. J Soc Iss 40:125–138.

Brown, A. L. (1979), Theories of memory and the problem of development: activity, growth, and knowledge. In: L. Cermak and F. I. M. Craik (eds.): Levels of Processing in Memory. Hillsdale, NJ: Erlbaum: 225–258.

Ceci, S.J., Ross, D. F., and Toglia, M. P. (1987), Age differences in suggestibility: narrowing the uncertainties. In: S. J. Ceci, M. P. Toglia, and D. F. Ross (eds.): Children's Eyewitness Memory. New York: Springer-Verlag.

Ekman, P. (1989), Why Kids Lie: How Parents Can Encourage Truthfulness. New York: Charles Scribner & Sons.

Franklin, R. and Hibbs, B. (1980), Child custody in transition. J Marit and Fam Ther 6:285–291.

Freed, D. J. and Faster, H. H. (1984), Divorce in the fifty states: an overview. Fam Law Quart 17:365–447.

Gardner, R. A. (1982), Family Evaluation in Child Custody Litigation. Creskill, New Jersey: Creative Therapeutics.

Goodman, G. S., Aman, C., and Hirshman, J. (1987), Child sexual and physical abuse: children's testimony. In: S. J. Ceci, M. P. Toglia, and D. F. Ross (eds.): Children's Eyewitness Memory. New York: Springer-Verlag: 1–24.

Goodman, G. S., Jones, D. P. H., Pyle-Taub, E., England, P., Prot, L., Rudy, L., and Prado-Estrada, L. (1989), Children in Court: The Emotional Effects of Criminal Court Involvement. New Orleans: American Psychological Association.

Goodman, G. S. and Reed, R. S. (1986), Age differences in eyewitness testimony. Law Hum Behav 10:317–332.

Greenberg, E. F. and Rappaport, J. (1984), Predictors of children's competence to participate in child custody decision making. Unpublished manuscript.

Johnson M. K. and Foley, M. A. (1984), Differentiating fact from fantasy: the reliability of children's memory. In: G. S. Goodman (ed.): The Child Witness. J Soc Iss 40:33–50.

Lombard, F. K. (1984), Judicial interviewing of children in custody cases: an empirical and analytical study. Univ Cal Davis Law Rev 17:807–808.

Marin, B. V., Holmes, D. L., Guth, M., and Kovac, P. (1979), The potential of children as eyewitnesses. Law Hum Behav 3:295–305.

Meadow, R. (1977), Munchausen syndrome by proxy. Lancet 2:343–345.

Morency, N. L. and Krauss, R. M. (1982), The nonverbal encoding and decoding of affect in first and fifth graders. In: R. S. Feldman (ed.): Development of Nonverbal Behavioral Skills. New York: Springer-Verlag: 181–199.

Moskowitz, L. (1978), Divorce-custody disposition: the child's wishes in perspective. Santa Clara Rev 18:427–452.

Myers, J. E. B. (1987), Child Witness: Law and Practice. New York: John Wiley & Sons.

Quinn, K. (1988), Children and deception. In: R. Rogers (ed.): Clinical Assessment of Malingering and Deception. New York: Guilford Press: 104–119.

Roe, R. J. (1985), Expert testimony in child sexual abuse cases. Univ. Miami Law Rev 40:97–113.

Runyon, D., Everson, M., Edelsohn, G., Hunter, W., and Coulter, M. (1988), Impact of legal interventions on sexually abused children. Advisor 2(2):6–7.

Siegel, D. M. and Hurley, S. (1977), The role of the child's preference in custody proceedings. Fam Law Quart 13:1–58.

Terr, L. C. (1981), Psychic trauma in children: observations following the Chowchilla bus kidnapping. Am J Psychiatry 138(1):14–19.

Terr, L. C. (1983), Time sense following psychic trauma. Am J Psychiatry 53(2):244–261.

Wallerstein, J. S. and Kelly, J. B. (1980), Surviving the Breakup: How Children and Parents Cope with Divorce. New York: Basic Books.

Weiss, R. (1977), Issues in the adjudication of custody when parents separate. In: G. Levinger and O. Moles (eds.): Divorce and Separation: Context, Causes, and Consequences. New York: Basic Books: 324–336.

Weithorn, L. A. (1984), Children's capacities in legal contexts. In: N. O. Repucci, L. A. Weithorn, E. P. Mulvey, and J. Monahan (eds.): Mental Health, Law and Children. Beverly Hills: Sage: 25–55.

Yuille, J. C. (1980), A critical examination of the psychological and practical implications of eyewitness research. Law Hum Behav 4(4):335–345.

VIII. SUGGESTED TEXTS FOR USE WITH CHILD WITNESSES

Anderson, D. and Finne, M. (1986), Margaret's Story: Sexual Abuse and Going to Court. Minneapolis, MN: Dillon Press.

Beaudry, J. and Ketchum, L. (1983), Carla Goes to Court. New York: Human Sciences Press.

Flynn, K. (undated), Some Questions You May Ask About Going to Court. Hennepin County (Minnesota) Public Affairs Department.

17

Legal Aspects of Mental Retardation

JAMES C. HARRIS, M.D.

I. CASE EXAMPLES

A. Case Example 1—Sexuality

John, a 13-year-old boy with Down syndrome is brought to your office by his mother and stepfather who claim that he was sexually involved with their 5-year-old natural son. They indicate that the 5-year-old told them that his brother, whom he sleeps with, was on top of him and pushed his penis against him. There has been considerable disagreement between the parents in regard to how to handle the boy with Down syndrome; the father rejects him, and the mother protects him. When examined, he is a short, moderately mentally retarded pubertal male with Down syndrome. He responds to direct questions, and through his answers to questions and supplemental drawings, he tells what happened.

B. Case Example 2—Criminal confession

William, a 19-year-old, mildly retarded male, is referred for evaluation after being convicted of fire-setting. His attorney is concerned about his enthusiasm in confessing not only to these fires but also to a series of other fires as well which took place in areas where he is not known to have access. Furthermore, although he was seen in the area where the first fires occurred (those he was convicted of setting), there is no witness who specifically saw him setting the fires. He has a history of aggressive behavior with his father and a history of two brief hospitalizations which took place following outbursts of temper and aggressive behavior. He has always lived at home with his parents and has completed a special education program at school without major incident. Since leaving school, he held two jobs briefly and was beginning a third job when the current episode took place which has resulted in his current hospitalization.

When interviewed he talks rapidly in the initial part of the examination about how the family television set caught on fire many years ago. When he thinks about the television set burning, he gets excited and feels the need to exercise to settle himself down.

C. Case Example 3—Right to drug treatment

Matthew, a 22-year-old, moderately mentally retarded young man, is brought for evaluation by his elderly parents. They bring a cardboard box filled with documentation about his previous evaluations. He has a very short attention span and is continuously active, so that he cannot be left alone at home. He asks questions constantly, thereby making it difficult for his mother to complete any of her own work. He has the delusional perception that he sees the director of his old group home, whom he says abused him, on the street or in crowds of people. He is quite frightened of being harmed by her. When his history is reviewed, it is apparent that he was well compensated behaviorally in the group home when taking 300 mg of Mellaril each day. However, because of the rule in the group home that psychotropic medications must be discontinued, his medication was stopped without consideration of his diagnosis of a paranoid disorder. He became aggressive and suspicious. Eventually he said he was "beaten" by staff members and was then discharged from the home because the staff said that his aggression had increased. Family members had noted bruises on a home visit. His family seeks help for his treatment and seeks advice in planning legal action against the group home for abusing their son.

D. Case Example 4—Use of antilibidinal agents

Raymond, a 19-year-old, profoundly retarded boy with the cri-du-chat genetic syndrome is referred for evaluation of self-injury (hand biting), sleep disturbance, and genital self-stimulation. When seen for evaluation, the patient was a dysmorphic, short, nonverbal, adolescent male. During the assessment he was aggressive toward both parents, particularly toward his father, whom he pinched on several occasions, when efforts were made to redirect him. When not attended to, he falls to the floor and attempts to masturbate through his clothing. His mother shows obvious embarrassment about his behavior. She is sleep deprived because he keeps her awake since he sleeps poorly at night and roams around the house. She is continually concerned that he will injure himself.

He is admitted to the hospital for treatment of his behavioral symptoms. However, the behavioral treatment is not successful, since he is constantly preoccupied with finding objects to use for masturbation. On home visits he reverts to his old patterns of behavior prior to hospitalization, and his masturbation is as frequent as it was before hospitalization. A trial of an antilibidinal agent, provera, is recommended after an 8-week inpatient hospitalization is not successful in controlling his behavioral problems. Staff members raise questions about his legal rights in regard to informed consent for the use of an antilibidinal agent.

E. Case Example 5—Sterilization

Jennifer is a 14-year-old, severely mentally retarded girl who is now menstruating regularly. She is brought to an outpatient clinic by her parents who ask that she be sterilized because of their concerns that she could become pregnant.

Her unmarried, older, mildly mentally retarded sister previously has delivered a child who is living in the family's home. Jennifer is attending a special education center for the severely mentally retarded, has a seizure disorder, and has a mental age of 4 years. When visitors come to the home she responds affectionately and likes to be held by them. Her parents are concerned that her affectionate behavior will be misinterpreted. They become increasingly insistent that she have a sterilization procedure.

F. Case Example 6—Execution of the mentally retarded

David, a 24-year-old man, who is mild to moderately mentally retarded and brain damaged (mental age 9–10 years) is seen for evaluation following the killing of the owner of a convenience store. The examiner is told that he had worked part time at the store and impulsively took merchandise. After arguing with the owner about his theft, he went to his family home and returned to the store with a gun and killed the owner after a second argument occurred. Is he competent to stand trial and participate in his own defense? The death penalty is a particular concern for his family. They ask if the death penalty can be applied to a mentally retarded person.

II. OVERVIEW OF MENTAL RETARDATION

A. Definition

The definition of mental retardation approved by the American Association on Mental Retardation (Grossman, 1983) is the most widely used and has been incorporated into DSM-III-R.

"Mental retardation refers to significantly subaverage intellectual functioning existing concurrently with deficits in adaptive behavior, and is manifested during the developmental period."

In this definition of mental retardation, significantly subaverage general intellectual functioning refers to the ability to learn and is measured by the intelligence quotient. Subaverage intellectual functioning is defined as an IQ of below 70 with a variation in measurement error of approximately 5 IQ points. However, the intelligence test alone is not an adequate assessment since an individual may come from deprived circumstances, and the test itself could be culturally biased. More specifically, IQ tests are not accurately measuring how an individual may function in society, although they may predict educational progress. The deficits in adaptive behavior are included to indicate that IQ tests alone are not an accurate measure of a mentally retarded person's functioning. Adaptive behavior has been defined as "the effectiveness or the degree with which the individual meets the standards of personal independence and social responsibility expected of his age and cultural group" (Grossman, 1983). This includes the areas of social skills and responsibility, communication, daily living skills, personal independence, and self-sufficiency (DSM-III-R, 1987). In addition, the low intelligence test score and lack of adaptive behavior must occur before the person is 18 years of age.

Mental retardation is not a disease or illness in itself. In mental retardation, thinking is not characteristically disordered, and perception is not distorted unless there is a concurrent mental disorder. It is made up of a heterogeneous group of conditions that range from genetic and metabolic disorders to functional changes that follow trauma to the nervous system at birth or later in the developmental period. Because of this heterogeneity each case must be considered independently according to whether or not there is an associated syndrome, e.g., Down syndrome, or an associated etiology, e.g., head trauma.

Although the mentally retarded may also have a diagnosis of a major psychiatric condition, their day-to-day problems ordinarily relate to difficulties in developmental functioning. Depending on the degree of cognitive ability, there may be deficits in abstract thinking, in social judgment, and in their fund of general information. Difficulties in these areas, if appropriate to the person's cognitive level, are not evidence of a mental disorder. (At the time of examination, it should be ascertained whether the individual was previously functioning in a higher level and has lost skills and regressed.) The mentally retarded person will develop over time and pass through the same developmental stages as a nonretarded person, but not reach the higher levels of cognitive functioning. Abilities are reduced in all areas of functioning including language, language communication, memory, attention, self-concept, suggestibility, knowledge base, control of impulsivity, moral development, and overall motivation. From a legal perspective, difficulty in logical thinking, planning strategies for action, and foresight are among the most important deficits. Furthermore, there is an intellectual rigidity in mental retardation which may be seen in impaired ability to learn from mistakes and difficulty in mentally generating a range of options to choose from in a new situation, particularly when stressed. A mentally retarded adult with a mental age of 6 years may be less flexible in thinking than a nonretarded 6-year-old. However, the adult mentally retarded person will have more life experience than a child of equivalent mental age on which to base his options.

B. Levels of severity of mental retardation

Mental retardation is divided into four degrees of severity reflecting the amount of intellectual impairment: mild, moderate, severe, and profound. Although an intelligence test is not the sole basis for determining mental retardation, these tests are the accepted standard to measure the degrees of severity of mental retardation. Profound mental retardation is an IQ of 20 or less (adult mental age less than 3 years), severe is an IQ of 20 to 34 (adult mental age 3 to less than 6 years), moderate is an IQ of 35 to 49 (adult mental age 6 to less than 9 years), and mild is an IQ of 50 to 69 (adult mental age 6 to 9 years) (*International Classification of Disease*, 10th edition). Intelligence scores are based on the assessment of a variety of relatively specific skills. Although these skills generally develop together, there may be wide discrepancies between sub-test scores (Jones, Barnett, McCormack, 1988); e.g., language functioning may be low and performance on tests of visuospatial skills higher. Because of this scattering of skills, the test profile must be considered in regard to adaptive functioning. Tests of adaptive behavior that are used together with intelligence tests include the AAMD Adaptive Behavior Scale (Lambert, Windmiller, and Segal, 1975) and the Vineland Adaptive Behavior Scales (Sparrow, Balla, and Cicchetti, 1984).

The overall prevalence rate of mental retardation is estimated to be approximately three percent of the school-aged population (Clarke and Clarke, 1975). In the adult population the prevalence of mental retardation is about one percent, since many of the mildly retarded may adapt in society following an appropriate education, and the more severely retarded with medical complications may not survive into adulthood. Eighty-five percent of the mentally retarded population fall into the mildly retarded range, and the remaining 15% are severely retarded. It is the mildly retarded who are most likely to be involved in criminal proceedings and may be found to be legally competent.

C. Multiaxial classification

The revised Third Edition of the *American Psychiatric Association Diagnostic and Statistical Manual of Mental Disorders* (American Psychiatric Association, 1987) includes mental retardation on the second axis, the designated developmental axis. Mental disorders in retarded persons are coded on Axis I, and multiple diagnoses may be listed. Medical conditions that relate to mental retardation are classified on Axis III. Psychosocial stresses which commonly occur in the lives of the mentally retarded are coded on Axis IV, and global adaptive functioning is coded on Axis V. This multiaxial approach then allows for the diagnosis of mental retardation, mental disorders that may be associated with mental retardation, and physical conditions which may be etiologically important in regard to mental retardation. The designation of the severity of psychosocial stresses that impinge on the retarded person and an overall global adaptive function rating complete this system. This diagnostic approach is descriptive in nature rather than etiologically based. Concurrent physical disorders or conditions can be indicated without necessarily suggesting that these conditions are etiologically related to a mental disorder in the mentally retarded person. Medical conditions, particularly if involving the brain, may be added vulnerability factors in increasing the risk of a mental disorder. In program planning, the multiaxial classification is of particular importance, since it designates each of the dimensions that is important in treatment planning and highlights those areas that are of most importance in evaluating the overall function of the mentally retarded person.

D. Normalization—the developmental model

Mental retardation is a permanent condition and is not curable, although the degree of habilitation that can be accomplished for the retarded person can be substantial (Wolfenberger, 1972). During the past 20 years a focus on a developmental model which acknowledges the capability for growth, of developing independence in social skills, and of new learning has been emphasized. The developmental model specifically addresses the fact that the retarded person's level of functioning is not static and that an individual's adaptive behavior may be improved through habilitation. Since the retarded person is capable of learning and adapting, legal approaches need to take into account that the retarded person may require additional education and effort but can learn new information.

The focus on normalization (Wolfenberger, 1972) for the mentally retarded has emphasized the importance of retarded persons' being entitled to services which are as culturally normative as possible to help them establish and maintain more appropriate personal behavior. Normalization emphasizes that the mentally retarded persons should live in the community, go to regular schools, seek competitive employment, and behave as closely as possible to the standards of the nonretarded persons at a comparable developmental age. Furthermore, they should be responsible for their own behavior, and others should not assume that because they are mentally retarded that they are not capable of doing so.

Special features of mental retardation that need to be taken into account in normalization are communication skills, previous life experiences, and any associated physical disorders. Many mentally retarded people have concurrent difficulties in language expression and articulation. Consequently, it may require a special effort to communicate with them and, in some instances, "signing" may be necessary to communicate. In other instances, the nonverbal retarded person with a physical handicap, such as cerebral palsy, may require a speech synthesizer or other language devices to assist in communication. The retarded person may have lacked certain life experiences because of poor programming which may then influence his ability to respond to new situations. Finally, physical disorders involving the brain and other organ systems are quite commonly found in mental retardation syndromes.

E. Sexuality

The mentally retarded may be stereotyped in regard to the expression of sexuality (Abram et al., 1988; Szymanski and Crocker, 1989). On the one hand, they may be considered to be sexually uninhibited, and on the other hand, considered to be eternal children or asexual and not have sexual interest and needs. Because of the first of these considerations as well as concerns about inheritability, sterilization of the retarded was practiced in the past, and some states still have such legislation. Although this is not the case, it was feared that the mentally retarded would indiscriminately procreate, leading to an increase in the incidence of mental retardation. Consequently, involuntary sterilization (Dickens, 1982) has been practiced, and marriages between retarded persons were often prohibited. In some circumstances, a retarded person was denied the opportunity to socialize and develop an intimate relationship with the opposite sex.

It is ordinarily after puberty that sexual interest becomes apparent; however, puberty may be delayed in some retarded persons secondary to the physical condition that underlies the retardation. Regardless of the age of pubertal onset, the most severely retarded individuals may show little interest in sexual behavior towards others. On the other hand, the mildly retarded and many of the moderately retarded may have normal pubertal development, demonstrate appropriate sexual interests, and establish sexual identities.

When the expression of their sexual interests is denied, sexual activity may be a response used to demonstrate their self-importance and be aimed at gaining acceptance from others. Sexual status may be important for their peer group, just as it is for those who are not retarded. The encouragement of a relationship with another and the learning of social skills are more important than specific instruction in sexual activity.

Mentally retarded persons, particularly women, may be exploited sexually. Their knowledge of sexuality is often not fully developed, because the usual sources of information may not be available to them. Peer relationships, printed reading material, and sex education in school are often limited or unavailable for the retarded. Furthermore, family members may be reluctant to review sexual matters with them. Mildly and moderately retarded adolescents frequently lack basic information on sexual anatomy, contraceptive issues, and venereal disease. Their knowledge of sexuality is related more to life experience and opportunity than to intelligence level.

III. LEGAL ISSUES

A. Scope of psychiatric involvement

The psychiatrist may be called upon to evaluate mentally retarded persons in a variety of situations that have legal implications. To properly conduct these assessments, background information is needed regarding the nature of mental retardation, an understanding of the legal rights of the mentally retarded (that have been clarified in the past 20 years), recognition that mental retardation is a vulnerability factor in mental illness, and awareness of developmental issues that relate to mental retardation (attachment, sexuality, aggression, moral development, attention processes, memory formation) (Kindred, 1976). The issue of brain damage in mental retardation and its relationship to aggression and social disinhibition, the use of psychotropic drugs and their complications (e.g., tardive dyskinesia) (Felding, 1980), and the recognition of the heterogeneity of mental retardation syndromes (e.g., Down, XYY) must be considered.

Psychiatrists may evaluate mentally retarded persons in a variety of settings, such as emergency rooms, where aggression toward self or others may be present, or where abuse of the retarded person is questioned; the court, where there may be questions of competency to stand trial or to act as a witness; the clinic, where an assessment of parenting skills or a diagnostic evaluation may be requested; and the school, where questions are raised about the least restrictive environment for education. Questions of legal rights are common; e.g., access to education, participation in decisions about medical treatment, access to medical records by retarded adults, the utilization of a guardian to guarantee the rights of an incompetent mentally retarded person. To adequately conduct these evaluations, the psychiatrist needs to be aware of the legal rights legislation that relates to the mentally retarded as well as the more traditional forensic concerns that relate to competency.

The psychiatrist must consider the special case that arises when a person who has been in an institution for much of his lifetime is deinstitutionalized and commits a criminal act without knowing that it is against the law. They have not learned the law during their institutional stay (Szymanski and Crocker, 1989). Furthermore, during the institutional stay, there may have been no opportunity to be involved in an illegal action.

B. The insanity defense

Formulations of the insanity defense traditionally base the defense on "mental disease or defect," the latter referring to mental retardation. Mental retardation then can be used as a basis for the insanity defense (Menninger, 1986). Ordinarily, the culpability of persons with mental retardation can be considered to be reduced, so mental retardation is considered to be a mitigating circumstance. Mental disorder and mental retardation both must be considered in decisions regarding the insanity defense. This distinction between them is clearly made in international classifications of disorders and diseases. However, this distinction is sometimes blurred in the court. This blurring may occur since cases brought for criminal action may involve both mental retardation and a mental disorder, both of which must then be taken into account in the assessment process.

When used with the mentally retarded, the insanity defense is most frequently considered in murder cases when the question of the culpability of a retarded person is raised. Culpability refers to the capacity of the accused to distinguish right from wrong. The legal standard that is applied most often is the M'Naghten rule, which requires that there be a lack of knowledge of the nature and wrongfulness of the committed act in order to be found to be not responsible. The American Law Institute has suggested the following modification of this rule: "A person is not responsible for criminal conduct if at the time of such conduct as a result of mental disease or defect, he lacks substantial capacity either to *appreciate* the criminality (wrongfulness) of his conduct or to conform his conduct to the requirements of the law." The difference in wording focuses on substituting the word "appreciate," which suggests both emotional and cognitive awareness, for the word "know." Knowing that an act is wrong may indicate only surface knowledge of its wrongfulness without a full appreciation of why it is wrong (Menninger, 1986). Furthermore, although knowing an act is wrong, because of excessive impulsiveness or enhanced suggestibility or acquiescence to authority, he may have difficulty in conforming his conduct to the law (Luckasson, 1988).

C. Competency

Issues related to competency include the basic legal competency to stand trial as a person responsible for one's own actions and the ability to be a competent witness (Smith, Kunjukrishnan, 1986). However, assessments must also be made of competency to manage one's own affairs, to care for one's self, and to care for another person (parenting). Basic elements of competency include (1) the ability to understand information presented regarding the consequences of the decision that is made; (2) the ability to consider alternatives before making a decision; (3) the manner in which the decision is made (weighing the alternatives and expressing a preference); and (4) the nature of and degree of commitment to the final decision. A competent decision then requires comprehension of the issue, autonomy in decision making, a rational reasoned process, an awareness of the future consequences of the decision, and the judgment to make choices despite uncertainty in the outcome. An accused person should not be allowed to waive a competency examination, and all parties involved in the process have a duty to raise the issue of competency if there is any doubt (*Pate v. Robinson*, 383 U.S. 375, 1966).

1. COMPETENCY TO STAND TRIAL

Competency to stand trial refers to the ability to comprehend the nature and quality of the legal proceedings and advise counsel in preparation and implementation of one's own defense (*Dusky v. U.S.*, 362 U.S. 401, 1960; Heller, Traylor, Ehrlich, and Lester, 1981; Golding, Roesch, and Schrieber, 1984). Persons accused of a crime cannot be tried for that crime unless they understand both the charge that is made against them and the consequences if they are convicted. Furthermore, the individual must be able to aid his lawyer in his defense. A mentally retarded person may have difficulties in each of these situations because of limited ability to understand the charges or their consequences due to reduced intelligence, lack of life experience, inadequate education, a tendency to overcompliance to please others, or a fear of the authorities.

In most states a defendant in a criminal trial who is thought to be incompetent is committed to a mental hospital for further assessment. If he is found to be incompetent, he will stay in the hospital for some time, after which he may be released or committed on civil grounds. There is the expectation that the individual may become competent at a later date when the illness is resolved. For the mentally ill who are not mentally retarded, this may be the case; however, the acquisition of later competency is more complicated in the case of mental retardation. Consequently, mentally retarded persons have been committed to institutions for life when accused of offenses that are minor. Had they been tried for them and convicted, they may not have been incarcerated at all. This situation has been considered by the U.S. Supreme Court in the *Jackson v. Indiana* case (406 U.S. 715, 1971). The ruling was than an incompetent offender could be committed to a hospital only for a reasonable period of time, after which he would be released or committed under a civil statute.

The patient was a mentally retarded deaf mute charged with robbery. A lengthy hospitalization was shown not to be justified on the grounds of restoring the retarded to competency. The court noted that due process requires that the nature and duration of commitment bear a relationship to the purpose for the commitment. If an individual is committed because of his incapacity to proceed to trial, he cannot be held more than a reasonable time to determine if there is a substantial probability that he will obtain the capacity in the foreseeable future. If it is not the case that he can achieve capacity, the State must institute customary civil commitment proceedings, as would be the case for other citizens, or release the defendant. If it is thought that the individual will be able to stand trial, continued commitment must be justified by evidence that progress is being made towards accomplishment of that goal. Understanding of these issues may lead to a change in the procedures by differentially processing and handling the mentally retarded/mentally ill.

2. COMPETENCY TO TESTIFY

In certain circumstances, mentally retarded persons may be asked to testify for the prosecution in a criminal case. The defense may argue that they are not competent to be witnesses and raise questions about their reliability. A witness is not specifically disqualified by law because he is mentally retarded, but an individual assessment of his competency to testify may be required. To do so, the prospective witness must understand that he may be punished for not telling the truth. He must be able to demonstrate the ability to recall and to report past events accurately. In this instance, the assessment of the retarded person to testify will require an evaluation of his language and memory capabilities, his personal understanding of the meaning of the alleged crime, the pressures exerted by others on him, and his capacity to differentiate reality from fantasy. The final determination of credibility of the retarded witness will be up to the court and jury. The evaluation of a potentially mentally retarded witness should include whether or not there is a past history of compulsive reporting of fantasy stories regarding the issue in question. The impact on him of testifying on the witness stand should also be considered, particularly if testimony is directed towards a family member or guardian who has a supervisory role for the retarded person (Szymanski and Crocker, 1989).

3. CONFESSION

Mentally retarded persons are at risk of giving a nonvoluntary confession (Praiss, 1989). A criminal confession in response to questioning while in custody cannot be used in evidence unless the defendant voluntarily, knowingly, and intelligently waived Miranda rights. These rights ensure that when a person is taken into custody he is informed of the Fifth Amendment right to remain silent and have counsel retained or appointed before an admissible confession can be obtained. A mentally retarded person requires a thorough explanation of these rights. Because of adaptive problems and intellectual limitations, care is needed in determining whether the waiver of rights is valid. Because of their special needs, a counsel should be sought as early as the pre-custodial stage. With early access to an attorney in addition to a familiar person, the mentally retarded person's waiver is best protected and more likely to be voluntary.

4. PARTIAL COMPETENCY/GUARDIANSHIP

The mentally retarded person may be competent to carry out some of his or her affairs, but not all of them. A person who is mentally retarded and who has difficulty in managing financial affairs (Kapp, 1981; Mesibov et al., 1980) but can handle other activities may have a guardian appointed to decide only financial matters. The view is that the retarded person is partially competent in handling his affairs. The assignment of a guardian may be determined by the degree of mental retardation. Mildly and moderately retarded individuals need to be judged on the basis of their adaptive functioning and not their IQ scores alone. However, severely and profoundly retarded individuals regularly will need the assignment of a guardian when they reach maturity.

5. PARENTAL COMPETENCY

The ability to care for a child on a day-to-day basis, to make future plans for the child, and to consistently set limits on behavior must be evaluated in the mentally retarded parent (Feldman, 1986). Mentally retarded adults may be overrepresented among neglectful parents but not necessarily among abusive parents (Schilling, Schinke, Blythe, and Brath, 1982; Seagull and Scheurer, 1986). Mental retardation, per se, is not automatically considered evidence for lack of competency in child care, although it is increasingly evident that successful parenting by a mentally retarded person is fraught with difficulty, particularly in the care of children beyond infancy (Whitman and Accardo, 1990). Children of mentally retarded parents are at risk for mental retardation, but a substantial number, 60%–70% in one study (Accardo and Whitman, 1990), were not retarded. Factual evidence of competency is necessary for mildly and moderately retarded parents; however, if the parent is severely and profoundly retarded, then the child will require placement. Considerable efforts may be needed to teach parenting skills to mentally retarded adults. This may be attempted either through group or through individual instruction with the additional provision of ongoing home support services. In some settings, both the parent and the child may be placed in a foster home. Here the foster parents can assume overall responsibility for the child's care and the natural parent can assist them in learning new skills. Issues of parenting by a retarded person are of particular importance when there are multiple children in the home and when the mentally retarded person has a normally intelligent child. The adolescent who is not mentally retarded may have particular difficulties in relating to a retarded parent.

D. Rights of the incompetent

Some mentally retarded individuals will be mentally incompetent from birth, and the protection of their constitutional rights is an ongoing consideration throughout their lifetime. The issues that come up most often relate to procreation, the issue of sterilization (Appelbaum, 1982), rights in regard to involuntary institutionalization, and the right of others to initiate medical intervention (Sundram, 1988) or to terminate life-sustaining treatment. A mentally incompetent, developmentally disabled individual is generally unable to exercise these rights. The procedural safeguards necessary to guarantee his rights even though he is incompetent are important to consider. How best to preserve the developmentally disabled person's autonomy despite his incompetency has been considered in several ways. Legislation focusing on the best interest test is one recent standard. This standard is contrasted with the substituted judgment test.

An incompetent mentally retarded person can not function normally in society or voluntarily consent in regard to decisions about his well-being. Others must make decisions for him which include: the choice to undergo or terminate life-sustaining treatment; the right to reproduce or procreate; and the right to remain in the community and not be institutionalized. These rights have been considered constitutionally protected (Roesch and Golding, 1979). However, the right of self-determination is exercised not by the retarded person but by another person—a parent or guardian appointed by the state through the courts.

The approach to the right of self-determination for incompetent individuals includes: (1) the best interest test and (2) the substituted judgment test. In the best interest test, the focus is primarily on the needs of an incompetent person. His expressed desires or intentions are considered but may be disregarded depending on the circumstances. In the substituted judgment test, the court renders the decision for the developmentally disabled person which it considers that the person would render for himself if he were competent. The substituted judgment test has been questioned, since it may lead to excessive involvement of the courts in matters that can be handled more personally and expeditiously by a guardian or family member. The best interest procedure may lead to better accountability and avoids the abstractions inherent in the court assuming how a person who has never been competent would make a decision.

Procedural safeguards which are available to protect the rights of the incompetent individual include: (1) the appointment of a guardian *ad litem*; (2) an adversarial hearing; and (3) limits on the control by the court. This last precaution considers whether the judge has the expertise to resolve the issues which arise.

a. Guardian *ad litem*

A guardian *ad litem* is appointed to represent an incompetent person. This guardian may be appointed by the court either on a motion to the court or following a statute. The guardian's responsibility is to defend the rights of an incompetent person and represent his best interests. He may also help resolve differences between medical and legal issues.

b. Adversarial hearing

A mandatory due process hearing may be required for specific issues regarding the mentally retarded, e.g., sterilization. In the due process hearing, several issues must be addressed. These include: (a) the opportunity to be heard; (b) the opportunity to question and cross-examine witnesses; and (c) the right to offer evidence. Such hearings may be necessary when there is a question as to whether a family is acting in the best interest of its mentally retarded family member and whether that retarded person's constitutional rights are not being protected.

However, in other instances, adversarial hearings have not been mandated; e.g., in the *Parham v. J.R.* case (442 U.S. 584, 1979), the Supreme Court upheld a Georgia law which permitted the parents of a mentally ill child to commit their child on their petition along with the recommendation of a psychiatrist, but without a formal hearing. The court indicated that the commitment was purely medical and suggested that a hearing "could exacerbate whatever tensions already exist between child and parent."

c. The role of the court

The judge must weigh the overall circumstances in regard to determining the rights of an incompetent litigant and those of family members. Family stability must be considered in reviewing the constitutional rights of the handicapped person. For example, a family might not be able to control a very aggressive child or may not be able to provide for the basic physical needs, such as dressing, toileting, and transporting their mentally retarded adolescent or young adult family member. The court would need to balance the constitutional interests of the child and the reasonable interests of the family who cannot properly care for the child at home.

E. Sterilization/antilibidinal agents

Legal issues in regard to the use of antilibidinal agents (Clarke, 1989) may come to the attention of the court in relation to legal rights and when sexual deviancy is at issue. The use of sterilization in mental retardation has also been an area of continuing concern. The Mental Health Law Project has recommended standards. These require representation by a disinterested guardian *ad litem*, independent evaluation of the individual, and the finding that the individual is not capable of and not able to develop the capacity to make an informed judgment. The individual also must be physically capable of procreation and likely to engage in sexual activity but permanently incapable of taking care of a child. Furthermore, there must be no alternatives to sterilization. The major concerns are to protect the individual's rights and to follow due process.

F. Responsibility in capital crimes

The Supreme Court has indicated that mental retardation must be considered as a mitigating circumstance in capital crimes. However, the Court has not ruled out the possibility that a mentally retarded person could be given the death penalty. The issue is most likely to arise with a mildly retarded person. The deliberations in the *Penry v. Lynaugh* case (109 S. Ct. 1934, 1989) discussed in the *Medical and Physical Disability Law Reporter* as considered by each of the justices of the Supreme Court (1989) do suggest that the death penalty would not be applied to a severely mentally retarded person. A number of states do have statutes that prohibit the death penalty for all mentally retarded persons. Because it is a mitigating circumstance, efforts may be made by an attorney to demonstrate that a person accused of a crime whose IQ is in the borderline range functions in the mentally retarded range. An evaluation of the specific profile on psychological tests and formal assessment of adaptive functioning may be critical in the assessment.

The AAMR position is that no mentally retarded person should be sentenced to death or executed. They suggest that such executions serve no purpose penologically, are disproportionate to the retarded person's culpability, do not consider degree of moral blameworthiness in the retarded, and are a cruel and unusual punishment for a handicapped person.

IV. CLINICAL ISSUES

A. Forensic assessment

It is a basic right of a mentally retarded person to be responsible for himself and to be held accountable for his own behavior (Szymanski and Crocker, 1989). Suggesting incompetency based on intelligence alone, without considering adaptive ability, diminishes the mentally retarded person as an individual. In criminal cases, the opportunity to stand trial offers the chance for probation, while being found incompetent may lead to an indeterminate sentence. When brought in for a forensic assessment, a mentally retarded person may be overwhelmed, particularly if there are legal proceedings that he does not understand. Time and patience will be needed to establish a sense of trust and rapport and to gain his assent to continue with the assessment. A mentally retarded person may not understand the officer's recitation when his rights are read to him, may not understand the nature of the offense that he is accused of, may not appreciate the consequences of the accusation, or know how to defend himself. A more gradual and considered approach that acknowledges his disability may render the individual competent. If one makes the necessary initial efforts at gaining the mentally retarded person's confidence, the assessment can be direct and detailed. The focus is on his self-care skills, his comprehension of the meaning of others' social behavior, and his facility in interpersonal communication. The psychiatric examination is comprehensive and deals with all these issues as well as with the specific legal questions of competency to stand trial and the kind of service programs needed by the individual. This added detailed information about therapeutic programming can then be used by the court in making the final disposition.

Mentally retarded persons are ordinarily taken by their caretakers for psychiatric assessment rather than being self-referred. Since the mentally retarded person often has difficulty in verbal expression, either in articulation or in expressive language; may have problems in memory; and is generally dependent on the caretaker, the caretaker's history is of paramount importance. A variety of special approaches may be needed in interviewing the retarded person. These include devices to augment communication (communication boards, computers, signing) and interviewing methods used for establishing therapeutic contact with younger normally intelligent children (drawings, stories, structured settings). In assessing the retarded person, one must consider, for example, his capacity to understand basic explanations for medical procedures, his degree of credibility and the ability to exercise independent decision making, the ability to advocate for his own rights, his ability to postpone immediate gratification for subsequent benefits, and his knowledge of managing his financial affairs. A past history of ability to carry out these activities is central and should be confirmed in the examination.

It is necessary to use several sources in addition to the family and retarded person himself for the history (e.g., schools, community programs, sheltered workshop staff, job coaches). When eliciting historical information, one must consider not only the specific behaviors of concern but also the circumstances under which the behavior is said to have taken place and how it was responded to by others. The caretaker's relationship with the retarded person must also be taken into account. The extent of parental involvement with the handicap and its meaning to them must be considered in the assessment. Their ability to see the referred person's strengths as well as his or her weaknesses should be investigated.

B. Parental competency

Assessment for parental competency requires a careful review of the individual's personal history and an evaluation of their child or children (Whitman and Accardo, 1989). If homemakers have been in the home, information needs to be gathered from the social agency in regard to how the homemaker was received. It is important to verify whether or not a homemaker who was placed to help with the children and the retarded adult is aware of the issues of mental retardation and to verify the degree of sensitivity shown towards the parents' ability and efforts. The parents may be familiar with how to provide physical care; however, they may have difficulty in regard to judgment when there are unexpected illnesses or when other new situations arise. The retarded parents' ability to appreciate the unique needs of a child and understand that the child's misbehavior may be a developmental issue en route to independence rather than a challenge to their authority will need to be considered. Some mentally retarded parents will be able to provide adequate physical care and nurturance for an infant but may have more difficulty with an older child, particularly an adolescent. The family system evaluation needs to consider what alternatives there are within the family for other family members to assist. This assessment must evaluate whether or not it is in the child's best interest to be placed outside the home at an early age rather than subsequently when the parents care-giving abilities are more strained.

C. Criminal liability

The majority of individuals with mental retardation are not prone to criminal or violent behavior. Those that are frequently have multiple risk factors, as pointed out by Lewis et al. (1988). They reported on 14 juveniles condemned to death in four states and found that one had an IQ score in the 60s and 5 were in the 70s. All had a history of head trauma in childhood with 9/14 requiring hospitalization. Twelve of the group had a history of abuse in childhood. The majority had severe deficiencies in abstract reasoning.

In the past it has been suggested that chromosomal abnormality may be associated with antisocial behavior (Telfer et al., 1968); however, this has not proven to be the case. Because of these misconceptions, when individuals with mental retardation become involved with the criminal justice system, through misunderstanding, they are at risk of being treated unfairly (Biklen, 1977; McAfee and Gural, 1988). The current evidence is that the mentally retarded may have a higher likelihood of being arrested for criminal behavior, especially for minor delinquent behavior. Crimes involving impulsive acts may be increased among mentally retarded individuals. One study found no increase in fantasy aggression among mentally retarded offenders but suggested possible difficulties in inhibiting impulses, a finding that needs replication. Firesetting has also been associated with mental retardation (Foust, 1979; Yesavage et al., 1983; Kearns and O'Connor, 1988). Rather than a specific cause of criminal behavior, mental retardation and its associated features are risk factors for legal difficulty. It is not mental retardation, per se, but the higher rate of associated behavioral and emotional problems in the mentally retarded that is of particular concern. The likelihood of emotional and behavioral problems is enhanced by frequent psychosocial adversity and central nervous system dysfunction. This increased prevalence of mental disorder further increases their vulnerability to acting antisocially. The issue of stigma must also be considered since "being different' and "being retarded" are factors that influence attitudes in the community. Often the mentally retarded are the first suspected of delinquency in their neighborhoods because of these attitudes in the community. In criminal proceedings mental retardation may be a mitigating circumstance that may lead to a reduction of the offender's personal culpability and moral blameworthiness for the act committed.

D. Confessions

Clinically, the mentally retarded person may be considered to be a normalized individual with limited learning capacity. Characteristics of mental retardation may impede voluntary and intelligent constitutional waiver of rights by a mentally retarded person. Competency must also be considered in regard to the reliability of a confession to a crime made by a mentally retarded person (Praiss, 1989). A mentally retarded defendant who has pleaded guilty may be referred to a psychiatrist to determine whether he was competent to do so. In some instances, mentally retarded persons have insisted that they were guilty and should be in prison. Here the individual may be responding to the attention accorded him at the time of the examination with the hope that this recognition might elevate his standing in the community as he may feel his self-esteem as an individual is enhanced by the proceedings.

Initially there may be confusion in the setting where the mentally retarded person is interviewed, such as a police station or courthouse. A retarded person may be compliant, seek approval, and have a desire to be accepted as well as demonstrate easy suggestibility. In this way, compliant mentally retarded persons are not a major problem for the police, but the police in the process of interrogation may be a major problem for them. Although there is no specific correlation between mental retardation and criminal behavior, a large number of the mentally retarded have been incarcerated. Despite the 2 to 3% of the general population who are retarded, up to 10 to 25% of the prison population has tested in the mentally retarded range. In some instances, mentally retarded people may be easily apprehended and less often paroled. When they are apprehended, they may assume blame to "please their accuser." Retardates may also be implicated and used by others who have encouraged them.

However, mental retardation does not necessarily exclude the ability to understand constitutional rights to remain silent or to obtain legal counsel. To reach the appropriate level of comprehension, rights must be slowly and carefully explained in terms that could be understood at that developmental level. It must be taken into account that adaptive impairments can cause retarded persons to become confused and more dependent in stressful circumstances. This may further inhibit their ability to understand new concepts and to make independent decisions. Consequently, a police officer's recitation of the standard Miranda warning may not be understood, and the person may not appreciate or have a requisite understanding of his rights and the consequences of waiving them; nor will the person necessarily be able to make a voluntary decision to waive those rights. A further complication is that even if police officers are trained to identify the mentally retarded and provide an appropriate setting and explanation of their constitutional rights and the consequences of abandoning them, the creation of a favorable environment of warmth and friendliness may, in itself, result in the retarded suspect's making a voluntary confession or being induced to make an involuntary confession after waiving his rights.

E. Psychiatric diagnosis

1. VULNERABILITY TO MENTAL DISORDER

A mentally retarded and mentally ill defendant raises concerns in regard to the relationship between the legal and mental health systems (Stark et al., 1988). The prevalence of psychiatric disorders in the mentally retarded population is three to five times that found in the general population (Reid, 1982). The more severely retarded the child, the greater the likelihood of disturbed behavior and interpersonal relationships (Szymanski and Tanguay, 1980). Recently, the term "dual diagnosis" has been used in describing psychiatric disorders in the mentally retarded. The mildly retarded individual is prone to the same range of psychiatric disorders as seen in the general population, but his vulnerability is increased as a result of his difficulty in social adaptation. The more severely and profoundly retarded children are more likely to have brain disorders which are often associated with genetic syndromes and metabolic diseases. Seizure disorders are the most common neurological problem seen in the mentally retarded population. However, birth trauma is also of considerable importance. Brain dysfunction is a vulnerability factor that increases the likelihood of behavioral and interpersonal difficulties; however, all behavior problems cannot be ascribed to brain dysfunction.

The mentally retarded are just as likely as others in the population to be diagnosed with major mental illnesses, such as depression and schizophrenia (Reid, 1982). Pervasive developmental disorders, which include autism and other forms of pervasive developmental disturbances in language and social behavior, are particularly important to recognize. Services for the latter group must include intensive training in social skills, since this is the major deficit.

2. THE PROBLEM OF PSYCHOSIS

Of major concern is the diagnosis of psychosis in the mentally retarded. The use of the diagnosis of organic psychosis for any disorganized behavior whose etiology may be unclear to the evaluator creates particular concerns. For example, talking to oneself, self-injury, self-stimulation, and unexplained aggression have been attributed to psychosis. Furthermore, the stereotypes and behavior mannerisms that are commonly seen in mental retardation, particularly in the autistic group, has been misinterpreted as symptoms of psychosis in the past. Historically, a special term, propfschizophrenie, was introduced to describe these manifestations. More recent investigations have demonstrated that standard diagnostic criteria can be used in the differential diagnosis of psychosis in mentally retarded persons. Although it may be difficult to differentiate particular subtypes of psychotic presentations, such as schizophrenia, in the nonverbally retarded, the moderately and mildly retarded who are verbal can describe symptoms such as delusions and hallucinations. For the nonverbal group disorganized behavior and substantial difficulties in interpersonal relatedness may require the use of undifferentiated or atypical diagnostic categories. The prevalence of psychotic conditions requires further research. A Swedish study demonstrated schizophrenia and paranoid disorders in four out of 51 mentally retarded persons.

One must consider the diagnoses of brief psychotic episodes and schizophreniform disorder in the mentally retarded. Individuals with brain dysfunction are more likely, with severe stress, to show these forms of psychotic manifestation, conditions which might resolve with appropriate supportive interventions. Stress leading to acute panic may result in substantial disorganization, which may result in the misdiagnosis of schizophrenia. These potentially transient psychotic episodes and the manifestations of post-traumatic stress in the mentally retarded need to be appreciated to avoid unnecessary labeling of a major mental disorder when the episode is an acute reactive one. Mentally retarded persons may not necessarily require any longer time to recover from an acute psychotic episode than a nonretarded person.

The diagnosis of schizophrenia may lead to referral to a mental hospital when the individual may actually have one of the other conditions mentioned. This may lead to longer periods of incarceration. When mentally retarded defendants are identified, they have the same right to treatment for their psychosis as do others who are not mentally retarded. To be found legally competent, treatment for the mental illness is necessary as well as training in the legal system routines and basic courtroom procedures. With treatment for the mental illness and with preparation for testimony, the mentally retarded person may be found to be competent. However, the training period should not begin until the acute psychotic symptoms are resolved. Therefore, mentally retarded, mentally ill defendants may require longer periods of time than nonretarded persons to be found incompetent to stand trial. The condition of mental retardation may require additional due process considerations in the court room, but it should not be automatically assumed that a mentally retarded person can be kept indefinitely incompetent to stand trial. The majority of retarded defendants, most of whom are mildly retarded, can achieve a basic understanding of courtroom procedures so as to present themselves favorably and assist their counsel.

3. MOOD DISORDERS

Mood disorders, particularly depressive disorders, are often not recognized in mentally retarded persons. In the past, it has sometimes been assumed that mentally retarded persons do not become depressed because they lacked the cognitive capacity to show self-blame. Furthermore, it was assumed that the mentally retarded did not develop low self-esteem because they were unaware of environmental expectations. In fact, the mildly and moderately retarded often have low self-esteem and can be diagnosed using modifications of the standard diagnostic criteria for depressive disorder or bipolar disorder. Modifications in the assessment procedures must be made, since difficulties in expressive language and difficulty in finding words to describe feelings may be associated with mental retardation. Diagnostic criteria may be difficult to apply since some require verbal reflection and others assume normal functioning prior to the depression. However, mood disorders may be demonstrated by sad expression, loss of interest in usual activities, and the characteristic changes in appetite and sleep. Unfortunately, individuals who are mentally retarded and depressed may go unnoticed if their behavior is not disruptive in the home or school setting. Individuals with Down syndrome may be more likely to develop depressive disorders (Harris, 1988).

The recognition of low self-esteem in the higher functioning retarded and the degree of demoralization that these individuals experience is one consideration. The recognition of mood disorders is another and is particularly important to recognize in regard to antisocial behavior. Irritability and agitation are early signs of a mood disorder that may go unrecognized or be mislabeled as bad behavior. The vulnerability to mood disorder and the fact of low self-esteem in many retarded individuals may be factors in their confessing to crimes that they did not commit. If they are stressed when incarcerated, subsequent stress in prison may provoke a retarded person to act in a self-destructive manner. Suicide is the most important complication of depression in the retarded.

Manic episodes may also occur in retarded individuals and be associated with antisocial behavior and sometimes with sexual dysfunction. Although the classic symptoms of flight of ideas, grandiosity, spending sprees, and delusions may not be demonstrated because of a lack of verbal skills, behavioral symptoms such as agitation, overactivity, self-injury, aggression, weight loss, sleep disturbance, and mood liability may be recognized.

4. ATTENTION DEFICIT DISORDER

Attention deficit disorder is another condition that occurs in the mentally retarded population and may go unrecognized if it is assumed that retarded people are necessarily impulsive and overactive. Symptoms of impulsivity, distractibility, and overactivity need to be assessed in view of the person's developmental level. The impulsivity and distractibility noted in this diagnostic condition are of particular importance, since an impulsive act may be an antisocial one. Attention deficit hyperactivity disorder or the diagnosis that is more commonly used in the retarded, undifferentiated attention deficit disorder, is an additional vulnerability factor. It may interact with adverse psychosocial situations to contribute to aggressive and antisocial behavior.

5. PERVASIVE DEVELOPMENTAL DISORDER

Pervasive developmental disorder represents a range of clinical conditions characterized by developmental disturbances, with particular deficits in language communication and social awareness. Both autistic disorder and a general category of pervasive developmental disorder not otherwise specified are classified. The majority of individuals with the diagnosis of an autistic disorder, 75% to 80%, fall within the mentally retarded range on cognitive testing. It is particularly important to recognize an autistic disorder in the mildly retarded population, since the deficits in language communication, and particularly in social interaction, may contribute to legal difficulties.

6. ORGANIC MENTAL DISORDER

The general diagnostic category, "organic mental disorder," is often used for the mentally retarded person. Before using this diagnostic category, more specific conditions must be considered. The presence of brain dysfunction must be demonstrated by history, through physical examination, and by psychological tests and laboratory examination. In some instances, organic mood disorder, or organic personality disorder, may be appropriately used especially following head injury. Behavior problems occur commonly following head injury where social disinhibition is a common sequela. This socially disinhibited behavior may lead to legal complications, especially aggression towards others and inappropriate sexual behavior.

F. Issues in treatment

Following multiaxial diagnosis, treatment is specified to the disorder or disorders which are identified, and a disposition may be recommended (Roesch and Golding, 1979; Quinsey and Maguire, 1983). Issues that commonly are addressed in an interdisciplinary assessment include appropriate use of psychopharmacological agents (Fielding et al., 1980) and concerns that relate to the use of adversive conditioning procedures (NIH Consensus Conference, 1990).

G. Sexuality

A minority of mentally retarded individuals may show socially unacceptable sexual behavior that brings them into conflict with the legal system. Early studies of criminology reported an increase in sexual offenses in the mentally retarded. These studies, however, are questionable on methodological grounds. This may be the result of ignorance or relate to a specific disorder in the individual. From a legal point of view, the major issues have to do with the rights of the individual in regard to sterilization (*In re Grady*: 170 NJ Super 98, 405 A. 2d 851, 1979) and the use of antilibidinal drugs (Clarke, 1989). The issue of sterilization most often comes up with the female mentally retarded person, and the use of antilibidinal agents for the male. More recently, the prevalence of mental retardation among male offenders is little different from the prevalence in the general population.

Pharmacological agents, particularly provera, have been used to reduce libido in mentally retarded individuals; for example, when excessive masturbation has prevented participation in programing and in cases of sexually deviant behavior.

Authors working in this area have suggested that a small reduction in sexual drive may be sufficient to enable a patient to avoid acting on an impulse that would lead to unacceptable behavior. Treatment with antilibidinal drugs, in addition to psychotherapy, is more effective than treatment with the antilibidinal agent alone. The drug treatment will reduce the intensity of the drive, but will not alter the direction of the drive.

H. Rights of the mentally retarded

Legislation providing for the rights of the mentally retarded to self determination has substantially increased. The Education for All Handicapped Act (PL-94-142), the Americans with Disability Act, reimbursement provisions under Title XIX, and amendments to the Vocational Rehabilitation Act have addressed restrictive treatment based on the handicap and focused on elimination of discrimination and provision of protections similar to those for other citizens.

V. PITFALLS

A. Inadequate assessment of mental age

The determination of the features of mental retardation requires individual testing and interpretation of results on tests, such as the WISC-R. Assessment of adaptive functioning may not be routinely carried out. Pitfalls include reliance on the group administration of tests rather than one-to-one testing and general descriptions of adaptive functioning when more formal measures, such as the AAMR Adaptive Scale or Vineland Social Maturity Scale are indicated.

B. Failure to understand the law or to provide counsel at early stage

1. THE MENTALLY RETARDED PERSON

Understanding of the law by the retarded person is a major issue. It is of particular importance in regard to understanding the Miranda warnings at the time of arrest. One approach to this pitfall is to provide for the presence of a familiar person and legal counsel available at an early stage to ensure that the retarded person is provided a requisite understanding of his constitutional right to remain silent and to retain counsel before these rights can be waived. There is a need for effective safeguards for these constitutional rights so that a mentally retarded citizen will not be vulnerable to misunderstandings about the justice system.

2. THE PROFESSIONAL

Failure by the professional to understand the nature of mental retardation, to understand issues related to competency, and to understand legal rights legislation takes on special importance in regard to the presentation of Miranda warnings and confessions. A common misunderstanding is the confusion of legal and psychiatric issues in case assessment.

C. Attitudes toward mental retardation

Mentally retarded persons may be stigmatized because of their appearance, social habits, and history of behavior with others in the community. Efforts are continually needed to clarify that, with normalization, behavioral difficulty can be reduced.

VI. CASE EXAMPLE EPILOGUES

A. Case Example 1

John, the young man with Down syndrome, is cooperative during the interview and through his drawings shows the sleeping arrangements in his home. There is no evidence of sexual interest toward the younger boy and no evidence that the boy with Down syndrome understands what happened as a sexual encounter. On the other hand, the younger boy showed sexual curiosity toward the older retarded boy compatible with his level of psychosocial maturation. The parents were counseled in regard to sexual development, and their concerns about mental retardation were addressed in the context of their marital difficulties. No charges were made against the mentally retarded boy. His need for attention and the younger boy's difficulty in adapting were explored in family sessions, and the two boys were given separate beds.

B. Case Example 2

William's assessment demonstrates that when this young man had agreed to charges of fire setting, he did not understand the implications of his confession. In order to please the authorities, he had confessed as an attention-seeking maneuver. Although it was true that this young man became excited by fires when he witnessed them, there was no evidence that he set them. He said that he would not set any fires. Since he had been found guilty, the charges could not be reversed, but a community program was worked out for him following an inpatient assessment. This included a behavioral program which addressed fire safety. His anxiety about witnessing the fire at home was dealt with as a symptom of a post-traumatic stress disorder, with reenactment of the event and mastery of the situation using desensitization techniques. The community program was developed with the eventual goal of supervised group home placement. A job coach was enlisted to oversee his community work effort.

C. Case Example 3

When Matthew was interviewed, he was noted to be overactive and easily distracted. He initially had difficulty cooperating with the examination. After considerable reinforcement, he was able to describe his fears about the group home staff. He insisted that he saw the group home director on the street watching him. A diagnosis of atypical paranoid psychosis was made although the question of post-traumatic stress disorder continued to be considered. With reinstitution of neuroleptic medication and weekly individual psychotherapy, his symptoms gradually resolved. It remains unclear whether he was physically abused or whether he developed a paranoid decompensation when his medication was discontinued which was associated with misinterpretation of the behavior of the staff toward him. The staff insisted that the bruises resulted from their attempts to restrain him. The family did not press charges. Three years later, he moved into another group home which could provide appropriate supervision and agreed to make no changes in his pharmacotherapy. He is doing well in the group home setting with ongoing psychiatric supervision.

D. Case Example 4

A meeting was held which included both of Raymond's parents, pertinent treating staff members from the inpatient unit, and the unit social worker. The psychiatrist explained the rationale for antilibidinal treatment and reviewed the medical literature in regard to its effects on sexual arousal and its potential side effects. The parents and each member of the treatment team signed a statement that outlined the risks, the benefits, and the risk-benefit ratio in choosing to use this medication. Antilibidinal treatment with provera was then initiated prior to hospital discharge after obtaining the informed consent from both parents who were deemed to be acting in his "best interest" since his masturbation prevented him from participation in a habilitation program. The family was seen in supportive psychotherapy, and assistance was given in identifying community programs. The parents and the patient's twin siblings were trained in behavioral overcorrection procedures to be used when he became aggressive at home. A bedtime behavioral program was instituted along with the periodic utilization of sleep medication. The use of provera was associated with a reduction in sexual drive and elimination of his attempts to fall to the floor to masturbate during the day. His new program was successfully instituted at his school following hospital discharge.

E. Case Example 5

Jennifer's family's concerns about the potential for pregnancy were addressed for both daughters. The mildly mentally retarded sister and her child were seen for an evaluation. A program in child care was established which involved the mother and her older daughter. Birth control procedures were reviewed and an oral contraceptive was chosen for the older sister, and she was enrolled in a social skills training program. The family was counseled in regard to the sexual interests of the younger daughter. It became clear that, like many severely retarded girls, she did not demonstrate sexual interest in others. However, she sought affectionate contact appropriate to her mental age without overt sexual interest. The family asked for a hysterectomy for the management of the younger daughter's menstrual hygiene. However, an outpatient behavioral treatment program was established utilizing appropriate prompts which allowed her to learn the necessary skills to participate in her own menstrual hygiene. No sterilization procedure was carried out.

F. Case Example 6

David, who was mentally retarded related to brain damage at birth and who currently has an IQ of 60 (mental age 9–10 years) on standard testing, was found competent to stand trial, and his confession was considered to be voluntary. On the Vineland Social Maturity Scale and the AAMR Adaptive Behavior Scale, he was found to be adapting in the same mental age range. At the trial, the psychiatric testimony determined that he was able to appreciate the wrongfulness of his behavior and able to distinguish right from wrong. No specific mental illness was diagnosed, and he was considered to be sane at the time of the crime. He was found guilty of murder, but with the mitigating circumstance of his mental retardation, the death penalty was not considered and he was given a life sentence with the possibility of parole.

VII. ACTION GUIDE

A. Mental retardation—essentials

1. Be familiar with the definitions of mental retardation (AAMR, DSM-III-R, and ICD-10).
2. Remember that assessment of adaptive function is a crucial aspect for evaluation.
3. Consider variability in cognitive profile on IQ tests, language functioning, and the presence of neurological conditions.
4. Keep in mind that mental retardation includes a heterogeneous group of individuals who range from mildly to profoundly retarded and includes specific syndromes as well as retardation secondary to traumatic head injury occurring during the developmental period.
5. Be cognizant of developmental level as well as IQ test data.
6. Record data using a multiaxial classification.

B. Competency

1. Consider the level of mental retardation in competency assessment.
2. Be aware of the definitions of competency and culpability as they relate to criminal responsibility.
3. Consider the stresses that may be involved when a mentally retarded person is asked to testify.
4. Carefully consider the circumstances in the elicitation of confessions.
5. Utilize all means to facilitate communication (e.g., communication boards, speech synthesizer, drawings) at the appropriate mental age level.
6. Be aware of the legal rights for the incompetent mentally retarded.
7. Consider the following in regard to competency:
   a. Lack of life experience,
   b. Inadequate education,
   c. Problems with over- or undercompliance,
   d. Fear of authority,
   e. Associated deficits.

C. Mentally ill/mentally retarded

1. Consider all DSM-III-R diagnoses that may be pertinent on Axis I.
2. Appreciate how diagnostic criteria may require modification for the mentally retarded.

3. Utilize all 5 DSM-III-R axes.
4. Remember to consider features of mental retardation when evaluating for suspected psychosis. Exercise caution in the diagnosis of schizophrenia.

D. Forensic assessment

1. Find and make careful use of multiple informants for data collection.
2. Be aware of issues of stigma in mental retardation.
3. Consider cognitive and adaptive limitations of the mentally retarded.
4. Remember that there may be considerable variability in profile.
5. Use specific measure of adaptive functioning such as AAMD scale and the Vineland.

VIII. SUGGESTED READINGS

A. GENERAL REFERENCES

Clark, A. M., Clarke, D. B., and Berg, J. M. (1985), Mental Deficiency: The Changing Outlook, 4th ed., New York: Free Press.

Kindred, M. (1976), The Mentally Retarded Citizen and the Law. New York: Free Press.

Stark, J. A., Menolascino, F. J., Albarelli, M. H., Gray, V. C. (eds.) (1988), Mental Retardation and Mental Health: Classification, Diagnosis, Treatment, Services. New York: Springer Verlag.

Szymanski, L. and Crocker A. (1989), Mental Retardation. In: Kaplan, H. I. and Sadock, B. J. (eds.) Comprehensive Textbook of Psychiatry, 4th ed. Baltimore: Williams & Wilkins.

B. DEFINITION AND CLASSIFICATION OF MENTAL RETARDATION

American Psychiatric Association. Diagnostic and Statistical Manual III (Revised) (1987), Washington, D.C.: American Psychiatric Association Press.

Grossman, H. J. (1983), Manual on Terminology and Classification in Mental Retardation, revised ed. Washington, D.C. American Association on Mental Deficiency.

Jones, J. M., Barnett, R. W., McCormack, J. K. (1988), Verbal/performance splits in inmates assessed with the multidimensional aptitude battery. J Clin Psychol 44:995–1000.

Lambert, N., Windmiller, R. N., Cole, E. et al. (1975), AAMD Adaptive Behavior Scale. Washington, D.C.: American Association on Mental Deficiency.

Sparrow, S. S., Balla, D. A., and Cicchetti, D. V. (1984), American Guidance Service. Circle Pines, MN.

Wolfensberger, W. (1972), The Principle of Normalization in Human Service. Toronto: National Institute on Mental Retardation.

C. CONSIDERATIONS IN FORENSIC ASSESSMENT

Foust, J. D. (1979), The legal significance of clinical formulations of firesetting behavior. Int J Law Psychiatry 2:371–387.

McAfee, J. K. and Gural, M. (1988), Individuals with mental retardation and the criminal justice system: the view from states' attorneys general. Ment Retard 26:5–12.

Menninger, K. (1986), Mental retardation and criminal responsibility: some thoughts on the idiocy defense. Int J Law Psychiatry 8:343–357.

Yesavage, J. A., Benezech, M., Ceccaldi, P., Bourgeois, M., and Addad, M. (1983), Arson in mentally ill and criminal populations. J Clin Psychiatry 44:128–130.

D. COMPETENCY/INCOMPETENCY

Golding, S. L., Roesch, R., and Schreiber, J. (1984), Assessment and conceptualization of competence to stand trial: preliminary data on the interdisciplinary fitness interview. Law and Human Behavior 8:321–334.

Heller, M. S., Traylor, W. H., Ehrlich, S. M., and Lester, D. (1981), Intelligence, psychosis, and competency to stand trial. Bull Am Acad Psychiatry Law 9:267–274.

Smith, S. M. and Kunjukrishnan, R. (1986), Medicolegal aspects of mental retardation. Psychiatry Clin North Am 9:699–712.

Sundram, C. J. (1988), Informed consent for major medical treatment of mentally disabled people. A new approach. N Eng J Med 318:1368–1373.

E. PARENTING

Accardo, P. J. and Whitman, B. Y. (1990), Children of mentally retarded parents. Am J Dis Child 144:69–70.

Feldman, M. A. (1986), Research on parenting by mentally retarded persons. Psychiatr Clin North Am 9:777–796.

Schilling, R. F., Schinke, S. P., Blythe, B. J., and Brath, R. P. (1982), Child maltreatment and mentally retarded parents: is there a relationship? Ment Retard 20:201–209.

Seagull, E. A. W. and Scheurer, S. L. (1986), Neglected and abused children of mentally retarded parents. Child Abuse Negl, 10:493–500.

Whitman, B. Y. and Accardo, P. J. (1989), When a parent is mentally retarded. Baltimore: Paul Brooks.

F. CRIMINAL LIABILITY/DEATH PENALTY

Lewis, D. O., Lovely, R., Yeager, C., Ferguson, G., Friedman, M., Sloane, G., Friedman, H., and Pincus, J. H. (1988), Intrinsic and environmental characteristics of juvenile murderers. J Am Acad Child Adolesc Psychiatry 27:582–587.

Lewis, D. O., Pincus, J. H., Bard, B., Richardson, E., Prichep, L. S., Feldman, M., and Yeager, C. (1988), Neuropsychiatric, psychoeducational, and family characteristics of 14 juveniles condemned to death in the United States. Am J Psychiatry 145:584–589.

Menninger, K. A. (1986), Mental retardation and criminal responsibility: some thoughts on the idiocy defense. Int J Law Psychiatry 8:343–357.

MPDLR. (1989), U.S. Supreme Court remands execution of man with mental retardation. Medical and Physical Disability Law Reporter. 13:334–338.

G. CONFESSIONS

Praiss, D. M. (1989), Constitutional protection of confessions made by mentally retarded defendants. Am J Law Med 14:431–465.

H. PSYCHIATRIC DIAGNOSIS IN MENTAL RETARDATION

Harris, J. (1988), Psychological adaptation and psychiatric disorders in adolescents and young adults with Down syndrome. In: S. Pueschel (ed.) Down Syndrome: Transition from Adolescence to Adulthood. Baltimore: Paul Brooks.

Kearns, A. and O'Connor, A. (1988), The mentally handicapped criminal offender. A 10-year study of two hospitals. Br J Psychiatry 152:848–851.

Luckasson, R. (1988), The dually diagnosed in criminal justice. In: Stark, J. A., Menolascino, F. J., Albarelli, M. H., and Gray, V. C. (eds.) Mental Retardation and Mental Health: Classification, Diagnosis, Treatment, Services. New York: Springer Verlag.

Reid, A. (1982), The Psychiatry of Mental Handicap. Boston: Blackwell Scientific Publications.

Szymanski, L. and Tanguay, P. (1980), Emotional Disorders of Mentally Retarded Persons: Assessment Treatment and Consultation. Baltimore: University Park Press.

I. SEXUALITY IN THE MENTALLY RETARDED

Abramn, P. R., Parker, T., and Weisberg, S. R. (1988), Sexual expression of mentally retarded people: educational and legal implications. Am J Ment Retard 93:328–334.

Appelbaum, P. S. (1982), The issue of sterilization and the mentally retarded. Hosp Community Psychiatry 33:523–524.

Clarke, D. J. (1989), Antilibidinal drugs and mental retardation: a review. Med Sci Law 29:136–146.

Dickens, B. M. (1982), Retardation and sterilization. Int J Law Psychiatry 5:295–318.

J. THE RIGHTS OF THE RETARDED

Kapp, M. B. (1981), Protecting the personal funds of the mentally retarded: new federal regulations. Hosp Community Psychiatry 32:567–71.

Mesibov, G. B., Conover, B. S., and Saur, W. G. (1980), Limited guardianship laws and developmentally disabled adults: needs and obstacles. Ment Retard Oct. 18(5): 221–226.

K. PSYCHIATRIC TREATMENT

Fielding, L. T., Murphy, R. J., Reagan, M. W., and Peterson, T. L. (1980), An assessment program to reduce drug use with the mentally retarded. Hosp. Community Psychiatry 31:771–773.

NIH. Consensus Conference on Treatment of Destructive Behaviors in Persons with Developmental Disabilities. (1990), Washington, D.C.: U.S. Government Printing Office.

Quinsey, V. L. and Maguire, A. (1983), Offenders remanded for a psychiatric examination: perceived treatability and disposition. Int J Law Psychiatry 6:193–205.

18

Psychiatric Commitment of Children and Adolescents

W. V. BURLINGAME, PH.D., AND MARCELINO AMAYA, M.D.

I. CASE EXAMPLES

A. Case Example 1

Margie, a 14-year-old junior high school girl, appears in the emergency room of a city hospital accompanied by emergency medical technicians who had been summoned to her junior high school by the guidance counselor. The girl's friends earlier informed the counselor that she had ingested a large number of aspirin tablets after two over-the-counter pregnancy tests had confirmed that she was likely pregnant. In the emergency room, the consulting psychiatrist concludes that Margie, in anticipation of her parent's reactions to the pregnancy, had impulsively attempted suicide. However, she will not disclose her parents' whereabouts, nor will she agree to meet with them, neither will she contract not to harm herself in the immediate future. Faced with a clinical impasse and continuing risk to the adolescent, the psychiatrist completes a petition for involuntary hospitalization.

B. Case Example 2

Paul is a 15-year-old boy who is irregular in keeping his outpatient psychotherapy and family therapy appointments at a community mental health center. Six months ago he was brought to the center by his stepmother due to a variety of conduct and related disturbances, consisting of running away, shoplifting, truancy, alcohol and marijuana use, defiance of parental rules and expectations, grade failure, and a generalized oppositionalism to adult authority. His natural parents, each of whom is now remarried, had experienced a highly conflicted marriage, and each has also had significant difficulties with substance abuse. The clinician suspects considerable unmet dependency needs occurring over some years, which results in underlying depression and rage, both of which are currently fueling the boy's acting out. On this occasion, the father and stepmother keep Paul's appointment because he states he will never come to the center again. The parents tell the clinician of intensified acting out and quite serious delinquencies, including breaking and entering and "joy riding" in a stolen car occurring over the past week. They feel that he is quite beyond their control, as well as that of his mother and stepfather. They relate that the juvenile authorities are intending to charge Paul for the delinquencies but will defer prosecution if Paul and his parents will secure inpatient evaluation and treatment. Immediately prior to the parents' departure to keep this appointment, Paul reluctantly agreed to an admission but has started to haggle over how long he might be hospitalized. The clinician, presented with willing parties but mindful of Paul's denial and prior resistance, contemplates residential and inpatient possibilities.

C. Case Example 3

Jenny is a 13-year-old girl who initially manifested significant separation difficulties in the first grade and had a spotty attendance record during the remainder of grammar school. After the Christmas holidays of her seventh grade year, she absolutely refused to return to school. Outpatient psychotherapy, family therapy, medication, special class placement, behavioral regimes, and two brief psychiatric hospitalizations have been to no avail. It is now the second week of September and it is clear that the parents and Jenny are again unable to keep her in the classroom for this, her second attempt at the seventh grade. The child psychiatrist who has been struggling with this case for nearly a year now seeks long-term hospitalization of Jenny. He knows that she will surely resist and oppose through all possible means and that her resistance to out-of-home treatment is a clear manifestation of her severe and disabling separation anxiety disorder.

D. Case Example 4

Tom is a 17-year-old high school boy who was involuntarily committed a week ago to a drug detoxification unit from the county jail. He had been arrested for a serious assault on another boy, the result of a fight which had erupted at a skating rink frequented by adolescents. The evaluation disclosed Tom's serious alcohol dependency abetted by stressors which included the loss of his girlfriend and the possibility that he might not graduate from high school due to his declining grades. It is now time for the hearing on his involuntary commitment. Detoxification has been completed, and it is doubtful that a finding of continuing dangerousness can be secured. Nonetheless, it is clear that continuing treatment is necessary lest he again deteriorate in the face of his ongoing dysthymia and his propensity to take refuge in alcohol. The attending psychiatrist and the judge are considering alternatives which will ensure his continuing participation in treatment but will allow him to return to his family and school.

II. LEGAL ISSUES

A. The historical context of children's rights

The above case examples demonstrate the range of treatment options necessitated in work with children and adolescents and suggest varying legal bases by which psychiatric hospitalization and treatment for children and adolescents is secured. In the absence of stringent constitutional mandates, the national picture lacks uniformity and remains enormously complex, necessitating a detailed understanding of the statutes governing hospitalization in the particular state in which the clinician practices. Despite the proliferation of psychiatric units for youth, psychiatric hospitalization of children and adolescents is a comparatively recent phenomenon, with significant numbers of admissions beginning to occur only in the 1950s and 1960s (which eventually led to the establishment of specialty treatment units for youth).

Only within the past two decades has the issue of psychiatric hospitalization and children's rights vis-à-vis their parents, guardians, caretakers, and caregivers been vigorously debated. Historically, in Greece, Rome, and medieval Europe, children essentially had no rights or legal status; they were viewed as chattel or property, typically of their fathers, and were considered, in a legal sense, largely in terms of their economic assets or liability. They came, however, to be included within that group of unfortunates (e.g., the insane and the retarded) who had no legal rights or could not act on their own behalf for whom the doctrine of *parens patriae* was enunciated. It was this benevolent and paternalistic tenet of English common law which obligated the monarch and the state to protect those individuals who could not protect themselves. For children, in the absence of responsible parents, it authorized the state to intervene in cases of dependency, neglect, abuse, abandonment, exploitation, and waywardness. For children who were hospitalized, inasmuch as their status as children conferred no constitutional rights, it was the parent or guardian who consented for psychiatric hospitalization in the same fashion as he or she might for surgery or other hospitalization.

B. *Gault* and *Parham*

By the 1960s, the stage was set for legal reform. The vagueness of the existing legal standards, when combined with the failure to fund child welfare programs adequately, had led to generations of abuse and little demonstrated efficacy. In *Gault* (1967), the Supreme Court overturned much of the procedural underpinning of juvenile justice, holding that the doctrine of *parens patriae* had been unconstitutionally applied. It ordered broad procedural and due process protections for children whose liberty interest was at stake (see Chapter 13).

Over the ensuing decade, the Court's reasoning in *Gault* was applied to instances of psychiatric hospitalization of minors. The plaintiffs cited the presence of numbers of children and adolescents in state operated institutions, including those who failed to receive appropriate care; whose need for treatment had been completed; who, in the case of wards of the state, failed to have other less restrictive placements pursued; who were unable to leave the institution due to the unavailability of other placements; who suffered societal stigma as a consequence of institutionalization; and, who may have been admitted due to the error inherent in admissions processes (with admitting officers believing parents and erring on the side of caution). All of these groups of youth were thought to have had their liberty interests compromised.

In a controversial and much criticized decision, a divided Supreme Court apparently reversed its earlier course and left largely intact Georgia and Pennsylvania statutes which authorized parents and guardians to consent for psychiatric admission with, of course, the concurrence of hospital administrators and clinicians. The Court held, ". . . the risk of error inherent in the parental decision to have a child institutionalized for mental health care is sufficiently great that some kind of inquiry should be made by a 'neutral factfinder' to determine whether the statutory requirements for admission are satisfied" (*Parham*, 1979, p. 606). In its attempt to balance the child's liberty interest, the parents' interests in having the child receive treatment, and the state's interest in the best utilization of its facilities, the Court did not mandate judicial or administrative review. Rather, the "neutral factfinder" could be the admissions officer who would conduct a careful inquiry, interview the child, and who had the authority to deny admission. Lastly, the Court required that ". . . the child's continuing need for commitment be reviewed periodically by a similarly independent procedure" (*Parham*, 1979, p. 606). And so, at the turn of the decade, parental and professional authority regarding admissions decisions received dramatic support, although a number of states had already enacted or established due process protections in the wake of less favorable decisions from lower courts.

C. Post-*Parham* trends and patterns of "voluntary commitment"

In the decade since *Parham*, the pace at which the states have effected due process protections for minors in psychiatric hospitals has clearly slowed, while admission rates have soared—as if the Supreme Court had opened the floodgates for admissions of adolescents, to private psychiatric facilities in particular. In a stinging indictment of the current scene, Weithorn (1988) cites "skyrocketing" admission rates, primarily of "troublesome" youth who she suspects are the same adolescents who have been deinstitutionalized from the juvenile justice system. Citing a variety of sources, she notes that, while public facilities have reduced admission rates, private psychiatric hospital admission rates have increased more than four-fold in the first five years following *Parham*. By 1980, the proportion of private hospital admissions had nearly doubled—to 61%, with private general hospitals probably acquiring the lion's share.

Weithorn further contends that these are not the most severely and acutely mentally ill youngsters, but are often those diagnosed as conduct disorders, a term which she finds ambiguous (probably the same as "status offender" or "juvenile delinquent"), merely permitting the "transinstitutionalization" of youth to the mental health system from juvenile justice. She posits that these youth are only mildly disordered, if not simply witnessing normal developmental processes, and that community-based outpatient treatment would be more effective were it available. Weithorn proposes that the advent of for-profit corporate hospital chains with relatively low cost psychiatric units has altered the financial incentives and that private hospital admitting staff, far from being "neutral factfinders," now have enormous conflicts of interest and stand to gain the most from the rising rates of admission. This circumstance is further abetted by insurance programs which favor inpatient over outpatient treatment or partial hospitalization.

At this juncture, it is not possible to respond to the range of conclusions and criticisms leveled by Weithorn. The absence of links in the continuum of care (e.g., outpatient, day treatment, and in-home services) certainly sets the stage for psychiatric hospitalization which might otherwise be prevented. The potential for conflicts of interests in the corporate hospital psychiatric units is obvious and begs for peer, judicial, or community review of psychiatric admissions of minors. The trends cited by Weithorn have not gone unnoticed by Congress, Medicaid overseers, professional associations, child advocates, and the popular press. Skirmishes continue at the state level, as in North Carolina, where attempts, which have been unsuccessful to this point, have been made to overturn the state's minor admissions law (which already mandates judicial review); the charge is that North Carolina's definition of mental illness in a minor is "unconstitutionally vague" and provides no standard for the court, even if guided by professionals. Aside from the courts, the issue of children in psychiatric hospitals is also securing attention in the popular media. Quite ironically, the same television channels that carry provocative advertisements for private hospital adolescent units also air national exposés of similar programs. The *Ladies' Home Journal* (Barrett and Greene, 1990) recently cited the plights of "thousands of routinely rebellious teenagers" who are committed to hospitals, "bombarded by strong medications," receive questionable treatment, and may be abusively controlled, at least until insurance benefits lapse.

Several sources (Burlingame and Amaya, 1985; Weithorn, 1988; Knitzer, 1982; Wilson, 1978) summarize state procedures for the voluntary admission of children and adolescents to psychiatric facilities. Because there is scarcely a constitutional "floor," state approaches to the issue are diverse and change constantly in the wake of local court decisions and legislative actions. As described, *Parham* gave insignificant pause to jurisdictions which were contemplating due process protections, although those which were already enacted have typically been left in place. Statutes vary, from some which empower the parent or guardian to admit a child without judicial or administrative review (Idaho) to those which mandate a full-blown potentially adversarial judicial proceeding for all admissions (North Carolina).

Statutes vary on a variety of other dimensions: those which, paradoxically, afford additional due process protections to youth in public facilities (established in the pre-*Parham* years, prior to spiraling private admissions) (California) versus those requiring such protections in private and public facilities alike (North Carolina); those which offer additional protections to wards of the state (District of

Columbia); those which require a preadmission hearing (Virginia) and those which defer the hearing for up to 10 days postadmission (North Carolina); those in which a hearing is initiated upon refusal of the child to consent to admission or when initiated by another party (several states) versus those in which a hearing is mandatory (North Carolina); those states which have experimented with an independent clinical/administrative review in lieu of an adversary court proceeding (Tennessee); those in which youth of specified ages may seek due process protections (in Illinois, minors age 12 may request judicial review) or may participate in their admission (in New Mexico, 12-year-olds may admit themselves, while those younger than 12 must cosign the admissions document with their parent and may seek judicial review if they subsequently object to the hospitalization); and those in which older adolescents may admit themselves, even over parental objection (many states).

D. Statutory criteria and standards of proof

As might be expected given the potpourri of state practice, statutory criteria for voluntary admission vary considerably. Some states provide ambiguous standards which can be attacked on the grounds of constitutional vagueness. For example, in Idaho, hospitalization by the parent or guardian must be "medically necessary," while in Arizona a child must "benefit from care and treatment of a mental disorder" (Weithorn, 1988). Obviously, given such statutory language, the courts can only be guided by professional expertise in contested cases, particularly those in which the child and parent oppose one another. Meanwhile, child advocates look with questioning eyes on the absence of more concrete statutory criteria with meaning to non-experts.

When states have seen fit to embody criteria in statute, they have tended to employ variations on the following three-pronged test, with an additional requirement for periodic review of the hospitalization: (1) there must be mental illness or mental disorder and need for treatment, although the definition of such may again be vague and circular or more rigorous through the use of behavioral criteria; (2) the treatment must occur in the least restrictive or intensive setting, although this criterion is occasionally diluted by permitting continuing hospitalization if less restrictive appropriate settings are not available; and (3) the necessary treatment must exist in the hospital to which the child is being committed, thus providing a measure of protection to patient and hospital alike in the case of overcrowded or otherwise compromised or limited facilities. At least one state has additionally indicated in its voluntary admissions statute for minors that a finding of dangerousness is *not* necessary, to alert judges and others not to employ the involuntary criterion of dangerousness with which they are typically more familiar.

The standard of proof, that is, the degree of certainty that a judge must find to concur with a parental admission or a finding of dangerousness in an involuntary proceeding, has varied and has been subject to constitutional test. Some states have required the most rigorous standard, "beyond a reasonable doubt," which is the standard for criminal cases and requires 90–95% certainty. The least stringent standard is "a preponderance of the evidence," the civil standard, which calls for 51% certainty or a finding of "more likely than not." Supreme Court action has held that, when liberty is at stake, a more rigorous but intermediate standard is appropriate, that is, "clear and convincing evidence," which requires 75% certainty.

E. Model statutes and AACAP guidelines

As the Georgia and Pennsylvania cases proceeded toward the Supreme Court, the major mental health professional associations provided *amicus* briefs. Although these differed somewhat from one another, they typically recognized the need for checks on unilateral parental and professional authority; they also called attention to the potentially damaging nature of the contested adversary proceeding, in which child could be pitted against parent (in reciting the tragic incidents leading to admission) and child against therapist (as the therapist details the evidence for mental illness or disorder). In the years following *Parham,* there have been a number of "model statutes," some emerging from the professional associations (Guidelines for the Psychiatric Hospitalization of Minors, 1982; American Psychological Association, 1984), as well as others (Wilson, 1978). In common, they call for an independent and neutral review process, typically carried-out under court auspices with legal representation for the child. The review would then ratify or overturn the decision to admit made by parents and professionals. The standards for commitment differ, but most tend to recognize the need for inpatient treatment for conditions which may not meet a dangerousness standard.

Aside from statutory reform, professional associations have also approached the matter of psychiatric hospitalization of children and adolescents from the point of view of policy and ethics. The most useful and comprehensive set of guidelines is that of the American Academy of Child and Adolescent Psychiatry (1987) which recommends psychiatric hospitalization when it is the least restrictive alternative for acute and severe conditions deriving from "psychiatric disease," in which the child or adolescent is at risk or severely dysfunctional. The Academy has also determined that it is unethical for its members to be affiliated with hospitals utilizing alarmist or misleading advertising.

III. CLINICAL ISSUES

A. Commitments and hearings

Inasmuch as state procedures vary in major ways, only general remarks can be offered regarding the issues associated with commitment processes. It is presumed that in most jurisdictions there is, at the least, a process for involuntary commitment which is utilized with minors as well as adults and that judicial proceedings exist in which the psychiatric commitment, voluntary or involuntary or both, is upheld or denied. Typically, there are notarized or sworn written statements associated with either proceeding which attest to the circumstances which the judge or magistrate then evaluates to determine whether statutory critera are met. From the outset, it is critical that committing clinicians be familiar with the criteria set-out in statute for commitment and that they verify and validate the presence of such behaviors and circumstances. This requirement inevitably results in some distortion of clinican interviewing and intervention in an emergency, since the clinician must not only be providing first aid and crisis intervention but must also be gathering data in anticipation of reviews by second parties to the commitment as well as by judges. Although the "hearsay" rules are often applied less stringently in psychiatric commitments, the clinician must convince himself and ultimately the court, in many cases, that there is indeed a suicide or assault risk or the presence of severe and acute mental disorder.

To proceed with the commitment, the clinician must be assured that the attempt is not whimsical, capricious, reckless, unduly convenient, or unnecessary, whether initiated by parents, community mental health authorities, or emergency room personnel. A careful clinician interviews not only the child and whatever family members are available but also others who may possess relevant information or were witness to the events (e.g., school and community mental health professionals). Needless to say, the authority-sensitive adolescent who is already in conflict with a variety of important adults is scarcely off to a good start in his hospitalization if he feels that he was judged unfairly by a committing clinician.

The advent of a hearing or rehearing following admission presents all parties with an additional set of potential dilemmas. In particular, there may be yet another clash between child and parents and a collision between the contesting child and the very clinician who is attempting to form an alliance with him on his behalf. Whenever possible, many clinicians would prefer to have the testimony or court affidavits provided by someone who is not caught in a dual relationship or seeming conflict of interest which operates at the expense of the therapeutic alliance. As in precommitment proceedings, the clinician must be careful to validate events; nothing plays into the defenses of a legalistic adolescent so much as inaccuracies which then become the crux of his "case" and allow him to distract himself from the core issues.

In general, it is probably preferable to prepare the child or adolescent, his family, and the respective attorneys for the proceeding by discussing in advance the anticipated testimony. Preparing the child for testimony on the issue of mental illness or mental disorder and the possible disclosure of diagnoses is critical for obvious reasons and may prevent some of the most deleterious effects of courtroom interactions. Attempting to enlist even the most aggressive public defenders on behalf of "the best interest of the child" may ultimately serve to reduce the intensity of the contested hearing. The adolescent who is prepared for the hearing by a clinician who reflects his own calmness, confidence, and integrity, despite the unpleasant encounter, is less apt to make the proceeding one more item in the adolescent's struggle with controlling adults. The decision to seek testimony from parents has many risk/benefit dilemmas in that the parent is often in the best position to document, in all its drama and tragedy, the child's condition; as noted, however, it may further stress the already damaged relationship with the child and cause significant, unfortunate additional distress for one or more parties. Whenever possible, it is often useful and convincing to the court to hear from referring clinicians and prior caregivers who can testify to unsuccessful attempts at treatment in less restrictive settings.

B. Clinical sequelae

The present authors have written at some length regarding the clinical events which surround judicial review of voluntary admissions (Burlingame and Amaya, 1985; Amaya and Burlingame, 1981). In summary, they have observed as follows:

> Even under the best of circumstances, a contested hearing may constitute a traumatic experience and may have a variety of potentially

destructive outcomes for the child, family, treatment personnel, and the milieu of the treatment unit. The following comprise a partial list of harmful results: the stress of a hearing may overtax the child's or adolescent's resources, precipitating a psychotic episode, regression, withdrawal, or aggressive acting out; severe declines in self-esteem may occur in response to testimony regarding diagnosis, personality structure, or dynamics; substantial anxiety and the utilization of excessive ego defense may occur in response to the premature revelation of personality dynamics, unconscious content, or family secrets; the already tenuous or damaged relationship between youth and parents may be further eroded in response to the open collision and conflict in court; the fragile relationship between youth and therapist may be ruptured by the court encounter in which the therapist opposes release and marshals suitable but threatening "evidence"; considerable amounts of treatment time may be lost as the child or adolescent prepares his "defense," putting emotional energies into securing release rather than addressing pathology; the authority and stature of treatment personnel and parent may be undermined, particularly for smaller children, by a confusing process in which important adults conflict with one another; treatment personnel may be intimidated, blackmailed, or compromised by the threats of youth, such that limits may not be set, rules may not be enforced in the milieu and living areas, and the patient's omnipotence may not be addressed; younger children, youth with defective reality testing, and those with primitive conscience formation may perceive themselves as on trial for all varieties of actual transgressions or other fantasied sins or misdeeds; the adolescent with a delinquent orientation and pathological omnipotence, who also denies personal responsibility and attributes causation for his dilemma to others, may be able to continue to attempt to manipulate others and avoid a necessary day of reckoning; the respective attorneys may debate procedural details and technicalities, which obscures the relevant behavioral and personality issues or provides the very unfortunate message that such issues do not matter; and, perhaps of greatest concern, there is considerable possibility that a seriously troubled youth may be unexpectedly and abruptly released without a plan or placement, through accident, judicial ignorance or whimsy, a technicality, or the unpreparedness or inexperience on the part of the treatment personnel (Amaya and Burlingame, 1981, p. 766).

The above recitation of unfortunate outcomes does not speak to the delay of treatment which occurs when a hearing is "continued" (because some necessary witness could not appear, for example); in this instance there is no closure, anxiety remains, and the incentives may be arranged for the youth to continue his defense and fail to engage in treatment. This circumstance painfully demonstrates that legal time frames can be enormously ill-fitting with treatment needs. In occasional proceedings and with particular public defenders, there is the circumstance in which the attorney affiliates emotionally with the contesting child and lends additional affective fuel to the process—which then establishes unexcelled opportunities for splitting or dividing on the part of patients with borderline personalities or conduct disorders. At the programmatic level, some facilities and units simply decide not to admit or retain contesting youth, thus reducing the treatment opportunities for this group which is often comprised of the most severely troubled of patients.

In spite of the array of worst case possibilities just presented, there are also uneventful hearings and useful outcomes. These occur, for example, when an irritated judge responds decisively to the narcissism, omnipotence, or denial of an acting-out adolescent. In such an instance, the adolescent's defenses are breached, and treatment may actually begin. At other times, the judge's positive statements reflecting his experience with the treatment unit and its professionals may lend support to the child and family in undertaking the arduous process of treatment. Although the negative outcomes are more memorable, in those states in which hearings are routine, most youth do not choose to contest their hospitalization, and many hearings are quite benign occurrences.

The present authors have also discovered that the decision to contest is correlated with diagnoses, with female histrionic personalities and schizophrenic adolescents of both sexes contesting disproportionately to other diagnoses. The authors' interpretation is that the hearing serves as yet another forum in which the histrionic personality can act out her dependency and need for visibility, while the devastation to self-esteem resulting from a first psychotic break drives the schizophreniform patient to deny the event and contest hospitalization.

Other variables which affect the decision to contest, and even the outcome, are highly situational and raise some doubts about the ultimate utility of judicial review as a protection for the liberty interest of a child or adolescent. Particular attorneys or public defenders are much more inclined to encourage children and adolescents to contest, reflecting their own views of psychiatric hospitalization. Some judges are responsible for most releases, while others almost never discharge the contesting child. Whether youth contest or not may be a function of whether they must endure an unpleasant trip across town with a psychiatric aide to an intimidating courthouse versus whether they travel as a group to an informal courtroom in the hospital, with a legitimate excuse from the psychiatric unit's school. In summary, although there has been persuasive evidence to the effect that there must be some check on the authority of parents and professionals to admit youth for psychiatric hospitalization in the absence of dangerousness, those who are familiar with judicial review cite a significant number of negative trade-offs and raise doubts regarding the efficacy of this as a mechanism.

IV. PITFALLS

A. Documentation

Major pitfalls in documentation, as have been suggested, include the failure to validate and verify incidents which demonstrate dangerousness or the presence of a disorder necessitating treatment. Commitments in which it becomes clear that there has been hyperbole or exaggeration in the documentation serve to undermine the credibility of clinicians in the eyes of the court and raise issues of bias and unfairness for the child or adolescent. Behavior which raises issues relative to matters of taste and morals (e.g., "sexual promiscuity" and "addiction to cult music") will need to be carefully tied to psychopathology if cited at all. The undue reliance on technical terminology or jargon is not usually useful, in that the court, ultimately, will render "a man on the street" judgment as to the need for hospitalization. In this regard, the failure to review behavioral data and events, when available, is a serious error and probably contributes more than any other substantive item to the release of patients by courts. The inability to provide convincing behavioral data, e.g., suicide gestures, self-injurious behavior, aggression, and acting-out, particularly in a hearing occurring months after hospitalization, is not necessarily disastrous; the clinician will, however, need to demonstrate that it is the treatment and the structure of the treatment program which is contributing to the improved mood, self-control, and judgment.

B. Technical errors

For those settings with judicial review and hearings regarding involuntary hospitalization, a variety of technical errors in the commitment process lead to the release of youth each year. Some may be as blatant as the child or adolescent being admitted by a person not holding custody, while others reflect errors in the process, for example, the failure to provide notice of hearing within the designated time format or errors on the commitment form, as in a misplaced signature. Obviously, these would seem to be avoidable, although they are often the inadvertent product of the crisis and turmoil surrounding a commitment. Nonetheless, when they constitute an abridgement of due process, they may establish a basis for dissolving the commitment and releasing the child.

C. Clinical errors and liabilities

To some extent these have been cited in III-B above. The child and family who have been prepared for the hearing, who anticipate the testimony, who are prepared for a redisclosure of traumatic incidents, and who are prepared for testimony regarding diagnosis and the presence of mental illness, will better tolerate a noxious proceeding. The adolescent who is dealt with openly and without defensiveness or anger on the part of a threatened clinician is less likely to experience the process as one more circumstance in which he has been victimized by a powerful adult. Testifying in positive terms regarding the child or adolescent's assets and gains may also serve to neutralize the harshness of accompanying testimony. With respect to accountability and liability, clinicians are rarely sued subsequent to their involvement in commitment processes. Often they are protected by "good faith" presumptions, which hold that when acting in good faith in the discharge of official duties (rather than acting vindictively or capriciously), they are immune from suit, even if error is found. Probably the most common form of error or malfeasance occurs when a beleaguered clinician, with no place for the child or adolescent to go, "bends" statutory criteria to make a case for commitment on the basis of dangerousness. Second parties to commitment processes, particularly those with no responsibility for the child, easily recognize such distortions and are faced with the decision whether to continue the charade or to return the child, often by law enforcement officers in the middle of the night, to an overwhelmed family (thereby dissolving the commitment). Although such distortions of the commitment process may not, in fact, lead to suit, they create distrust and resentment within the continuum of care and may become the basis for irritated clinicians bringing ethics complaints against their colleagues to professional associations and licensing bodies.

D. Process pitfalls

These, also, have been noted in III-B above. They include the failure to have parties present who can testify to actual events if hearsay is an issue. They also include the failure to have parents, guardians, prior caregivers, and the like present to document the ongoing nature of the psychopathology and the inappropriateness of alternative dispositions.

The most common disturbances in treatment resulting from untoward hearings have been described earlier as clinical events. The sequelae can often be minimized following the guidelines suggested herein, although some are clearly unavoidable. The following communication from a colleague illustrates a not uncommon course of events. Although not easily circumvented in this situation, the pitfall is one of being caught in multiple roles with the patient.

Recently, a patient assigned to a Psychology Intern that I supervised contested his admission in court. I represented the hospital at the hearing, and the judge ruled in favor of the boy's continued treatment. The whole event, however, was quite distressing to the patient, who attempted to run away when he reentered the court's waiting room. He threw an ashtray and had a physical altercation with the technicians who tried to subdue him. Two months later, I became his therapist when the trainee's placement ended. We spent several sessions dealing with his still intense feelings regarding the court hearing. He remained angry that I had written negative things about his behavior and testified that he was mentally ill. He was also embarrassed that I had witnessed his outbursts following the hearing. It was remarkable to me that, two months later, his memories of the hearing were so vivid and constituted a significant barrier to the development of a therapeutic relationship. The situation was eventually worked through, but given the short-term nature of our treatment, it was unfortunate to give up time to deal with this reaction to the court hearing. It was so clear that the events surrounding the hearing constituted one more assault on his damaged self-esteem. In fairness, many patients proceed through the court process with few complications. But, there have been occasions when I have had to "mop up the mess" therapeutically with patients who experienced the court process as a loss of control, a public humiliation, or an adversarial interaction, not just with the judicial system but with their therapists and other treatment team members. In particular, it is extremely difficult to write a court document that will be specific and decisive enough to ensure a favorable ruling from the judge, yet benign enough to be heard by the patient without negative reactions (Margolis, 1990).

V. CASE EXAMPLE EPILOGUES

A. Case Example 1

For Margie, the impulsive suicide attempt provided an escape from the wrath she anticipated from her parents regarding her probable pregnancy. By refusing to identify her parents and by refusing to contract not to harm herself, she created a situation in which the consulting psychiatrist petitioned for involuntary commitment in view of "imminent danger to self." A magistrate and a second physician concurred, and in her state, this allowed her to be placed on the hospital's locked psychiatric unit until 10 days had elapsed. At that point a hearing would be held to determine further disposition. The girl was thus detained and provided short-term treatment, potentially over both her and her parents' opposition. This procedure is typically referred to as an "involuntary commitment" or "involuntary hospitalization." It exists almost universally throughout the United States and may be used with children, adolescents, and adults alike, given a finding of dangerousness to self or others. In Margie's case, the hospitalization permitted intensive family treatment, in particular, to resolve the estrangement between her and her parents and her meeting of dependency needs through peers. Her dysthymia remitted quickly, and outpatient treatment structures were secured such that she was discharged just prior to the hearing. By that time, she and her family were established with outpatient therapists, and the decision for a therapeutic abortion had been made.

B. Case Example 2

In the case of Paul, the 15-year-old conduct-disordered boy who was willing to consider inpatient evaluation and treatment in lieu of prosecution within the juvenile system, the clinician arranged for his admission for 4 months of evaluation and treatment on an inpatient psychiatric unit specializing in the treatment of adolescent conduct disorders. The boy was admitted on the signature of his custodial parent. This procedure, in which the parent or guardian consents for treatment, even over the potential opposition of the adolescent and without judicial scrutiny or review and any finding of dangerousness, continues to exist in a number of states and is constitutionally viable although often criticized. In other states, older adolescents may admit themselves, and in some way they may co-sign with the legally responsible person. This form of admission is typically termed "voluntary hospitalization" or "voluntary commitment," although this is something of a misnomer, since the act may be voluntary on the part of the parent or guardian, but not necessarily on the part of the child or adolescent.

C. Case Example 3

For Jenny, the 13-year-old girl with a disabling separation anxiety disorder, the treating child psychiatrist sought long-term inpatient treatment. Following evaluation by an appropriate facility, she was eventually admitted for extended inpatient treatment. In her state, however, the decision to hospitalize made by parents and hospital required review in district court to determine whether a mental disorder necessitating such measures existed. In this case, professional staff testified at an initial hearing and subsequent rehearings to the presence of a severe and disabling separation anxiety disorder and the need for continuing treatment; this position was countered by Jenny's claims and those of her attorney to the effect that the difficulty had been overcome and that she "deserved a chance to prove herself." She remained in treatment through several contested hearings until discharged after 9 months of treatment. The court was empowered by statute to release her at any of the hearings but was convinced by the weight of medical testimony and sanctioned continued treatment. This case illustrates one of the myriad forms of due process protection which serve as checks on parental and professional authority and currently exist in a number of states.

D. Case Example 4

For Tom, the 17-year-old adolescent whose detoxification had been completed, the attending psychiatrist recommended, and the judge considered, accepted, and ordered an "outpatient commitment." This procedure, now available in a number of states, permits a presiding judge to order outpatient treatment, in this case, individual psychotherapy and substance abuse counseling. The failure to attend sessions would cause Tom to be detained by law enforcement personnel and returned to an inpatient setting to await another hearing. As a treatment option, it offered this boy, who was desperately attempting to master developmental tasks of middle and late adolescence, the autonomy and freedom to do so, while providing supportive treatment and a legal "safety net."

VI. ACTION GUIDE

A. General principles

1. Become familiar with state statutes governing voluntary and involuntary commitment of children and adolescents, particularly the relevant statutory criteria.
2. Maintain as guiding principles in the voluntary and involuntary commitment of children, "the best interest of the child" and "least restrictive appropriate alternative."

B. Procedures relative to commitment hearings

1. In addition to meeting traditional clinical documentation requirements, gather data relevant to the statutory criteria for hospitalization.
2. Provide the court with behavioral incidents, whenever possible, which illustrate psychopathology and the need for treatment.
3. Verify incidents which are to be used in court documents and testimony to support commitment.
4. Be alert to sources of procedural error which might overturn commitments.
5. Secure corroborative information from community agencies, e.g., public schools, departments of social service, and juvenile authorities, to support commitment.
6. Document and introduce data regarding prior attempts to treat in less restrictive modes.

7. Consider securing primary testimony from another clinician or administrator, thus reducing the risk of contaminating the role of therapist.
8. Prepare for the hearing by collaborating with the attorney who is representing the hospital or advocating for commitment.
9. To the extent that it is ethically permitted by legal canon, educate opposing lawyers regarding the needs of the child and family.
10. Exercise caution in the use of technical terminology and jargon in testimony, and be prepared to translate these, as well as all clinical concepts and diagnoses, into lay terms.
11. Exercise caution in providing testimony relevant to matters of taste and morals, particularly if such is used to support contentions regarding psychopathology.
12. Provide testimony and documentation regarding the child or adolescent's assets and strengths, as well as any indications of progress and favorable prognosis.
13. Prepare the child or adolescent for court by reviewing anticipated testimony and recommendations.
14. Prepare the parents for court by informing them of anticipated testimony and recommendations, as well as by assisting and supporting them in providing their testimony.
15. Provide for catharsis, ventilation, and debriefing following courtroom proceedings, and be alert to the increased likelihood of acting-out or self-injurious behavior on the part of the child or adolescent.
16. Advocate for the release of the child or adolescent when the clinical purposes for hospitalization have been achieved and transition to a less restrictive and less intensive setting is appropriate.

C. Miscellaneous

1. Advocate for responsible advertising on the part of hospitals offering inpatient treatment for children and adolescents.
2. Educate judges, bar groups, and legislators regarding deficiencies in the continuum of care for children and adolescents, as well as problems in commitment processes.
3. Recognize the potential for conflicts of interest, particularly in admissions to private and similarly constituted psychiatric units, and seek formal or informal independent peer review and consideration of issues by ethics bodies and professional associations.

VII. SUGGESTED READINGS

Amaya, M. and Burlingame, W. V. (1981), Judicial review of psychiatric admissions. J Am Acad Child Adolesc Psychiatry 20:761–776.

American Academy of Child and Adolescent Psychiatry (1987), Child and Adolescent Psychiatric Illness: Guidelines for Treatment Resources, Quality Assurance, Peer Review and Reimbursement. Washington, D.C.: American Academy of Child and Adolescent Psychiatry.

American Psychological Association (1984), A Model Act for the Mental Health Treatment of Minors. Washington, D.C.: American Psychological Association.

Barrett, K. and Greene, R. (1990), Mom, please get me out. Ladies' Home Journal 57(5):98–107.

Burlingame, W. V. and Amaya, M. (1985), Psychiatric commitment of children and adolescents. In: D. Schetky and E. Benedek (eds.) Emerging Issues in Child Psychiatry and the Law. New York: Brunner/Mazel, 229–249.

Guidelines for the psychiatric hospitalization of minors. (1982) Am J Psychiatry 139:971–974.

In re Gault, 387, U.S. 1, 1967.

Knitzer, J. (1982), Unclaimed Children. Washington, D.C.: Children's Defense Fund.

Margolis, A. (1990), Personal communication.

Parham v. J. R., 442, U.S. 584, 1979.

Weithorn, L. (1988), Mental hospitalization of troublesome youth. Stanford Law Review. 40:773–838.

Wilson, J. P. (1978), The Rights of Adolescents in the Mental Health System. Lexington, MA: Heath.

19

Maternal-Fetal Conflicts: A Modern Dilemma

MIRIAM B. ROSENTHAL, M.D.

I. CASE EXAMPLES
II. MATERNAL FETAL CONFLICT ISSUES: OVERVIEW
III. NONCOMPLIANCE WITH MEDICAL TREATMENTS IN PREGNANCY
IV. REFUSAL OF SURGICAL INTERVENTIONS IN PREGNANCY
V. REFUSAL OF PSYCHIATRIC TREATMENTS BY PREGNANT WOMEN
VI. DECISION MAKING AND PREGNANCY
VII. ALCOHOL AND SUBSTANCE ABUSE IN PREGNANCY
VIII. THE ROLE OF MENTAL HEALTH PROFESSIONALS IN MATERNAL FETAL CONFLICTS

I. CASE EXAMPLES

A. Case Example 1

A 21-year-old woman with juvenile-onset, insulin-dependent diabetes is 32 weeks pregnant when first seen by the psychiatric consultant to obstetrics. She had had numerous bouts of ketoacidosis during this pregnancy and had been in and out of the intensive care unit three times. She was transferred from the unit to the obstetrical floor. Her obstetrician wanted her to remain in the hospital for the duration of this pregnancy and believed that leaving might well increase the risk of death to her fetus and to herself. She wanted to go home, to her husband and two young children, ages 1 and 2 years. She insisted on signing out against medical advice. She was mentally competent. A court order was obtained for her to stay. However, working with social service, a caring nursing service, and staff, a compromise was reached. She was given some home visits, and she was willing to return. She was also noted by the psychiatrist to be depressed, and treatment of that helped her comply with the diabetic regime. She delivered a healthy baby.

B. Case Example 2

A 20-year-old woman with an IQ of 71 was first seen by the psychiatrist after the death of her newborn baby in the toilet at term. This was her third pregnancy. Her first had been born in a hospital where she had gone for abdominal pain and was found to be 32 weeks pregnant. She was 16 years old at the time. She was admitted to the hospital with toxemia and delivered a healthy infant. She denied knowing she was pregnant until coming to the hospital. Her second infant died in the toilet in a hospital emergency room at term, where she had gone for abdominal pain, again denying that she knew she was pregnant. Her mother and husband also denied knowing she was with child. The following year, she had a third baby born in the toilet at home, again denying the pregnancy. She was not psychotic, had no mental illness, and was convicted of voluntary manslaughter and sentenced to 7–25 years in prison. She had no past history of violence, antisocial behaviors, or drug or alcohol use. She had taken good care of her one living child.

C. Case Example 3

A 21-year-old woman had had 2 pregnancies. She had given the first one up for adoption at age 17. She denied knowing she was pregnant with the second one until giving birth in the toilet to a full term infant who died. She admitted to the use of cocaine, which was detected in the baby. She was convicted of voluntary manslaughter and sentenced to 5–25 years in prison. The judge stated that this was a warning to all women who used illegal drugs.

D. Case Example 4

This Georgia case is that of a woman with a complete placenta previa (the placenta covered the outlet from the uterus) who refused a cesarean section and blood transfusions. Her doctors believed that there was a 99% chance that the unborn baby would not live and a 50% chance that the mother might die also. A court order was obtained by the hospital and the court decided that the "unborn child" should have legal protection and that the mother must have "all medical procedures deemed necessary by the attending physicians to preserve the life of the defendant's unborn child." The mother refused on religious grounds. She disappeared from the hospital and gave birth vaginally. Both mother and baby did well (Annas. 1982).

E. Case Example 5

A well-publicized case was that of A.C., a 27-year-old woman, dying of leukemia and 26 weeks pregnant. She had agreed to treatments that would prolong her life in order to give her fetus a better chance for survival, but she did not agree to permission for a cesarean section. The chance for a viable fetus was about 50–60%, with a less than 20% risk for serious handicaps. The patient, her family, her husband, and her physician all concurred in not wanting a section done. The hospital brought the matter to the court, and a judge ordered the surgery to be done. The newborn infant died 3 hours after the cesarean section, and the mother, 2 days later. Eventually, a higher court reversed the decision. The Appeals court ruled that the lower court should not have ordered the surgery because there was not enough evidence that the mother wanted it. The court indicated that the right to "bodily integrity" is not removed because one is sick. If one is competent, his or her wishes should be respected unless there is some major complicating factor which must be considered (*Washington Post*, April 27, 1990).

F. Case Example 6

A 27-year-old woman in the 28th week of pregnancy did not believe she was pregnant, but rather, that a tumor was growing inside of her. She had command hallucinations which told her to cut it out. She was refused admission to both state and private hospitals because she was not deemed sufficiently ill. She refused medications. Her family agreed to provide constant care for her.

G. Case Example 7

A 24-year-old woman was 30 weeks pregnant and had the diagnosis of schizophrenia. She refused medications at a time when she was having hallucinations and delusions. She was involuntarily admitted to a state psychiatric hospital for the duration of her pregnancy for the protection of her fetus.

H. Case Example 8

A 30-year-old woman became pregnant with triplets with the use of fertility drugs after several years of infertility. This was a very desired pregnancy. She and her husband understood that there might be a better chance of survival if there were only two fetuses. She also understood the risks. A selective termination of one fetus was done, a second died. The third fetus survived.

II. MATERNAL FETAL CONFLICT ISSUES: OVERVIEW

There has been an increasing emphasis in the United States on the rights and privileges of unborn children, i.e., fetuses. Since most women do want the best possible outcome for their offspring, this is often not a problem. In some settings, however, the very unique relationship of mother to fetus has set up a conflict of interests where the former is seen as an adversary rather than a protector of the other. Obstetricians, family practitioners, and nurse midwives have always and will continue to have as their goal the delivery of a healthy infant to a healthy mother.

It was thought that good care of the pregnant woman would lead to the best results. Dr. Nicholas Eastman, Professor of Obstetrics at Johns Hopkins Hospital, wrote in 1953: "The paramount aim of obstetrics is the preservation of maternal health." In contrast to this concept, one reads in the preface to the latest edition of *Williams Textbook of Obstetrics,* "The quality of life for mother and her infant is our most important concern. Happily, we live and work in an era in which the fetus is established as our second patient with many rights and privileges comparable to those previously achieved only after birth" (Nelson, 1988). There are many reasons for this change in emphasis. These include the most remarkable advances in technology that enable us to visualize the fetus, to treat the fetus, and to make labor and delivery safer (Petchesky, 1987). The fetus is seen by the parents via ultrasonography. Fathers are thought to bond earlier with their offspring whom they can see during the pregnancy. The sex of the fetus may be known. Advances in the understanding of fetal physiology provide more knowledge about the effects of drugs, alcohol, smoking, diet, environmental toxins, and exercise on the developing organism.

Amniocentesis, ultrasound, and fetal monitoring give valuable information about the fetal condition and may indicate the need for fetal treatments, including surgery. For many women and couples, there is the fantasy that they will have the perfect baby if only the doctor and the parents do the right things. This rise in technology and expectations comes at the same time as the ending of the baby boom, a rise in infertility, and a public yearning to protect unborn children. The state has been asked to take a position in this arena.

The government has declared its interest in the fetus from the time of viability as set down by the Supreme Court in *Roe v. Wade* (1973). Viability is defined as the potential to live outside the uterus even with artificial aid. It is generally considered to be present from the third trimester which begins after 24 weeks of pregnancy. Abortion is legally permitted in *Roe v. Wade* until viability and afterwards in certain circumstances, such as severe congenital anomalies. Abortion is certainly considered a maternal fetal conflict, but will not be discussed here, since the mother's choice in those instances should be respected. *Roe v. Wade* does support the rights of the mother and considers the interests of the mother to be primary.

The malpractice climate has also affected the mother-fetus conflict in that medical personnel often behave in defensive ways to protect themselves from lawsuits.

This chapter will address some of the current issues in maternal fetal conflicts and in the consequences of the increasing trend to see fetal interests as separate and apart from the mother's. Such conflicts may arise if the mother refuses certain treatments recommended by her doctors, refuses prenatal care, or refuses to change certain behaviors which may be harmful to the fetus, such as use of drugs or alcohol, smoking, or poor dietary habits. Finally, the role of the psychiatrist in the maternal fetal area is discussed with some recommendations for the involvement of such mental health professionals.

III. NON-COMPLIANCE WITH MEDICAL TREATMENTS IN PREGNANCY

The competent patient who can give informed consent is usually free to make decisions about his or her medical treatments with the physician, even though at times the decision may be contrary to the recommendations of the medical staff. For the pregnant patient, this freedom becomes more problematic, especially when the fetus has reached viability (Case Example 1).

A competent patient who refuses compliance with the medical regime prescribed by her doctors presents a dilemma. Physicians are obliged to do as much as possible to enhance the health of mother and fetus and to do no harm, but there needs also to be a recognition and respect for the patient's autonomy. The time factor in Case Example 1 was not as pressing as it often is in instances that have to do with labor and delivery, and the staff working with her and her family were able to achieve compromises and better compliance with the prescribed management.

Another area where lack of compliance has lead to bad outcomes for mother and infant is lack of prenatal care. This is considered one of the major factors in the etiology of low birth weight and prematurity which have a major effect on the health of infants and children. That the United States was 19th among industrialized nations in infant mortality in 1987 is due in large part to the many low birth weight infants who weigh 2500 gm or less and who are 40 times more likely to die than heavier babies (Klerman, 1990). While women who do not obtain medical care during their pregnancies are often considered indifferent to their offspring, there are many reasons women, especially those who are poor, do not get such care. Among these are: inability to pay, shortage of clinics that will care for women without insurance or who receive public assistance, and private physicians who often will not take Medicaid patients. There is a shortage of nurse midwives to provide prenatal care. Other reasons may relate to social factors such as inadequate transportation, inadequate child care, inconvenient clinic hours, harsh staff attitudes, cultural barriers, and patient attitudes toward medical establishments. There is an added fear on the part of patients suffering from psychological disorders and alcohol or substance abuse that their children may be taken away. A small number of women deny their pregnancy and learn about it at the time of labor and delivery for the first time. They often encounter negative and punitive attitudes when they do come for medical assistance.

In Case Examples 2 and 3, the women did not obtain prenatal care, denied knowledge they were pregnant, and their babies died. The families with whom they lived shared no responsibility, not even an abusive spouse who supplied the woman with drugs. Both of these women were considered by the courts to have abused their infants and were punished accordingly.

IV. REFUSAL OF SURGICAL INTERVENTIONS IN PREGNANCY

There have been instances in recent years in which a woman close to or at term has refused recommended surgical interventions thought necessary by her physicians to protect the life of her unborn baby and/or herself.

Case Example 4 illustrates the uncertainty which is often inherent in medical advice. It also illustrates the issue of the courts having to make judgments very quickly in emergency situations in which they will usually side with medical authorities. (*Jefferson v. Griffin Spalding County Hospital Authority,* February 2, 1981). The case was appealed to the Supreme Court of Georgia who upheld the verdict, citing *Roe v. Wade,* asserting that the state had an interest in the fetus after viability. A recent study by Kolder (1987) described such instances of court-ordered interventions and described a survey of attitudes of obstetricians who directed fellowship training in maternal fetal medicine. About half of the directors believed that using the courts to force such necessary treatments was justified. It was interesting to note that most of the patients discussed were in teaching hospitals, were receiving public assistance, did not have English as their first language, and were not known to their doctors prior to coming to the hospital for treatments. Many were minority or Hispanic women. The importance of the doctor-patient relationship in helping patients with decision making is well illustrated in these cases. However, there are examples such as Case Example 5 where even the patient's physician was not able to influence the hospital's decision. However, the Appeals court revised the lower court's decision, which will influence further such situations.

Mahowald (1989) summarizes some of the ethical arguments for and against court-ordered surgical interventions for pregnant women. Opposing such forced procedures are: (1) the doctrine of informed consent for competent patients who may accept or refuse the procedure based on their understanding; (2) the right of the patient to her own bodily integrity; (3) the personhood of the fetus is not really settled; (4) cesarean sections or other surgical procedures are not without risks from bleeding and anesthesia, and the state has the duty to protect the individual from bodily harm; (5) an individual can not be forced to have her body invaded to help someone else; (6) the obstetrician's first duty is to the woman; (7) finally, the diagnosis and/or the prognosis may be wrong as in the Jefferson case.

Less compelling are the arguments for forced surgical procedures. The fetus does have the right to life. Obligations exist to save the life of the mother which may be in jeopardy. The ethical principle of beneficience says that the practitioner has the responsibility to do all that he or she can to benefit the mother and her fetus, the soon-to-be infant.

V. REFUSAL OF PSYCHIATRIC TREATMENTS BY PREGNANT WOMEN

For the psychiatric patient requiring psychotropic medications, pregnancy may present a problem. The effects of the drugs on the fetus are still not well known, especially in the first trimester, as the fetal organ systems are developing. Many of the reported adverse effects of these drugs are anecdotal with the exception of some such as the cardiac defects caused by lithium. There may be other effects in the third trimester. Therefore, the prescription of such drugs may be a conflict for doctors, and the taking of such medications a dilemma for the patient. Risk-benefit ratios need to be assessed. Therefore, some of the issues that rise during pregnancy may be extremely difficult (Spielvogel, 1986; Applebaum, 1982).

Case Examples 6 and 7 illustrate some of the difficulties encountered in the treatment and management of the pregnant psychiatric patient. They also point out the inconsistency of such management. These patients were very similar in their presentation. The issues of competency, the right to refuse treatment, and informed consent of patients and their families prior to decision making are involved.

VI. DECISION MAKING AND PREGNANCY

Many of the decisions that must be made in pregnancy highlight the conflict between mother and fetus. The first of these decisions is perhaps the ultimate one in the conflict, i.e., deciding whether or not to continue the process. Throughout recorded history, women have had to make the decision about when and if to choose an abortion, and they will continue to do so, whether it is legal or not. It is assumed, therefore, that if a woman decides against abortion and for the continuation of the pregnancy, she has certain obligations to her fetus. Implicit in this obligation is the assumption that the decision to continue the pregnancy was a conscious and deliberate choice, which often it is not. Some women first realize they are pregnant when it is too late to terminate it. They may not be aware of their choices or know how to obtain an abortion.

In the case of genetic abnormalities or multiple gestations, the question of termination may rise, and the decision may be very difficult. The pregnancy is often very much wanted and the meaning of the genetic abnormality uncertain.

There has been difficulty for parents who have the choice now of selective termination in multiple gestations. In addition to spontaneous pregnancies with two or more fetuses, many of the new reproductive technologies result in multiple fetuses. These pregnancies occur after periods of infertility in patients strongly wanting children. They are told, however, that chances of survival for the fetuses will be diminished if over a certain number are growing.

Having chosen to continue the pregnancy, women are constantly faced with choices about their treatment, their lifestyle, their behaviors which may affect the fetus, and choices about labor and delivery. They are given information and advice which may not have absolute outcome certainty. While most medical staff respect patient autonomy, there are times when their judgment diverges from that of the pregnant woman and decisions must be made, often quickly. Time may be important, especially during labor and delivery. Some theoretical concepts in decision making may be useful. Five patterns of coping with decisions have been described by Janis (1982). They are:

1. Unconflicting inertia in which all new information is ignored and the patients and doctors may continue with the same pattern.
2. Unconflicted change in which any new course of action is undertaken without careful consideration; panic may take over and replace careful consideration.
3. Defensive avoidance where there is evasion of decision making altogether and the burden of the responsibility is shifted to someone else.
4. Hypervigilance when there is panic even more than with the unconflicted change; there is a frantic search for the answers which may not be definite.
5. Vigilance and logic where adequate knowledge and consideration are used to come to a conclusion.

Psychiatrists are often involved in such decision making, helping individuals to see their choices and choose a course of action. In working with patients, it is important to be able to help patients make informed decisions, and that requires that they be competent to make choices about their treatments. An individual is considered competent to make treatment decisions if she can understand the nature of the conduct in question and be able to understand its quality and consequences. One can be mentally ill and still be able to make decisions about the treatment in question. However, anxiety, depression, delirium, extreme fear, or severe obsessional ruminations may get in the way of informed decision making. Some of the factors involved in assessing competency for decision making (not a legal concept) are knowing there are choices, (having the cognitive capacity to understand the options and their advantages and disadvantages as well as the relevant facts); the absence of any major psychopathology that could affect beliefs about the decision (the woman who thought her pregnancy was a tumor that should be cut out); having the absence of any interfering motivational factors such as intense rage; having the absence of helplessness dependency on another person; and finally, having the awareness of how others may view the decision, including societal attitudes, and still understanding the reasons for making the decision even if it deviates from these attitudes (Mahler, 1988).

VII. ALCOHOL AND SUBSTANCE ABUSE IN PREGNANCY

One of the most difficult areas of maternal fetal conflict today is in the area of alcohol or substance abuse and pregnancy. Should pregnant women be held accountable for their behaviors which may in some way endanger the fetus? How should such accountability be enforced without bias, and in what circumstances?

Instances illustrating this conflict are in the media almost daily in regard to the use of drugs and alcohol, especially the former, although the latter is a major public health hazard as well.

There is currently believed to be an epidemic in this country of drug use, especially cocaine. It is estimated that about 15% of pregnant women are using cocaine, and the effects on the baby may include neurological, endocrinological, cardiac, and respiratory problems, prematurity, and organic brain disease. In July, 1989, a woman in Florida was convicted of "delivering cocaine to her newborn child through the umbilical cord." She had delivered three other cocaine-affected babies and all four were in the custody of relatives. She was given 14 years of probation (Curriden, 1990). Since then, there have been at least 14 other cases of women prosecuted for drug abuse in pregnancy which have harmed their offspring. They have been charged with felonies, child abuse, criminal neglect, delivering drugs to a minor, and endangering an unborn child. A poll done by the *Atlanta Constitution* showed that 71% of 1,500 people asked for their views favored punishing women who used drugs which harmed the baby. Forty-five percent favored criminal charges being brought against women whose use of alcohol or cigarettes harmed their babies. Civil libertarians are very concerned about such intrusion by the state into the lives of pregnant women. They believe there is a violation of the right to privacy and due process. They believe poor women may become more and more afraid to seek adequate prenatal care. They would like to see more drug rehabilitation programs which at this time are frequently unwilling or unable to accommodate pregnant women. There is also the belief that there is considerable bias against minority and poor women who are more frequently brought to the attention of the authorities than are white women and those with financial resources. This is true, although a study in Pinellas County, Florida, showed that cocaine use was similar in all populations (Chasnoff, 1990). Drug use in pregnancy is a health problem, not a legal problem.

At this time, legislators in several states are attempting to deal with this problem. In Illinois, the Infant Neglect and Controlled Substances Act of 1989 says it is a felony to "inflict or create a substantial risk of physical injury to a newborn infant" with illegal drug use by mother in pregnancy. A temporary guardian can be appointed for a newborn if the mother or baby is found to have illegal drugs in the blood or urine. The mother can be detained in a medical facility, not prison. There is the question of testing of the pregnant woman and her fetus and the newborn, without her permission. Committees of the American Bar Association are studying these issues (Curriden, 1990).

VIII. THE ROLE OF MENTAL HEALTH PROFESSIONALS IN MATERNAL FETAL CONFLICTS

The dilemmas presented in the preceding sections represent a number of areas where mental health professionals and psychiatrists, in particular, may be especially useful to their colleagues in obstetrics and to the patients. These can be summarized as follows: there can be considerable usefulness in helping with counseling regarding decision making and understanding options, especially when there is ample time. Psychiatrists can participate in the assessment of competency and help with informed consent. They can collaborate with their colleagues in the care of psychiatrically ill pregnant patients. Their expertise should include the effects of psychotropic drugs in pregnancy. They should understand the effects of certain behaviors in women in pregnancy, how they affect the fetus and how they can be modified, to the benefit of mother and fetus. There should be active involvement in encouraging the establishment of alcohol and drug rehabilitation programs that will serve the needs of all women, rich and poor. There should be advocates for appropriate legislation that will support treatment programs rather than prison sentences when appropriate. Extremely important is research collaboration with obstetricians, clinicians, ethicists, attorneys, and others interested in this area of mother-fetal interaction.

One of the tasks that the consulting psychiatrist in obstetrics is often called upon to do is to assess the pregnant woman for her future role as a parent. If she has some children and has parented them well, this task may be easier than if it is the first pregnancy. Some of the guidelines are:

1. Has the mother been abused as a child physically, sexually, or emotionally?
2. Has the mother had a close relationship with her mother and experienced some nurturing?
3. Has the mother a supportive relationship with the father of her baby or some other family members or close friends?
4. Does the mother abuse alcohol or drugs?
5. Does the mother have some cognitive impairment or evidence of mental illness that would impair her competency and judgment? Is she depressed?
   AFTER BIRTH in hospital:
6. What are the nurses' observations of the mother's interactions with her newborn infant?
7. Does the mother have the capacity to put her needs at times secondary to those of her infant and to act in synchrony with the infant?

Mental health people need to remember that pregnancy, like puberty or menopause, represents life crises for women and men, a developmental task where significant changes can occur, given adequate support and care. There is the exciting challenge of helping to get new life off to a good start by doing the best possible for the woman carrying the fetus.

SUGGESTED READINGS

Annas, G., (1982), Forced cesarians: The most unkindest cut of all. Hastings Cent Rep June.

Applebaum, P. and Gutheil, T. (1982), Clinical aspects of treatment refusal. Compr Psychiatry 23:560–566.

Bouton, K. (1990), Painful decisions: The role of the medical ethicist. New York Times Mag, August 5.

Bowes, W. A. and Selgestad, B. (1981), Fetal versus maternal rights; Medical and legal perspectives. Obstet Gynecol 58:209–214.

Chasnoff, I., et al. (1990), The prevalence of illicit drug or alcohol use during pregnancy in mandatory reporting in Pinellas County, Florida. N Engl J M 322:1202–1205.

Chervenak, F. (1985), Perinatal ethics: A practical analysis of obligations to mother and fetus. Obstet Gynecol 66:442–446.

Curriden, M. (1990), Holding mom accountable. Amer Bar Assoc J March.

Englehardt, H. T. (1985), Current controversies in obstetrics: Wrongful life and forced fetal surgical procedures. Am J Obstet Gynecol 151:313–318.

Harrison, M. (1990), Drug addiction in pregnancy: The interface of science, emotion and social policy. Paper presented at American Psychiatric Association Meeting, May 17.

Hoffman, J. (1990), Pregnant, addicted and guilty. New York Times Mag, August 19.

Janis, I. L. Decision making under stress. (1982), in: Goldberger, L. and Breznita, S. (eds.): Handbook of Stress: Theoretical and Clinical Aspects. New York, N.Y.: MacMillan Free Press. 69–87.

Johnson D. (1987), A new threat to pregnant women's autonomy. Hastings Cent Rep, August 33–40.

Jurow, R., et al. (1984), Cesarian delivery for fetal distress without maternal consent. Obstet Gynecol 63:596–598.

Klerman, L. (1990), Prenatal care. In: Wymelenberg S (ed.): Science and Babies, Private Decisions, Public Dilemmas. Washington, D.C.: National Academy Press.

Kolder, V., Gallager, J. D., Parsons, M. T. (1987), Court ordered obstetrical interventions. N Engl J Med 316:1192–1196.

Landwirth, J. (1987), Fetal abuse and neglect: An emerging controversy. Pediatr 79:508–514.

Lieberman, J. R., Mazor, M., Chaim, W. and Cohen, A. (1979), The fetal right to live. Obstet Gynecol 53:515–517.

MacKenzie, T. and Nagel, T. (1986), When a pregnant woman endangers her fetus. Hastings Cent Rep, February 24–25.

Mahler, J., and Perry S. (1988), Assessing competency in the physically ill. Guidelines for psychiatric consultants. Hosp and Comm Psychiat 39:856–861.

Mahowald, M. (1989), Beyond abortion: Refusal of cesarian section. Bioethics 3:106–121.

Mogul, K. (1985), Psychological considerations in the use of psychotropic drugs with women patients. Hosp Community Psychiatry 36:1080–1085.

Mother's Right is Placed Over Fetus' Care. The Plain Dealer Newspaper, April 27, 1990.

Nelson, L., and Milliken, N. (1988), Compelled medical treatment of pregnant women. JAMA 259:1060–1066.

Petchesky, R. (1987), Fetal images: The power of visual culture in the politics of reproduction. In: M. Stanworth (ed.): Reproductive Technologies. Minneapolis: U. Minn. Press.

Pollitt, K. (1990), Fetal rights—A new assault on feminism. The Nation, March 26.

Robertson, J. A. (1983), Procreative liberty and the control of conception, pregnancy and childbirth. VA Law Rev 69:405–464.

Roe vs Wade, 410 U.S. 113 (1973).

Roth, L., et al. (1982), The dilemma of denial in the assessment of competency to refuse treatment. Am J Psychiat 139:910–913.

Schetky, D. (1989), Ethical issues in the care of the unborn. Newsletter: Am Acad of Child and Adoles Psychiat, Summer.

Spielvogel, A, and Wile, J. (1986), Treatment of the psychotic pregnant patient. Psychosomatics 27:487–492.

Stillman, R. (1986), Smoking and reproduction. Fertil Steril 545–566.

Woman get access to jobs with risk. New York Times, May 19, 1990.

20

Psychic Trauma and Civil Litigation

DIANE H. SCHETKY, M.D.

I. CASE EXAMPLES

A. Case Example 1

Becky, a shy, overweight, 14-year-old was a passenger in a motorboat that collided with another one. She was thrown overboard, became entangled with the propeller, and lost consciousness. She suffered extensive facial lacerations, nerve damage to her arm, and spent two weeks in the hospital. Her attorney who was filing suit for physical damages wondered if she might also have a case for psychic trauma and sought psychiatric consultation.

B. Case Example 2

Jesse was 10 when he was repeatedly fondled by a male teacher at school. Psychiatric consultation was sought 5 years later regarding pending litigation against the school. Questions had to do with causality, effects of abuse, and treatment needs. Jesse gave a very convincing and detailed account of the abuse. His subsequent course had been stormy with academic failures, substance abuse, self-destructive behaviors, psychiatric hospitalization, and conflicts around his sexual identity. His mother portrayed him as a model child before the abuse and minimized the possible role of the family in her son's ensuing psychopathology.

C. Case Example 3

Jared, age 6, was attacked by his neighbor's pit bulldog and required plastic surgery to his face. Upon return home from the hospital he developed nightmares, was afraid to play alone out of doors, and became terrified whenever he saw a dog. His parents promptly took him to a child psychologist who initiated play therapy. His mother stated that she had no intentions of suing, and the neighbor offered to pay for necessary treatment. Jared's attorney calls you requesting an assessment of his treatment needs.

II. LEGAL ISSUES

A. Tort law

1. DEFINITION

A tort is a civil wrong for which an individual may sue to recover damages. Tort law may only be invoked if it can be shown that there was violation of a duty owed to the injured party by the defendant. In a typical tort claim the plaintiff alleges that another person's negligence or willful behavior caused an injury or loss to the plaintiff's person or property. Tort actions may be classified as intentional or unintentional.

a. Intentional torts

An intentional tort occurs when an individual deliberately sets out to harm another through acts of omission or commission. Included in this category are the intentional infliction of emotional distress, slander, and in some cases "undue familiarity" suits. In such cases the plaintiff has the burden of proving the intent or state of mind of the defendant.

b. Unintentional torts

This category includes acts that are negligent but not willful, such as medical malpractice and personal injury cases. Negligence is defined as "conduct which falls below the standard of care established by law for the protection of others against unreasonable harm" (Restatement [Second] of Torts 282, 1964). The standard of care is regarded as that which would be expected from a reasonably careful and prudent person under the circumstances. In a medical malpractice case the standard refers to the standard of practice within that community.

2. PURPOSE

The intent of tort actions is to obtain financial compensation for losses or injuries suffered by the plaintiff as a result of another person's negligence.

3. ESSENTIAL ELEMENTS

There are four components to a negligence tort that must be demonstrated in order for the plaintiff to prevail. These include establishing that:
   a. There was the existence of a duty of care between the plaintiff and defendant;
   b. There was a breach of that duty, i.e., negligence on the part of the defendant;
   c. That the plaintiff suffered compensable damage;
   d. That the ensuing damage was caused by the negligence.

4. COMPENSATION

The sole remedy provided by a tort claim is a monetary award to the plaintiff. The money is intended to compensate the victim for injuries suffered and to help restore him to his prior level of functioning. Damages may be broken down into 1) Compensatory damages, i.e., for pain and suffering; 2) Special damages for medical and psychiatric care, property damage, and loss of income; and 3) punitive damages that may be awarded in an intentional tort. Compensatory damages are the most difficult to determine, e.g., how does one put a price tag on the grief and loss sustained by a child in a suit claiming the wrongful death of a parent.

5. CONTRIBUTORY AND COMPARATIVE NEGLIGENCE

Awards may be limited if the plaintiff is found to be at fault, i.e., has assumed unreasonable risk or contributed to his own injury. Exceptions to this principle exist, as in no-fault automobile insurance policies and workman's compensation laws that provide compensation for injuries arising in the domain of employment.

6. PREEXISTING CONDITIONS

The concept of the "eggshell skull" plaintiff deals with predisposing conditions that might render a plaintiff more vulnerable than the average man to certain stresses. Thus under law, the defendant is still held liable for the disproportionate harm that the eggshell plaintiff suffers. In other words, the defendant must take the plaintiff as he finds him.

B. Evolution of case law regarding claims for psychic trauma

It is only recently that courts have allowed recovery for damages that are purely psychic in nature. In the past it was feared that recovery for psychological suffering would open the floodgates to fraudulent claims. In the early 20th century recovery for psychic trauma was permitted for the first time but only if there were concomitant physical losses. This then gave way to the "zone of danger" principle that permitted recovery by plaintiffs who were at risk of physical injury owning to their proximity to a dangerous circumstance, yet only suffered psychic trauma. The next extension of this was to allow recovery by a person who had a special relationship to the one injured or killed, if they witnessed the trauma but were not in the zone of danger. Thus, in *Dillon v. Legg* (68 Ca. 2nd 728, 1968) a mother and daughter who, although not in danger themselves, witnessed the negligent death of another daughter were allowed to recover damages.

C. Issues for the plaintiff

1. STATUTE OF LIMITATIONS

The statute of limitations refers to the period of time in which an action must be brought in order to be enforced. By limiting the time period, the defendant is in a better position to defend himself, and presumably the memories of witnesses have not yet faded. The statutory limit usually runs from when the injury is discovered and until the period of limitations has expired. The period of statutory limitations varies from state to state and according to the type of action. The statute is tolled for minors and does not begin to run until they reach the age of majority. Other conditions that may extend it include insanity, imprisonment, or being comatose.

2. COSTS

The plaintiff who brings suit is liable for the costs of the suit in contrast to criminal proceedings. Attorneys may accept a case on a contingency fee if there appears to be a good chance of recovery.

3. STANDARD OF EVIDENCE

In civil litigation, a lower standard of evidence, preponderance of evidence, is used, rather than the beyond a reasonable doubt standard used in criminal proceedings. The burden of proof lies with the plaintiff.

4. TENDERING OF RECORDS

If the plaintiff introduces his mental or physical health as an issue, he, in so doing, waives claims of confidentiality regarding his medical records. The plaintiff's relevant medical records will be made available to the defendant's attorney to aid in his defense of the case.

D. Civil court procedures

1. FILING COMPLAINT

Court procedures are initiated by the filing of a complaint that is a written statement drafted by the plaintiff's attorney describing the nature of the claim. The party being sued is then served with a summons and copy of the complaint. The defendant is expected to respond to the complaint within a specified period.

2. MOTION TO DISMISS

After the defendant's attorney reviews the claim he may file a motion to dismiss based on the legal insufficiency of the claim. A motion for summary judgment attempts to dispense with the claim based on showing that the facts cannot be proven. A motion for judgment on the pleadings questions the legality of the proceedings. These measures may serve to weed out cases that lack merit. The judge then analyses the situation and decides whether there is a sufficient legal basis for sustaining the complaint.

3. DISCOVERY

Discovery is a process whereby the defense is provided with the tools necessary to discover the facts of the case before proceeding to trial. These may include the identification of witnesses, review of relevant records, facts of the case, and the opinions of expert witnesses. An oral deposition involves questioning the witness under oath. In deposing an expert witness the defendant's attorney will attempt to establish how firm the expert's opinion is and how well he defends it. Alternatively the defense may present witnesses with a list of questions termed interrogatories to be answered in writing and under oath. Discovery permits each side to approximate their chances of winning and promotes out-of-court settlement.

4. PRETRIAL CONFERENCE

A pretrial conference involves a meeting between the judge and involved attorneys in which the issues are informally reviewed. In most civil cases out-of-court settlement will be reached by this point. In the event that settlement is not reached the next task is to define the scope of the trial in terms of the issues to be raised, the number of witnesses that will testify, and the decision whether to have a jury trial or to have a judge hear the case.

5. JURY TRIAL

Jurors are chosen randomly from the community, often from the motor vehicle registry. Once a case has been assigned to a courtroom, jurors are further screened through the process of voire dire. They are questioned by the attorneys about their qualifications and possible biases. Each attorney is allowed a number of peremptory challenges for which no cause need be given for excusing a juror. Once the jury is selected, the jurors are administered an oath and impaneled.

The trial begins with an opening statement by the plaintiff's attorney in which the facts of the case that he intends to establish are outlined. The defendant's attorney may then follow with his views on the case.

Witnesses are then called, sworn in, and asked questions under direct examination by the plaintiff's attorney. The defendant's attorney then cross-examines the witnesses. Additional evidence may be presented in the form of documents, photographs, written medical reports, and sometimes physical evidence. Attorneys then conduct redirect examinations of their witnesses. Leading questions are permissible on cross examination, as they are felt to test the credibility of the witness.

Rules of evidence must be followed regarding the admissibility of evidence. These include relevancy and exclusion of hearsay evidence, i.e., that evidence which does not come from personal knowledge of the witness. Rules of evidence also govern the limits on the subject matter of the witness' testimony. If following the presentation of evidence the plaintiff's attorney feels they have not substantiated the claims, he may move for a non suit. If the motion is granted, the trial ends and the plaintiff loses. If the motion is denied, the case then proceeds with the defense presenting its arguments, witnesses and exhibits.

After the evidence has been presented from both sides either party may appeal to the judge for a directed verdict. If the case seems perfectly clear the judge may decide the case at that point and the moving party wins without the case going to the jury. If the case goes to the jury, each lawyer presents his closing arguments and summarizes the relevant law and the testimony heard. The judge then instructs the jurors how to proceed.

The jury adjourns to the jury room where they deliberate until they arrive at a verdict. In civil cases this requires that there be consensus of at least three quarters of the jurors. The jury also decides on the amount of damages to be awarded.

6. APPEALS

The losing party has a right to appeal the case to the next highest court. The issues considered at the appeal are limited to questions of law raised at the trial.

III. CLINICAL ISSUES

This section will focus on issues unique to civil litigation. For information on the clinical evaluation and written report, the reader is referred to Chapter 2.

A. Questions to be asked

1. DEGREE OF IMPAIRMENT

The first task is to determine whether the plaintiff is suffering from a mental disorder and if so how impaired he is. Sometimes after-effects of abuse may be subtle, i.e., inability to trust, feeling damaged, conflicts around sexuality, yet the patient may have no diagnosable mental illness. Nonetheless, these findings may constitute impairment. In contrast, some patients may demonstrate full-blown symptoms of post-traumatic stress disorder following a trauma that are easily recognized by the psychiatrist. The defendant's attorney may argue that these symptoms are purely subjective and ask what concrete evidence the expert has for such symptoms, or he may try to attribute them to an unrelated trauma.

2. CAUSALITY

Having established impairment, the next step is to determine whether there exists a proximate relationship between the trauma and the symptoms reported or observed. It is useful to ask, "But for this trauma would the patient have developed these symptoms?" Hoffman and Spiegel (1989) caution that the relationship between severity of trauma and ensuing harm is not necessarily linear. A severe reaction to a minimal trauma may occur if the injury is sudden and unexpected, defensive action is blocked, and the injury occurs in a safe, familiar environment. For instance, a couple was awakened by a psychotic intruder in their home and found him sodomizing their dog. Although neither of them was harmed, both developed symptoms of post-traumatic stress disorder and felt violated by the intrusion into their home. Symptoms may also be modified by constitutional factors, prior experience, the family and the community's responses, and the need to be looked after.

3. CREDIBILITY

a. Factors affecting credibility

Credibility may be affected by the plaintiff's conscious or unconscious wish for secondary gain. Symptoms may be exaggerated or held onto because they render attention or because of the hope of financial gain. The latter is unusual for children, but they may be influenced by parental attitudes. Plaintiffs or parents may give a skewed history minimizing the impact of other traumas or emotional problems in their lives. Hoffman and Spiegel (1989) point out that it is not the history of prior conditions that prejudices the plaintiff's claim so much as it is the attempt to conceal them.

Credibility will be enhanced by consistency as the history is repeatedly told and by corroborating findings, ability to give details, symptoms that seem understandable in the context of the trauma, and affect appropriate to the situation. Exceptions exist to the latter, as when the patient uses dissociative defenses or when a child has told her history so many times that she becomes comfortable with it.

b. Conversion disorders

The psychiatrist needs to ask if the child's presentation is consistent with a recognized medical or psychiatric disorder. Persons with conversion disorders are usually compliant, dependant, cooperative with evaluations and suggestible. Symptoms in conversion disorders are symbolic, triggered by an unconscious psychological conflict, are not under voluntary control, and become a source of secondary gain. The picture may be complicated if the psychic trauma being litigated has triggered the conversion disorder. For instance hysterical seizures have been described as a sequela to child sexual abuse. The important distinction to make in such a case is that the child's distress is real, but is psychic not physical.

c. Malingering

The malingerer consciously feigns illness, often resists examination, may exaggerate symptoms, and is consciously using symptoms for secondary gain. Like persons with conversion disorder, their symptoms do not fit any known diagnostic entity. However, in contrast to conversion disorder, there is no alteration in physical functioning. Typically there will be a discrepancy between alleged complaints and what the plaintiff can do.

d. Factitious disorders

The patient with a factitious disorder has a need to be in the sick role and will intentionally feign symptoms or induce physical findings. In contrast to malingering, economic gain is not an issue. In Munchausen by proxy syndrome a parent will induce symptoms in a child for her own "gratification." In as much as these parents have much invested in having a sick child they are unlikely to litigate.

4. Implications of injury on ensuing development

Traumas need to be understood in the context of the child's development. For instance, a 4-year-old boy witnesses his mother's rape. He confuses violence with sexuality and feels guilty for not protecting her. He goes on to develop problems separating from her and in his fantasies he imagines repeated assaults. Without help these issues may interfere with his entering into latency and developing a healthy male identity. The child who is sexually assaulted may have that trauma reactivated when he reaches puberty and has to deal with his own sexuality and sexual identity. Thus, many children may require therapy not only at the time of the trauma but at subsequent nodal points in their lives.

5. Treatment needs and costs

Assessing the need for treatment involves considering prior functioning as well as predisposing, contributing, and perpetuating conditions, the child's level of development and current functioning, the nature of the trauma, and the response from the child's environment. The type, frequency, and duration of treatment indicated should be discussed. It is important not to short change the plaintiff with therapeutic optimism. If the child's trust has been undermined, or if the child has been forced to keep secrets, treatment may proceed very slowly. It is also appropriate to discuss the possibilities of additional problems ensuing based upon what we know of long term follow-up studies on, for instance, child sexual abuse (Schetky, 1990).

The cost of future therapy can be estimated based on prevailing rates in the area where the plaintiff resides, taking inflation into consideration.

6. Prognosis

Prognosis should consider what is known about the plaintiff in terms of strengths and weaknesses, resilience, diagnosis, availability of and likelihood of using treatment, and availability of other supports. In addition, the expert can refer to long term outcome studies. If the plaintiff has already received treatment by the time the case comes to trial, this is often a good indicator of how she will respond to future treatment.

B. Effects of litigation on therapy

One should be aware of the effects that litigation may have on psychotherapy. It used to be feared that patients in litigation would hold onto their symptoms to gain compensation for them. Current thinking (Mendelson, 1982) challenges this notion, and there is little to support this in the child psychiatry literature. Unfortunately, many attorneys continue to defer getting treatment for their clients until the case has settled. This does a great disservice to children and their families, many of whom cannot afford psychotherapy. Typically, years elapse before these cases are settled, and untreated symptoms may interfere with the child's ensuing development.

In some instances, the shadow of litigation and prospect of having to testify may sidetrack therapy and prevent the child from dealing with other issues. The approaching trial may also serve as a catalyst reactivating issues of trust, guilt, and lack of control over his life (Schetky and Benedek, 1989). Not uncommonly, children fear that they are on trial and that they may be sent to jail and do not readily make distinctions between plaintiff and defendant. Having to confront the offender in the courtroom may exacerbate symptoms of post-traumatic stress disorder, but also may help the child begin to master her fears. Litigation may enable the child to direct anger where it belongs and to have her feelings validated.

The downside is, of course, that litigation often has a terribly disruptive effect on the child's life. This is particularly so when there are many delays and the case drags on. The child is subjected to repeated interrogations and disruptions in schooling and everyday routines. These constant reminders of the trauma make it difficult for her to put it behind her.

IV. PITFALLS

A. Superficial evaluation

The psychiatrist may be so convinced by the patient's account of the trauma and ensuing symptoms that he fails to consider what other factors might be at play. The defense attorney, in contrast, will leave no stone unturned and may confront the expert with potentially embarrassing material that undermines his position. At this point the psychiatrist needs to consider whether the new information alters his opinion and be prepared to back down if necessary.

B. Credibility

Credibility can be evaluated by considering other possible explanations for a child's statements or behavior and by exploring contradictions in the history or statements made. Sometimes we may be misled, as when parents or attorneys deliberately withhold information from us. The psychiatrist needs to avoid being drawn into collusion with them and see the problem as theirs not his. A parent's deception will undermine the case and gain points for the other side.

C. Issues for treating psychiatrist

Treating psychiatrists may be forced to testify to damages, and this creates a boundary violation in therapy. In cases of delayed post-traumatic stress disorder, the defense attorney may attempt to attribute the symptoms to therapy and to the treating psychiatrist as a defensive maneuver.

V. CASE EXAMPLE EPILOGUE

A. Case Example 1

Becky remained unconscious in the hospital for several days and upon awakening could not recall the accident. Her friends and family rallied around her, and her parents noted that she seemed more outgoing than before the accident. In spite of her nerve injury, she was playing basketball again, counter to predictions. She was dealing well with her facial disfigurement and had decided to postpone plastic surgery. The psychiatrist who evaluated her could find no evidence of post-traumatic stress disorder or other symptoms of emotional distress related to the accident. In the absence of memory, there was no basis for the development of post-traumatic symptoms. She related her findings to the referring attorney who accepted them and did not pursue a claim for psychic trauma.

B. Case Example 2

At the time of her deposition the psychiatrist learned from the defendant's attorney that prior to the sexual abuse the plaintiff had been treated for enuresis and diagnosed as having attention deficit disorder. Additional information came to light, including the fact that two siblings, who the attorney was quick to point out had not been sexually abused, had substance abuse problems, and the plaintiff's mother probably did as well. The psychiatrist had failed to ask about familial substance abuse. While these new facts did not alter her opinion about the plaintiff's credibility, they did put more weight on a contributory role of ongoing family problems in the boy's continued behavioral problems. The case settled out of court.

C. Case Example 3

During 6 months of therapy Jared's symptoms gradually remitted. Shortly before termination, Jared got a puppy dog that he loves. Jared did well for the next 6 months but then began having trouble keeping up in first grade. Psychological testing documents a learning disorder. The psychologist reports that Jared developed acute post-traumatic stress disorder following the dog bite, that he has responded well to therapy, that he has an unrelated learning disability, and that the prognosis for his trauma-related symptoms is good. The case settles out of court, and the owner of the dog agrees to pay for the cost of related medical and psychiatric care to date.

VI. ACTION GUIDE

A. Avoid shortcuts

Shortcuts and premature conclusions can only lead to embarrassment further down the line.

B. Maintain objectivity

It is easy to become attached to one's opinion and convinced of the accuracy of one's findings. It is foolish to adhere rigidly to one's opinion in the face of new contradictory information.

We need to keep an open mind, be receptive to new information, and strive for an objective stance that weighs all possibilities.

C. Don't get too invested in outcome

This is easier said than done when one has invested hours in a case. The risk of overinvolvement is that of losing objectivity and appearing too emotional on the witness stand. Remember that the jury, not the psychiatrist, is the ultimate finder of fact.

D. Keep current on literature

Trauma research is rapidly evolving. We need to be aware, for instance, of neurophysiological factors in post-traumatic stress disorder that may account for the chronic and episodic nature of symptoms and that have profound implications for treatment.

VII. SUGGESTED READINGS

FORENSIC ISSUES:
Goodman, G. S. and Rosenberg, M. (1987), The Child Witness to Family Violence. In: Sonkin, D. J. (ed.): Domestic Violence on Trial: The Legal and Psychological Dimensions of Family Violence. New York, N.Y.: Springer.

Grilliot, H. (1983), Introduction to Law and the Legal System. Boston: Houghton Mifflin.

Hoffman, B. F. (1986), How to Write a Psychiatric Report for Litigation Following a Personal Injury. Am J Psychiat 143(2):164–169.

Hoffman, B. F., and Spiegel, H. (1989), Legal Principles in the Psychiatric Assessment of Personal Injury Litigants. Am J Psychiat 146(3):304–310.

Lindy, J. and Titchener, J. (1983), "Acts of God and Man": Long-Term Character Change in Survivors of Disaster and the Law. Behavioral Sciences and the Law. 1(3):85–96.

Malmquist, C. P. (1985), Children Who Witness Violence: Tortious Aspects. Bull Am Acad Psychiat Law 13(3):298–304.

Mendelson, G. (1985), Compensation Neurosis. Med J of Australia, 142:561–564.

Quinn, K. M. (1982), Children and Deception. In: Rogers, R. (ed.): Clinical Assessment of Malingering and Deception. New York, N.Y.: Guilford Press.

Resnick, P. (1982), Malingering in Post-Traumatic Disorder. In: Rogers R. (ed.): Clinical Assessment of Malingering and Deception. New York, N.Y.: Guilford Press.

Schetky, D. H. and Benedek, E. P. (1989), The Victim of Sexual Abuse in the Courtroom. Psychiat Clinics of N A, June.

Scrignar, C. B. (1988), PTSD: Diagnosis, Treatment and Legal Issues, 2nd ed. New Orleans: Bruno Press.

Slovenko, R. (1973), Traumatic Neurosis. In: Slovenko, R.: Psychiatry and Law. Boston: Little Brown.

PSYCHIC TRAUMA:

Bleser, G. C., Green, B. L. and Winget, C. (1981), Prolonged Psychosocial Effects of a Disaster: A Study of Buffalo Creek. New York, N.Y.: Academic Press.

Burgess, A. W. and Holmstrom L. L. (1974), Rape Trauma Syndrome. Am J Psychiatry 131:981–986.

Eth, S. and Pynoos, R. (1985), Developmental Perspective on Psychic Trauma in Childhood. In: Figley (ed.): Trauma and Its Wake. New York, N.Y.: Brunner/Mazel, Inc.

Eth, S. and Pynoos, R. (eds.) (1985), Post-Traumatic Stress Disorder in Children. Washington, D.C.: APPI.

Figley, C. R. (ed.) (1985), Trauma and Its Wake: The Study and Treatment of Post-Traumatic Stress Disorder. New York, N.Y.: Brunner/Mazel, Inc.

Figley, C. R. (ed.) (1986), Trauma and Its Wake, Vol II. New York, N.Y.: Brunner/Mazel, Inc.

Garmezy, N. and Rutter M. (1983), Stress, Coping and Development in Children. New York, N.Y.: McGraw Hill.

Giller, E. L. (1990), Biological Assessment and Treatment of Posttraumatic Stress Disorder. Washington, D.C.: APPI.

Green, A. (1983), Dimensions of Psychological Trauma in Abused Children. J AACP 22:203–207.

Horwitz, M. (1983), Post Traumatic Stress Disorders. Behavioral Sciences and the Law 1(3):9–24.

McCann, L. and Pearlman, L. A. (1991), Psychological Trauma and the Adult Survivor. New York, N.Y.: Brunner/Mazel, Inc.

Reiker, P. and Carmen, R. (1986), The Victim to Patient Process: The Disconfirmation and Transformation of Abuse. Am J Orthopsych 65(30):360–370.

Schetky, D. H. (1990), Literature Review of Long Term Effects of Child Sexual Abuse. In: Kluft, R. (ed.): Incest Related Syndromes. Washington, D.C.: APPI.

Schetky, D. H. and Green, A. H. (1988), Child Sexual Abuse: A Guide for Healthcare and Legal Professionals. New York, N.Y.: Brunner/Mazel, Inc.

Terr, L. (1983), Chowchilla Revisited: The Effects of Psychic Trauma Four Years after a School Bus Kidnapping. Am J Psychiat 140:1542–1550.

Terr, L. (1984), Time and Trauma. Psychoanalytic Study of the Child 39:633–665.

Terr, L. (1990), Too Scared to Cry: Psychic Trauma in Childhood. New York, N.Y.: Harper and Row.

Van der Kolk, D. (ed.) (1987), Psychological Trauma. Washington, D.C.: APPI.

Wilson, J. (1989), Trauma, Transformation, and Healing. New York, N.Y.: Brunner/Mazel, Inc.

Wyatt, G. E. and Powell, G. J. (1988), Lasting Effects of Child Sexual Abuse. Newbury Park: Sage Publications.

21

Peer Review

DIANE H. SCHETKY, M.D.

I. CASE EXAMPLES

A. Case Example 1

Several patients in your practice have been put on Ritalin by Dr. Jones, a local pediatrician. Following your evaluation of these children you conclude that the Ritalin was inappropriately prescribed and that dosages were excessively high and poorly monitored. You are concerned that this is a repeated pattern in her practice.

B. Case Example 2

An attorney asks you to review a custody evaluation prepared by Dr. Wise, a noted child psychiatrist. Dr. Wise has evaluated the mother and her child but not the father. He concluded that the father is an antisocial personality and that the mother is a more fit parent than her husband.

C. Case Example 3

Your state licensing board asks you to evaluate Dr. Lonely who has applied to have his license reinstated. His license was suspended 2 years previously when he was convicted of unlawful sexual contact with an adolescent female patient. He states he has worked through the relevant issues in his therapy and feels that he is able to resume his practice.

II. LEGAL AND ETHICAL ISSUES

A. Definition and functions of peer review

Peer review is a process designed to uphold the standard of practice within the profession and to determine whether a physician is professionally qualified to perform his or her duties. As medicine enters a decade fraught with complex ethical decisions, it is becoming an increasingly important means of monitoring ethical behavior. A third function of peer review is to help determine how limited health care dollars should best be spent. This involves determining that services rendered are appropriate and delivered in the most cost effective manner. Peer review occurs in a variety of contexts, both formal and informal, which will be reviewed in this chapter.

B. Reporting violations of ethical code or statute

The clinician should be familiar with the ethical codes of his professional organization and the laws governing the reporting of unethical or unprofessional behavior in his state. For instance, laws governing the reporting of substance abuse by a physician vary from state to state and according to whether one is in a treating relationship with that physician. If incompetence is related to substance abuse, aging, or emotional problems one may be required to report to an Impaired Physicians Committee or licensing agency.

A particularly difficult situation arises if a patient reveals unethical behavior by a former therapist. In such situations, the treating therapist must weigh the obligation to protect other patients at risk against the patient's right to privacy. One solution to this dilemma is to urge the patient to file an ethics complaint, though some patients may not be able to do so until well along in therapy. Patients may also reveal impairment in a physician parent or spouse to a therapist. The therapist should beware of whether there are statutes in his state requiring him to report or to warn or protect patients of such a colleague.

C. Immunity standards

The American Psychiatric Association (APA) code of medical ethics states, "a physician shall deal honestly with patients and colleagues, and strive to expose those physicians deficient in character or competence, or who engage in fraud or deception (Sec.2)." Physicians who file a report against a colleague in good faith are usually immune from damages.

Immunity for physicians acting as part of an official peer review organization is governed by local laws. Generally, as long as one is acting without malice there is little risk of being sued for damages. State laws that protect members of peer review groups from civil liability allow members to review cases in a more open setting without the fear of intimidation or reprisal. Federal law provides immunity from civil or criminal liability arising in the course of duties to those in a fiduciary relationship with a review organization performing federal reviews, providing that they exercise reasonable care.

In order to encourage physicians to report acts of substandard care by peers and to participate in peer review, Congress, in 1986, passed the Health Care Quality Improvement Act. The first part of the act provides broad, but not total, immunity from damages to hospitals and medical staff members involved in credentialing decisions in the event that a disappointed physician should sue them. For the immunity to apply, it must be demonstrated that the action was taken (1) in the "reasonable belief" that it would promote quality health care, (2) that "reasonable effort" was made to determine the facts, (3) that fair hearing procedures were followed, and (4) that there was "reasonable belief" that the action was warranted (Miles, 1987).

The second part of the act requires that hospitals report to the Board of Medical Examiners or DHHS (Department of Health and Human Services) or both, actions taken against the privileges of staff members. Hospitals are required to request information from the DHHS's data bank when a physician applies for staff privileges and at least once every two years thereafter (McNair, 1987).

The act provides protection from damages, not from being sued and does not apply to civil rights actions or those brought about by the U.S. or state's attorney general. Furthermore, it only applies to physicians and to decisions based on a physician's professional conduct and competence. While the act was designed for hospital credentialing committees, it also applies to other organizations of physicians, such as medical society ethics committees, as long as these committees follow a formal peer review process.

D. Antitrust issues

An important case that became the impetus for the Health Care Quality Improvement Act (HCQIA) was that of *Patrick v. Burget* (800 F. 2nd 1498, 1986). The case arose in 1981 when the members of the only hospital in Astoria, Oregon, sought to terminate Dr. Patrick's staff privileges, claiming his medical care was substandard. Patrick sued, claiming the motives of those initiating the complaint were financial and that they were trying to eliminate competition. Patrick successfully invoked the Sherman Antitrust Act and was awarded $650,000. Under antitrust laws this sum tripled to $1.95 million. The appellate court reversed the decision holding that the Peer Review Committee's conduct was immune from antitrust scrutiny because the state action doctrine exempts actions of the states from antitrust scrutiny.

In 1986, the case went to the Supreme Court, which overruled the appellate court. It found that state action doctrine did not protect Oregon physicians from federal antitrust liability for their activities on hospital peer review committees. They noted that the case did not satisfy the two prongs necessary for making this determination, i.e., (1) that the challenged restraint of Patrick's professional practice was not state policy and (2) that there was no state supervision of the anticompetitive conduct. In sum, the ruling made it clear that the state must be involved in supervising the peer review and that merely reporting to the Board of Medical Examiners does not suffice.

A later challenge involving an antitrust suit, *Bolt v. Halifax Hosp. Med. Center et al.* (851, E. 2nd 1273, 1988), arose in the 11th Circuit District Court in Florida. A physician alleged that three hospitals had acted in a "community conspiracy" to deprive him of the opportunity to practice in his area of Florida. The court of appeals dismissed the actions against the hospital on the grounds of "state action" immunity. It held that the Supreme Court decision in *Patrick* did apply to this case because there was adequate state supervision in Florida's peer review system, as evidenced in the peer review decisions.

E. APA procedures for handling complaints of unethical conduct

Ethics committees exist to uphold professional standards, to provide fair consideration by professional peers of charges lodged against members, and to attend to the educational and rehabilitative needs of colleagues who have deviated in their conduct. If a complaint of unethical conduct arises within the APA, the complainant needs to send a signed complaint to the District Branch (DB) of the accused member for investigation. The DB Ethics Committee then decides whether to pursue an investigation. Upon completion of an investigation, results and recommendations are forwarded to the APA's Ethics Committee for review.

If it decides an ethics violation has occurred, the accused member is notified in writing. Sanctions include expulsion from the APA, suspension, reprimand, or admonishment. Admonishment and reprimand are the least serious sanctions and do not affect membership rights, nor are they reportable under the Health Care Quality Improvement Act. However, they may have to be reported on applications for hospital privileges, licensure, and liability insurance. Suspension deprives a member of the right to hold office in the APA, vote, or serve on committees, but the member remains eligible for APA member benefits. If the decision is for expulsion, it is then reviewed by the APA Board of Trustees who notify the DB and member of their final decision. The name of any member who is expelled is reported in *Psychiatric News*.

Decisions regarding unethical conduct may be reported to any medical licensing authorities, medical societies, hospitals, clinics, or institutions when such disclosure is deemed appropriate to protect the public. In the event that a member resigns during the course of an investigation, this is reported by the DB or APA.

A DB may impose conditions of practice on a suspended member, such as ongoing supervision or educational requirements. Details of the supervision are left to the discretion of the DB. Once a DB imposes conditions it is expected to monitor compliance. A member who fails to satisfy the conditions may be expelled. Psychotherapy, in contrast to supervision, may be recommended but not imposed upon a member.

F. Rights of the accused

The accused physician must be given notice of the action proposed, the reason for it, his rights at the hearing, and his right to an attorney. He also has the right to call witnesses and to question adverse witnesses. At the completion of the hearing, he is entitled to receive the written recommendation of the panel that heard the case. The accused has the right to appeal the decision to the APA Ethics Appeals Board. The appeals board may make one of several decisions: (1) affirm the decision and sanction, (2) affirm the decision but alter the sanction, (3) reverse the decision of the DB, or (4) remand the case to the DB with instructions as to what further information or action is needed. If the decision is for expulsion, it is then reviewed by the APA Board of Trustees who notify the DB and member of their final decision.

G. Confidentiality

Proceedings and records of peer review organizations are usually considered confidential and are exempted from discovery without a showing of good cause. Confidentiality assures more candid and critical discussion of the issues involved. Peer review privilege was first adopted in Illinois in 1961, and most states have since followed suit. However, in Missouri and Oregon the laws providing this privilege were declared unconstitutional. Ott (1986) points out that much of peer review records, such as unsubstantiated allegations, are nothing more than hearsay and as such would be inadmissible, even in the absence of privilege. Nevertheless, confidentiality offers reassurance to reviewers in an uneasy professional task.

III. CLINICAL ISSUES

A. Varying contexts of peer review

1. HOSPITALS

Peer review in hospitals is required as part of hospital quality assurance programs under the Joint Commission on Accreditation of Health Care Organization requirements. It includes ongoing quality assurance programs that review and evaluate patient care and respond to recommendations put forth by these reviews. In addition, external reviews may occur as part of accreditation in which case outsiders are brought in to conduct the reviews of physician practices and credentials or of programs.

2. PROFESSIONAL SOCIETIES

Peer review by these groups occurs in response to complaints of misconduct and is designed to maintain standards of the profession and to protect the public from unscrupulous or substandard practices. Peer review may occur within the Ethics Committee, as described above, or within The Impaired Physician's Committee. At times the jurisdiction of these committees may overlap, as when impairment contributes to unethical behavior. These committees are also helpful sources of information for physicians.

3. STATE LICENSING BOARDS

State Licensing Boards are involved with the initial qualifying of applicants for licensure, with disciplinary actions, and with requests for reinstatement. When rules or conditions of licensure are violated, the board has several options. These include issuing warnings or censure, suspending a license, and stating terms of probation. Thus, the penalties that may be imposed by this body are of a higher order than those imposed by the APA. Psychiatrists may be involved as board members or more likely as consultants when psychiatric evaluation of the licensee is requested. Questions may be asked about the degree of impairment, type of therapy indicated, and whether the physician in question poses a risk to patients. The information obtained during such an evaluation does not go beyond the licensing board, but it may lose this status if brought out in a public hearing.

4. INSURANCE COMPANIES

Private reviews occur when individuals or organizations contract to conduct utilization reviews and quality of care assessments for insurance companies. The reviews serve to help contain the cost of health care and to monitor the quality of health care offered by providers. Increasingly, at least within child psychiatry, emphasis is being placed upon the severity and complexity of the illness rather than upon the diagnosis as the criteria for determining intensity and duration of services. Guidelines for peer review of child and adolescent treatment have been described in detail by the AACAP (1989).

Guidelines for conducting peer review are also contained in the Tax Equity and Fiscal Responsibility Act (TEFRA) of 1982 that revises the Federal Professional Standards Review Organization (PSRO) program of the Social Security Act. The new statute requires that review organizations be willing to contract with private and third party payers, e.g., Medicaid. As a condition for reimbursement, providers must agree to release patient data to review organizations that have contracts with DHHS. Under the new law, organizations may contract with peer review organizations that operate for profit as well as with not for profit peer review organizations (Hastings, 1983). TEFRA provides for confidentiality of Medicaid and Medicare records, with a few exceptions, and stipulates that such records may not be subject to subpoena or discovery.

The private review and confidentiality of records is covered by state statutes and common law. A critical issue has been whether such records are discoverable in court proceedings. As noted by Hastings (1983), "Wherever the statute is ambiguous, a court is likely to find that the greater equities lie with the injured patient."

The sanctions available to private review organizations include withholding of payment for inappropriate services and in some instances notice to licensure boards and medical societies of inappropriate care.

5. EXPERT WITNESSES

A more informal type of peer review occurs in forensic cases when an expert is asked to critique evaluations or depositions of another colleague. This occurs at the request of an attorney who seeks to impeach the opinions or credentials of the other side's expert. This is a perfectly legitimate activity providing one acts with fairness and remembers that one has not seen the patient in question. It may be important to reveal to the jury the flaws in the expert's qualifications and testimony. For instance, credentials may be misrepresented, the expert may lack expertise in the area in question, or he may present a biased report or conclusions that are not supported by the observations described.

6. JOURNALS

Yet another type of peer review occurs through the editorial boards of journals and outside reviewers who serve as consultants to them. The goal of this type of peer review is to maintain quality. Traditionally this sort of review is confidential and receives little outside surveillance. Recently, in the wake of the publication of fraudulent research, the peer review process of scientific journals has come under more careful scrutiny. Some have argued that such review needs to be more objective, open, and accountable. Relman and Angell (1989) remind us, "If peer review cannot guarantee the validity of research, still less can it be relied on to detect fraud." They conclude that in spite of its limitations, it remains a "powerful means of protecting and improving the quality of what is published."

B. Standard of practice

In determining whether an ethical violation has occurred psychiatrists are guided by the APA's *Principles of Medical Ethics with Annotations Especially Applicable to Psychiatry* (1983). Many cases fall into the gray area, particularly if one does not know how a particular behavior has affected another party. At times it is not possible to gain access to all information because of the constraints of confidentiality. For instance, a physician was suspected of rubber stamping disability evaluations, yet confidentiality prevented the ethics committee from gaining access to them.

If possible malpractice is an issue, the standard then becomes a matter of what is the acceptable standard of care within the community where the physician practices. Increasingly, the concept of "community" is becoming nationwide. Specialists are held to a higher standard of care than non-specialists. The Academy of Child and Adolescent Psychiatry notes, "Psychiatry has pluralist approaches, and the guidelines for purposes of peer review should not be made the standards against which practice is judged in courts of law concerned with malpractice" (AACAP, 1989).

C. Standard of proof

The APA does not specify what standard of proof should be used in conducting ethics hearings, and this decision is left to the discretion of individual committees. Borenstein (1987) argues for the use of the clear and convincing evidence standard, feeling that beyond a reasonable doubt is too stringent and that preponderance of evidence is too low given the serious potential consequences of being convicted of an ethical violation. He notes that once his DB ethics committee agreed on their standard of proof the committee became much more efficient and effective.

D. Institutional ethics committees

Institutional Ethics Committees (IECs) address themselves to a broad spectrum of medical and societal issues. A major concern is whether to offer or withhold treatment from patients unable to make these decisions for themselves. These committees are also involved with education, policy making, and consultations. The latter are usually prospective, but may include retrospective ones, and in this regard IECs may overlap with some functions of ethics committees. The focus of IECs is generally on issues and current patient care, and they tend to function in an advisory capacity. In contrast, medical peer review committees are generally retrospective, focus on the standard of practice, and are disciplinary in nature. Another major difference is that IECs are interdisciplinary and include lay persons as well as paramedical personnel. The matters of confidentiality and immunity are ill defined in IECs and most tend to operate without legislative intervention.

IV. PITFALLS

A. Conflicts of interest

Peer reviewers must serve impartially. This is best achieved when one does not have a personal or competitive professional relationship with the member under review. For instance, a member of the DB Ethics Committee agreed to investigate a psychiatrist then learned that they were adversarial witnesses in a sexual misconduct case. She disqualified herself feeling that this encounter might tinge her views about the member under investigation. Those serving as reviewers should not be in direct economic competition with the member being investigated, for obvious reasons. This can be a problem if one is practicing in a state or county where there are few psychiatrists. Outsiders should be consulted to avoid bias and antitrust liability.

B. Confidentiality

Cases that come before peer review may be disturbing and high profile in the media. Peer reviewers need to confine their emotional responses to the peer review committee and avoid any temptation to allude to these cases with colleagues or family members. Should non-physicians be involved with peer review they need to be reminded about the importance of confidentiality.

C. Countertransference issues

It is important to avoid holier than thou attitudes and to try to think in terms of how a reasonable, ethical physician would have handled a matter. If the peer reviewer has himself transgressed in the past, he needs to avoid overidentifying with the member in question and not try to rationalize his behavior.

The peer reviewer needs to guard against punitive responses that may emanate from countertransference issues. For instance, Dr. Smith who lost a son to suicide, may still be angry over the failure of professionals to prevent his death. These feelings are resurrected when his committee is asked to hear a case in which a psychiatrist failed to warn parents that their daughter, who made a serious attempt, was suicidal. If Dr. Smith has not resolved his own issues about his son's death he probably should disqualify himself from hearing this case.

V. CASE EXAMPLE EPILOGUES

A. Case Example 1

You decide to call Dr. Jones and express your concerns. She is defensive on the phone but thanks you for calling. She continues to overmedicate with Ritalin. You then decide to file a formal complaint with her medical society. Eventually, a hearing occurs and her state medical society admonishes her. It further stipulates that she must take a course on pediatric psychopharmacology as a condition of continuing to prescribe Ritalin.

B. Case Example 2

You review records and are perturbed to read that Dr. Wise has taken everything the mother told him about her husband as fact. There is no evidence that he sought any corroboration of her statements. Also, he seems to have minimized the many positive statements the child made about his father. Evidence of possible bias is further suggested by Dr. Wise's pejorative statements about the father. His recommendations seem dogmatic, and at no point does he qualify his opinions as having been derived from a limited data base. His diagnosis on the father appears to be premature and irresponsible considering that he has not attempted to interview him. You agree to testify about your opinions on the case.

C. Case Example 3

You evaluate Dr. Lonely and find that he has only been in therapy for 6 months. Thus far, the focus of his therapy has been educational and behavioral. Dr. Lonely states that his only motive in the inappropriate sexual contact with his patient was the wish to give her the affection she was not receiving at home and to help her feel lovable. He persistently avoids referring to the contact as having been sexual, instead using euphemisms. He offers many intellectual explanations about why such behavior could be harmful to patients. At no point does he indicate that he gained any insight into his need to act upon his own sexual needs. He does not seem to have processed the many factors in his past and present life that contributed to his being at risk for abusing patients. You decide to recommend that relicensure is premature and that he needs further psychotherapy.

VI. ACTION GUIDE

A. Know your immunity

You should be familiar with your state laws regarding peer review and aware of your possible liability exposure and protection. When contracting with a review organization, it is useful to inquire whether there are indemnification or "hold harmless" provisions that prevent the reviewer from being held liable for actions of the insurer. Hastings (1983) recommends that the insurer, not the review organization, make the final determination regarding sanctions. This puts a greater responsibility and potential for liability upon the insurer while diminishing the risk exposure of the reviewer.

B. Avoid financial conflicts of interest

Physicians who are in direct economic competition with the physicians being reviewed should not serve as reviewers. This avoids appearances of possible conflict of interest. If there are too many conflicts of interest among peer review committee members, a DB may need to appoint an ad hoc investigating committee to conduct the investigation or bring in an outside consultant.

C. Establish criteria for staff privileges

Criteria for staff privileges should be delineated prospectively and applied to all physicians. This makes them easier to defend in a lawsuit (Pudlin, 1989).

D. Let hospital board make ultimate decision

By funneling final decisions to the top it becomes more difficult for a plaintiff to prevail in an antitrust suit. Careful overseeing by hospital boards lessens the likelihood that the plaintiff may claim that peer reviewers are acting out of competitive self-interest (Pudlin, 1989).

E. Understand the role of the expert witness

Training programs should address basic forensic issues such as the nature of the adversarial system, the role of the expert witness, and how the expert can maintain objectivity and professional integrity. Brent (1982) advises, "The testimony provided should be similar regardless of whether one is testifying for the plaintiff or defense, otherwise one is presenting partisan testimony."

F. Don't avoid peer review

Stay knowledgeable about the issues, remain involved, and be willing to serve. We can learn from one another's mistakes, and peer review improves our own practices and the practice of psychiatry in general. Furthermore, in the public interest, the legislature and courts generally favor protection of honest reviewers.

VII. SUGGESTED READINGS

American Academy of Child and Adolescent Psychiatry. (1985), Code of Ethics. Washington, D.C.: AACAP.

American Academy of Child and Adolescent Psychiatry. (1989), Guidelines for Treatment Resources, Quality Assurance, Peer Review and Reimbursement. Washington, D.C.: AACAP.

American Academy of Psychiatry Law (1989), and the Ethical Guidelines. Revised ed.

American Psychiatric Association. (1985), Opinions of the Ethics Committee on the Principles of Medical Ethics. Washington, D.C.: APA.

American Psychiatric Association. (1985), The Principles of Medical Ethics with Annotations Especially Applicable to Psychiatry. In: *By-Laws*. Revised ed. Chapter 10:1–15. Washington, D.C.: APA.

American Psychiatric Association. (1985), Procedures for Handling Complaints of Unethical Conduct. In: *By-Laws*. Washington, D.C.: APA.

American Psychiatric Association. (1991), Video: Reporting Ethical Concerns about Sexual Involvement with Patients. Washington, D.C.: APA.

Borenstein, D. (1987), Standards of Proof for Ethics Committees of Professional Organizations. Hosp and Comm Psychiat 38(7):711–717.

Brent, R. L. (1982), The Irresponsible Expert Witness: A Failure of Biomedical Graduate Education and Professional Accountability. Pediatrics 70(50):754–762.

Ciccone, R. and Clements, C. (1984), Forensic Psychiatry and Applied Clinical Ethics: Theory and Practice. Am. J. Psychiat 141(3):395–399.

Cranford, R., Hester, A., and Ashley, B. (1985), Institutional Ethics Committees: Issues of Confidentiality and Immunity. Law Med Health Care 13(2):52–60.

Ellman, E. (1989), Monitor Mania: Physician Regulation Runs Amok. Loyola U of Chicago Law J 20:721–774.

Gainer, P. and Miles, J. (1988), The Impact of *Patrick v. Burget* on Peer Review. The Medical Staff Counselor 2(4):13–20.

Hastings, D., Borsody, E., and Green, P. (1983), Legal Issues Raised by Private Review Activities of Medical Peer-Review Organizations. Jour Health Policy Law 8(2):293–313.

Herman, S. and Levy, A. (1989), Does Peer Review Have a Place in Child Custody Evaluations? Child-Today 18(3):15–18.

Jorgenson, L., Randles, R., Strasburger, L. (1991), The Furor over Psychotherapist-Patient Sexual Contact: New Solution to an Old Problem. William and Mary Law Rev 32(3):645–732.

McNair, R., Jr. (1987), The Health Care Quality Improvement Act of 1986: Reporting Practitioner Malpractice and Discipline. The Medical Staff Counselor 1(2):10–18.

Miles, J. (1987), The Health Care Quality Improvement Act of 1986. The Medical Staff Counselor I(2):1–9.

Ott, R. (1986), Peer Review: The Essence of a Profession. State Health Legislation Report 14(4).

Pudlin, H. P. (1989), Eight Precautions for Peer Reviewers. PA Med 92(4):34–36.

Relman, A. and Angell, M. (1989), How Good is Peer Review? NEJM 321(12):827–829.

Sun, M. (1989), Peer Review Comes under Peer Review. Science 244 (May) 910–912.

Walzer, R. (1990), Impaired Physicians: A Legal Update. Jour Legal Medicine. (2):131–198.

Index

Page numbers in *italics* denote figures;
those followed by "t" denote tables.